Perioperative Nursing Core Curriculum

D1296791

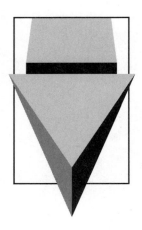

EDITED BY
Rosemary Ann Roth, RN, MSN, CNOR, CNAA

Nursing Director, Surgical Suite
The Genesee Hospital
Rochester, New York

W.B. SAUNDERS COMPANY
A Division of Harcourt Brace & Company
Philadelphia   London   Toronto   Montreal   Sydney   Tokyo

Perioperative Nursing Core Curriculum

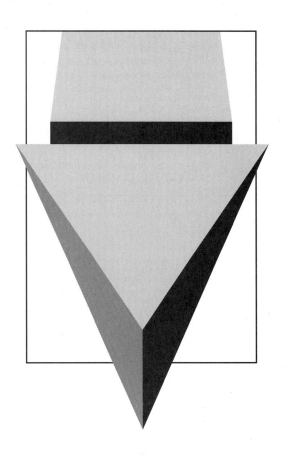

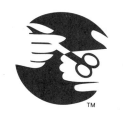

ASSOCIATION OF OPERATING ROOM NURSES, INC.

W.B. SAUNDERS COMPANY
A Division of Harcourt Brace & Company

The Curtis Center
Independence Square West
Philadelphia, Pennsylvania 19106

q
RD32.3
.P46
1995

Library of Congress Cataloging-in-Publication Data

Perioperative nursing core curriculum / Association of Operating Room Nurses, Inc.
    p. cm.
  Includes index.
  ISBN 0–7216–5197–6
   1. Operating room nursing.   2. Operating room nursing—Problems, exercises, etc.
I. Association of Operating Room Nurses.
  [DNLM: 1. Operating Room Nursing—education—United States. WY 18.2 P445 1995]

RD32.3.P46 1995   610.73′677—dc20
DNLM/DLC
                                      95–10280

PERIOPERATIVE NURSING CORE CURRICULUM   ISBN 0–7216–5197–6

Copyright © 1995 by W.B. Saunders Company

All rights reserved. No part of this publication may be reproduced or transmitted in any form or by any means, electronic or mechanical, including photocopy, recording, or any information storage and retrieval system, without permission in writing from the publisher.

Printed in the United States of America

Last digit is the print number: 9   8   7   6   5   4   3   2   1

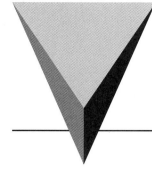

Contributors

Cyndi Abbott, RN, PhD, CNOR
Director, Perioperative Nursing Services
Ireland Army Community Hospital
Ft. Knox, KY
Practice Scenario 2: Asepsis: Protecting the Patient, Personnel, and Environment

Willa M. Abbott, RN, BSN
Clinical Director, Operating Room
North Carolina Baptist Hospitals, Incorporated
Winston-Salem, NC
Practice Scenario 2: Anesthesia and Perioperative Nursing Care

Deborah Alpers, RN, MS, CNOR, CNA
Nurse Manager, Operating Room, St. Luke's Episcopal Hospital
Texas Medical Center
Houston, TX
Practice Scenario 1: Surgical Patient Intraoperative Positioning

Carol Dungan Applegeet, RN, MSN, CNOR, CNAA, FAAN
Director, Center for Nursing Practice
Association of Operating Room Nurses, Inc.
Denver, CO
Chapter 1: History of Surgery and Perioperative Nursing

Donna Benotti, RN, CNOR
Clinical Staff Nurse IV
Summit Medical Center
Oakland, CA
Practice Scenario 1: Professional Perioperative Nursing Development

Linda Brazen, RN, MSN, CNOR, C
Continuing Education Coordinator
Association of Operating Room Nurses, Inc.
Center for Perioperative Education
Denver, CO
Chapter 10: Perioperative Clinical Education

Pur 3/18/96
DBCN ACY-4438

MAR 26 1996

Connie Diane Brown, RN, BSN, CNOR

Clinical Program Coordinator, Operating Room
Baylor University Medical Center
Dallas, TX
Chapter 4: Sterilization/Disinfection: Equipment and Instruments

Lois M. Bruning, RN, BSPA, CNOR

Woodstock, GA
Chapter 5: Environmental Safety in the Surgical Suite

Barbara Crim, RN, MBA

Director of O.R. Education
Baylor University Medical Center
Dallas, TX
Practice Scenario 1: Sterilization/Disinfection: Equipment and Instruments

Gayle Drinville-Shank, RN, CNOR

Staff Nurse, Operating Room
Primary Children's Medical Center
Salt Lake City, UT
Practice Scenario 1: Surgical Wound Management

Diane Ebbert, RN, MSN, ARNP, CNOR

Clinical Instructor/Clinical Nurse Specialist
University of Kansas
Kansas City, KS
Practice Scenario 1: Planning Perioperative Patient Care

Elizabeth M. Edel, RN, MN, CNOR

Perioperative Clinical Nurse Specialist
St. Luke's Episcopal Hospital
Houston, TX
Practice Scenario 2: Surgical Patient Intraoperative Positioning

Nancy Girard, PhD, RN, CS

Assistant Professor
University of Texas Health Science Center at
San Antonio School of Nursing
San Antonio, TX
*Practice Scenario 1: Asepsis: Protecting the Patient, Personnel, and
   Environment*

Shirley Hazen, RN, MN, CNOR

Clinical Educator
Wichita State University
Wichita, KS
Practice Scenario 2: Planning Perioperative Patient Care

Edith M. Hill, RN, BSN, CNOR

Perioperative Nurse Clinician, Operating Room
The Genesee Hospital
Rochester, NY
Practice Scenario 2: Environmental Safety in the Surgical Suite

MAR 26 1990

Susan V. M. Kleinbeck, RN, MS, CNOR

Doctoral Candidate, School of Nursing
University of Kansas
Kansas City, KS
Chapter 6: Planning Perioperative Patient Care

Theresa K. Kulb, RN, BSN, CNOR

Independent Nurse Consultant
Bloomington, IL
Practice Scenario 1: Environmental Safety in the Surgical Suite

Judy Little, RN, BSN, CNOR, CST, CCST

Perioperative Staff Educator
Nurse Manager, Operating Room
University of Utah Health Science Center
Salt Lake City, UT
Practice Scenario 2: Surgical Wound Management

Martha March, RN, BSN

Clinical Supervisor, Operating Room
North Carolina Baptist Hospitals, Incorporated
Winston-Salem, NC
Practice Scenario 1: Anesthesia and Perioperative Nursing Care

Sandra M. Maree, CRNA, MEd

Director, Nurse Anesthesia Program
North Carolina Baptist Hospitals, Incorporated
Winston-Salem, NC
Chapter 7: Anesthesia and Perioperative Nursing Care

Mae Taylor Moss, RN, MSN, MS

Vice President, Perioperative Services
St. Luke's Episcopal Hospital
Houston, TX
Chapter 8: Surgical Patient Intraoperative Positioning

Sheila A. O'Connor, RN, MS, CNS, CNOR

Nurse Manager, Perioperative Services
St. Luke's Episcopal Hospital
Houston, TX
Chapter 8: Surgical Patient Intraoperative Positioning

Doris A. Porter, RN, BSN, MS, CNOR

Consultant, Perioperative Education
Same Day Surgery Systems
Burbank, CA
Practice Scenario 2: Professional Perioperative Nursing Development

Leana Revell, RN, MSN, CNOR

Associate Professor
San Antonio College
San Antonio, TX
Chapter 3: Asepsis: Protecting the Patient, Personnel, and Environment

Kathie G. Shea, RN, BSN, CNOR

Nurse Educator, Surgical Services
Summit Medical Center
Oakland, CA

Chapter 2: Professional Perioperative Nursing Development

Donna Wahoff-Stice, RN, MSN, CNOR

Perioperative Clinical Nurse Specialist
University Hospital
Salt Lake City, UT

Chapter 9: Surgical Wound Management

Debbie Woodard, RN, BSN, CNOR

Clinical Program Coordinator, O.R. Education
Baylor University Medical Center
Dallas, TX

Practice Scenario 2: Sterilization/Disinfection: Equipment and Instruments

Karen Zaglaniczny, CRNA, PhD

Associate Director, Nurse Anesthesia Program
Henry Ford Hospital
Detroit, MI

Chapter 7: Anesthesia and Perioperative Nursing Care

Reviewers

Sheila L. Allen, RN, BSN, CNOR
Nursing Department
Baton Rouge General Medical Center
Baton Rouge, LA

Susan N. Bushard, ADN, BA, Human Services, CNOR
Operating Room
Hennepin County Medical Center
Minneapolis, MN

Karen L. Engledow, RN, CNOR
Perioperative Educator
Mother Frances Hospital
Tyler, TX

Patricia Ann Hercules, MS, BSN
Nursing Education Department
The Methodist Hospital
Houston, TX

Edith M. Hill, RN, BSN, CNOR
The Genesee Hospital
Rochester, NY

Patricia P. Kapsar, RN, MBA, CNOR
Nursing Department
Bethesda General Hospital
St. Louis, MO

Paula Anne Latz, RN, MSN, CNOR
The Methodist Hospital
St. Louis Park, MN

Vickie B. Moore, RN, BSN, CNOR
Operating Room
Virginia Baptist Hospital
Lynchburg, VA

Helen Starbuck Pashley, RN, BSN, CNOR
Student, Writer, and Editor
Evergreen, CO

Jacklyn J. Takahashi Schuchardt, RN, MSN, BSN, CNOR
Staff Developer
John Muir Medical Center
Walnut Creek, CA

Cynthia Spry, RN, MA, MSN, CNOR
Director, Surgical Services
United Hospitals
Newark, NJ

Patricia Sanger Stein, RN, BSN, CNOR
Surgical Services
St. Paul-Ramsey Medical Center
St. Paul, MN

Karen Zaglaniczny, CRNA, PhD
Nurse Anesthesia Program
Henry Ford Hospital
Detroit, MI

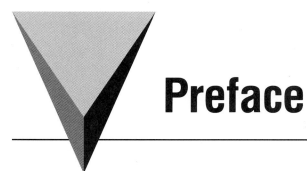

Preface

This book is intended for registered nurses hired immediately after graduation from accredited nursing schools and for registered nurses without previous perioperative nursing experience. In addition, perioperative clinical educators, managers, clinicians, and perioperative nurses who function as preceptors also will be interested in this book. The concepts of the *Perioperative Nursing Core Curriculum* are applicable to perioperative nursing in any location or facility, at any point on life's continuum, and across specialty practice.

The overall theme of the book is competency and standards focused. The use of the term "competency" is intended to be congruent with the Joint Commission on Accreditation of Health Care Facilities' *Agenda for Change* and is not necessarily based on AORN's *Competency Statement in Perioperative Nursing*.

The *AORN Standards and Recommended Practices* manual is intended to be used in conjunction with this book. The combination of the two manuals allows the reader access to current concepts.

The book is organized into ten chapters. The first two chapters build the foundation and describe the development of the specialty of perioperative nursing. These chapters are

Chapter One—History of Surgery and Perioperative Nursing

Chapter Two—Professional Perioperative Nursing Development.

The next three chapters address the technical aspects of perioperative nursing. These chapters are

Chapter Three—Asepsis: Protecting the Patient, Personnel, and Environment

Chapter Four—Sterilization/Disinfection: Equipment and Instruments

Chapter Five—Environmental Safety in the Surgical Suite.

The next four chapters address the professional aspects of perioperative nursing practice—from the application of the nursing process to the nurse's responsibility in the care of the surgical patient and family. These chapters are

Chapter Six—Planning Perioperative Patient Care

Chapter Seven—Anesthesia and Perioperative Nursing Care

Chapter Eight—Surgical Patient Intraoperative Positioning

Chapter Nine—Surgical Wound Management.

The last chapter (Chapter Ten—Perioperative Clinical Education) is written for the experienced perioperative nurse who is functioning as the clinical resource for the novice perioperative nurse. The content addresses principles of adult education and helps to focus on the educational process in the operating room.

The three phases of perioperative nursing practice, with a concentration on the intraoperative phase, are addressed in the text and in the practice scenarios at the end of the clinical chapters.

Each chapter identifies the prerequisite knowledge that the learner needs to assimilate from the chapter content. This knowledge includes the AORN *Standards of Practice and Recommended Practices for Perioperative Nursing.* A general chapter outline and specific learner objectives for each chapter are also included.

The text is written in a narrative format using boxes and tables to highlight information. The contributors have been encouraged to include a "controversy box" to present opposing views on a questionable area.

A glossary of terms and a list of suggested readings provide the learner with additional resources. Chapters two through nine conclude with practice scenarios that apply the concepts learned to perioperative patient care situations. These scenarios focus on the specific content and may not address all the intraoperative nursing interventions that an experienced perioperative nurse might utilize.

The chapters and practice scenarios were written by clinically experienced perioperative nurses with expertise in the specific areas addressed. The editor wishes to thank these nurses for their time, effort, and patience with the process of the book's development.

ROSEMARY ANN ROTH, RN, MSN, CNOR, CNAA

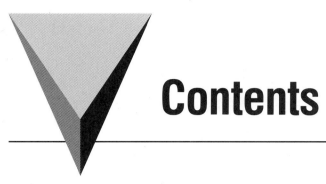

Contents

Chapter One

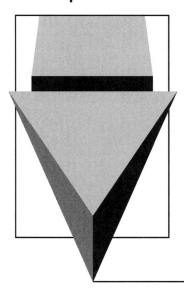

History of Surgery and Perioperative Nursing

Carol Dungan Applegeet, RN, MSN, CNOR, CNAA, FAAN

Prerequisite Knowledge   Basic nursing education. To understand current perioperative nursing practice and to be able to plan for the future, the registered nurse must have an appreciation for the foundations of surgery and operating room nursing.

Chapter Outline

Learning Objectives

1. Describe the societal and cultural influences on the progress of medicine and nursing in ancient civilization.

2. Identify the sentinel events leading to the development of the surgical specialty.

3. Describe the evolution of the perioperative nursing practice.

First Surgical Renaissance 4000 B.C. – 1500 A.D.

MEDICAL/SURGICAL TREATMENTS IN ANCIENT CIVILIZATIONS

The early stages of nursing and medicine were interwoven. In 4000 B.C., "nurses" worked with priests and medicine men relying heavily on witchcraft and magic to insure cures. Primitive medicine was based on widespread belief in supernatural powers rather than natural laws. All medical interventions were centered on religious beliefs, and "physicians" were actually priests. Amulets, ritual mutilations (e.g., circumcisions), and body painting were frequent. When trephining of the skull to liberate evil spirits, cesarean section to deliver babies, and subincision of the penis were successful, it was assumed to be based on supernatural powers rather than technical skill. People regarded disease as the work of the devil, and cleanliness as a virtue. Although the value of cleanliness was recognized, people relied on supernatural influences, magic formulas, charms (amulets), and exorcisms to clean the body and soul of disease and disorders.

The Babylonians recorded their medical notes on clay tablets. The oldest surviving legal code, the Code of Hammurabi of Babylon (2250 B.C.), contained laws specifying fees for surgical and medical practice and punishment for malpractice (Ackerknecht, 1968; Jamieson, 1959). Egyptian physicians also were priests, whereas surgeons were merely men who dressed combat wounds and set bones. An ancient Egyptian medical textbook devoted exclusively to surgical treatment presented case histories and established the notion of disease. For the first time, physician-priests had a system to establish a diagnosis and examine the patient, determine a prognosis, and apply therapeutic measures. Meanwhile, Inca and Mexican ancient civilizations were developing real skills (surgery, trephination, excision of tumors, amputation). The heads of ants were used as clamps in sutures! (Ackerknecht, 1968).

The first real mention of nursing principles and practices comes from India around 800 B.C. Nurses were young men who belonged to the Brahmin subcast or priest order, and they worked in hospitals. Susruta, a Hindu surgeon, first noted nurses as assistants in surgery (Jamieson, 1959). Buddha brought hospitals to India, so it is not surprising that medical treatment was based on a mixture of religious, astrologic, and scientific elements. Virtually all therapeutics were accompanied by prayer or spells.

Indian surgical interventions began with a prayer, and the patient was positioned in the right direction while the priest-surgeon consulted astrology. Wine was the anesthetic. One of eight techniques was then used: incision, excision,

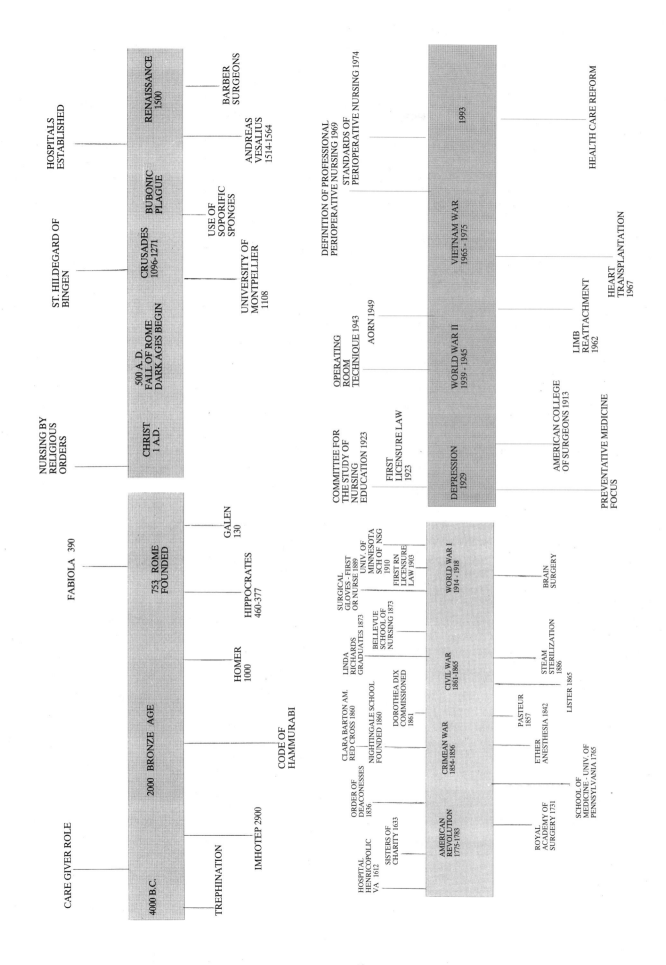

scraping, puncturing, probing, extraction, provoking secretion, or suturing. Over 100 instruments were available, including tongs, rectal specula, bougies, hooks for nasal polyps, and magnets. The surgeon cauterized with hot irons and performed chemosurgery with caustic salves. Surgeons pierced earlobes, extracted cataracts, sutured intestines, excised tumors, and attempted repair of hydroceles and hernias (Ackerknecht, 1968).

Ancient Chinese medical/surgical development took a different turn, although China was a literate society and its medical literature was extensive. Ancient Chinese culture gives us yang and yin, male and female natures, drug lore, and acupuncture. Surgery never developed as a specialty, however, because the ancient Chinese had an aversion to blood shedding and a belief that mutilation continued in life after death. Physicians were not considered part of the scholastic group (Ackerknecht, 1968).

Ancient Greek civilization gave us the beginning of modern medical terminology. The word *surgeon* was derived from Greek, *cheir* meaning hand and *ergon* meaning work. The Greeks believed in many gods who produced and cured disease. Hygeia was the goddess of health, and Panacea was the restorer of health. Apollo was regarded as the god of disease and healing until the 5th century B.C. when he was replaced by Asclepias, who was originally a legendary physician and a patron of the guild of physicians. Hippocrates, known as the Father of Medicine, lived from 460 to 377 B.C. and was greatly influenced by philosophers. Greek physicians treated fractures, dislocations, wounds of the head, ulcers, fistulae, and hemorrhoids in a conservative, rather than surgical, manner. During this era, over 200 instruments were made of hardened steel. Galen, a famous Greek surgeon, wrote at least 22 volumes on surgical care. Although he was a good surgeon to gladiators, he left surgery in favor of medicine. Surgery was deemed to be manual labor, beneath the dignity of a gentleman. Thus developed the beginning of the schism between medicine and surgery (Ackerknecht, 1968).

The vocation of nursing came into being at the beginning of the Christian era. The nursing vocation was seen as a divine call for religious or charitable service, and a professional was defined as an individual who openly professed religious beliefs in religion or made a vow of a life of service. The church's influence on nursing was unquestioned. Deaconesses, virgins, and widows provided care. Deaconesses were the forerunners of the modern nurse. Virgins assisted with the distribution of alms and care of the church vestments. Fabiola is credited with being the first nurse of the Christian era (390 A.D.). Having founded the first free public hospital under the auspices of Christianity, Fabiola sought out the poor and sick in the streets and cared for them.

MEDIEVAL PERIOD

Surgery reached its lowest depths in medieval times. The Council of Tours in 1163 took surgery out of the hands of physicians with the pronouncement *Ecclesia abhorrent a sanguine* (the church does not shed blood). This edict lasted for 700 years. Since the church forbade wearing beards, barbers emerged, and surgery was left to the barbers, bathkeepers, hangmen, sow-gilders, and quacks. Barber-surgeons did bleeding, cupping, leaching, and tooth extractions, and they treated surgical wounds with hemp as the only anesthetic. Surgical texts disappeared from medical libraries, and the separation of surgery and medicine begun with Galen continued (Ackerknecht, 1968). Only in Italy and southern France did some physicians continue to practice surgery.

The greatest accomplishment of the Middle Ages was the hospital. It was not a medical institution, however, but a facility offering hospitality and refuge to the old, disabled, and homeless. The transformation of the first hospitals from charity institutions to medical facilities occurred in the 13th century when the administration of the hospitals was taken over by the city (Ackerknecht, 1968).

Three hospitals existed outside monastic walls. They were the Hôtel Dieu of Lyons, Hôtel Dieu in Paris, and Santo Spirito of Rome. Women worked in them as bed makers (Griffin, 1973).

Nursing's darkest period was between 1600 and 1752. In Paris at the Hôtel Dieu, the oldest purely nursing order of nuns was overworked and repressed. They cared for the sick and wounded during the crusades, and their male counterparts, the Knights Hospitallers, nursed the sick when they were not fighting. The military ideal of order and discipline was established, and women nurses were organized as auxiliary units of the orders. When the crusades ended, both male and female nurses cared for lepers and continued to fight disease, but the emphasis was on rank and deference to superiors rather than on patient care. The nursing dress of the day was distinctive, reflective of monastic life common during the crusades (Jamieson, 1959).

Second Surgical Renaissance 1500–1842

RENAISSANCE PERIOD

The Renaissance period was heralded by the introduction of gunpowder, the invention of printing, the discovery of a sea route to India and America, the introduction of an economy based on money, and the spread of Greek scholars all over Europe. New mores arose, peasants staged uprisings, England started to become a world power, new universities were developed, and there was a religious explosion of reform and counterreform, along with revisions in the art world. Witch hunting became prevalent. There was a rebirth of the clinic and surgery, and the application of chemistry to medicine began. The title, Greatest Renaissance Surgeon, was given to Ambroise Paré who treated gunshot wounds and reintroduced ligature in 1552 (Ackerknecht, 1968).

Medical education was pursued within the university, but nursing education was not allowed within the hallowed halls. Nursing techniques remained unchanged under the guardianship of the secular orders, even though paid services for hospital care emerged, and nursing became pivotal to hospital functions. People saw nursing as domestic service—not a profession. Respectable women did not undertake nursing because of the deplorable conditions, and the status of nursing further declined with the decline of monastic life (Griffin, 1973). In 1633, the Order of Sisters of Charity was established. It was the most widespread and most beloved of the nursing orders (Jamieson, 1959).

SEVENTEENTH CENTURY

During the 17th century, superstition was still widespread, and quackery was still very much in evidence. Medical education lacked focus on clinical skills and continued to teach harmful bloodletting and purging. Physicians (addressed as doctors) with university degrees were considered the elite, and they preferred studying, teaching, and debating to taking care of patients. Surgeons (addressed as misters) were considered socially inferior to physicians. Few had university degrees, and they were trained through apprenticeship and hospital instruction. Barber-surgeons continued to use razors to open veins and let blood (Marks, 1973).

The century was heralded by the advent of physiologic and microscopic research. The compound microscope was invented in 1600; the circulation of blood was explained by William Harvey (1578–1657); and the physiology of the lymphatic, digestive, and respiratory systems was discovered (Ackerknecht, 1968). The discovery of circulation led to intravenous injections and transfusion, but patient outcome was so poor that transfusion was abandoned until the 19th century.

Gentleman surgeons, not physicians, made the journey to the New World. Prior to 1700, only three or four physicians in Virginia had medical degrees, and they practiced alongside the surgeons of the day. The only difference was the extent of their education. Until the 19th century, hospitals were for the homeless, strangers, and mentally ill. The first American hospital was built in 1612 in Henricopolic, Virginia. Its 80 beds were attended by keepers, male nurses, who were on hand to take care of patients. The hospital is believed to have burned in 1622 during an Indian massacre. In December 1658, a New Amsterdam surgeon became concerned about the lack of proper medical care for ailing soldiers and employees of the Dutch West India Company, and he petitioned the provincial council to establish a hospital on Manhattan Island. The hospital opened prior to July, 1660 and was torn down in 1680.

EIGHTEENTH CENTURY

The preoccupation with body systems continued in the 18th century with the study of disease. Hospitals improved, and individual hygiene was emphasized. Surgery became fully emancipated, and advances were achieved in surgical technique and anatomy. By 1776, the thermometer was perfected, blood pressure measurement was possible, and limited inoculation and vaccination were available. Mental illness was recognized as a disease, not the result of possession by evil spirits (Ackerknecht, 1968).

By the time of the American revolution, 400 physicians with university education practiced in the United States. Surgeons practiced after serving an apprenticeship and getting hospital experience, the forerunners of internships and residencies. Following the Revolutionary War, the surgeon was the most needed doctor on the frontier. Instrumentation included amputation instruments, trephining instruments, pocket instruments, and crooked and straight needles. Some surgeons carried a scalpel and forceps. Instruments of iron and steel were made by blacksmiths, and instruments with ivory and carved wooden handles were often stored in velvet cases.

Nursing continued to develop an identity, albeit a poor one, during this time as well. Nurses still tended to be female camp followers with no training. Charles Dickens' writing at the time described nurses as illiterate, heavy-handed, and alcoholic. Nurses were believed to lack moral standards and were unfeeling and unsympathetic. Nursing was occasionally done by prison inmates on 10-day passes. In 1752, the term *matron* referred to the head of nursing staff and *sister* designated the head nurse. The term *sister* is still used in the United Kingdom and some European countries today.

In America, between 1775 and 1777, the Colonial Congress adopted legislation to establish Army hospitals with the provision that the number of nurses must be proportional to the number of sick and wounded. At the close of the Revolutionary War, five hospitals had been established: the Bellevue Almshouse in New York, New York Hospital, Blockney and Pennsylvania Hospitals in Philadelphia, and Eastern State Hospital for the insane in Williamsburg.

Third Surgical Renaissance 1843–Present

NINETEENTH CENTURY

During the 19th century, medicine moved from science by intention to science in fact. Developments in medicine, technology, and science were paralleled by the growth in industry, capitalism, and politics. The basic sciences advanced in microscopic anatomy, physiology, pathology, and pharmacy, giving medicine knowledge of the intricate structures of the human body.

Research advanced as well. There was an increased emphasis on bacteriology as the study of disease-causing microorganisms. In 1857, Louis Pasteur, a chemist, showed that fermentation was the work of microorganisms, but microorganisms were not identified as the causative factor in disease in 1877. Robert Koch isolated tuberculosis and cholera bacilli. Main body functions such as respiration, circulation, digestion, metabolism, nervous action, internal secretion, and reproduction were understood. Surgical advances included extirpations of the thyroid by Roux, ulcers by Récmier, and the rectum by Lisfranc. Lembert developed the intestinal suture.

By the 1830s, as a consequence of economic development and new scientific advances, surgeons were seen to be also practicing medicine in England. This period marked the beginning of the realignment of medicine and surgery in France. Specialties developed during this time included pathology, dermatology, psychiatry, and pediatrics (Ackerknecht, 1968; Marks, 1973).

Hospitals were dirty and overcrowded and had the image of houses of death because of the high number of infections. Ether and antisepsis used in the home became inconvenient. To accommodate the need for privacy and overcome the fear of hospitals, surgeons moved operations to medical boarding houses that provided hotel and nursing services. Doctors built small hospitals in suburbs. Surgery became a profit-making venture for hospitals. After 1900, most surgeries moved to hospitals. Profit-making hospitals of the early 1900s were mainly surgical centers, small, with no ties to medical schools. They relied on fees from patients in the upper and middle classes. Their rate of patient survival was the lowest. The Mayo Clinic was opened in the 1880s by William and Charles Mayo, surgeons with reputations for skill, invention, and low mortality rates (Marks, 1973).

In 1831, the Ohio General Assembly passed a statute that provided a fine not to exceed $1000 and/or imprisonment for up to 30 days for wantonly exhuming a corpse. The Zanesville, Ohio Daily Courier reported on November 18, 1878:

> In all parts of the country are established medical colleges. In fact, a second class city is not thought to be complete unless a medical college is established within its limits. Here collect ignorant professors to lecture to still more ignorant pupils. Surgery! Not one in a hundred knows anything about surgery. But bodies must be secured to make the brainless youths believe the brainless professors know something about surgery. These brainless youths, who will soon be turned out to prey, like a set of harpies, upon the people, must be taught, however, to make sport over the remains of some body, which has been stolen from where relatives and friends have tenderly placed it. It is a most disgraceful thing that people are preyed on by ignorant blockheads who sail under the name of physicians (Marks, 1973).

Several states passed laws to prevent the grave-robbing with penalties imposed. However, laws were also enacted that required that the decision to donate one's body to science be made prior to death (Marks, 1973).

Apart from the reunification of medicine and surgery and the social reacceptance of the surgeon, three factors were responsible for the growth of surgery in the 19th century: localism, anesthesia, and asepsis. Localism was the treatment of disease in a local area of the body with reliance that it would not grow again in the same or another spot. The advent of anesthesia made it practical to operate on people without the overriding issue of the treatment of pain during surgery. The advent of asepsis then made it possible to control infections postoperatively (Ackerknecht, 1968).

Ignaz Semmelweis suspected the cause of puerperal fever to be related to unwashed hands of the practitioners, and he instituted handwashing with a chlorine solution to reduce mortality rates. Before the sensational work of Joseph Lister, most wounds became infected, and the mortality rate for deep and extensive wounds was 70% to 80%. Lister tackled the infection problem by analyzing the differences between simple and complicated fractures and then surmising that air might contribute to septicemia. After Lister began applying carbolic acid to all open fractures, he saw dramatic decreases in infections. He then began to spray all instruments, wounds, and operators with carbolic acid, and antisepsis was born. Lister's techniques were eventually replaced by those of Semmelweis, and instruments were disinfected with steam, while hands and the surgical field were disinfected with other chemical agents. In 1886, Ernst von Bergmann devised a method of steam sterilization in Germany (Ackerknecht, 1968).

In the early 19th century, it was customary to intoxicate a patient with alcohol or opium prior to surgery. Before the middle of the 19th century, true anesthesia did not exist. In 1840, a British surgeon, James Esdaile, used hypnosis as an anesthetic technique, but it was not taken seriously because chemical anesthetics were being discovered in the United States. Ether was first given in Massachusetts General Hospital on October 16, 1846. The patient had a benign vascular tumor of the neck, and because of his fear of pain he agreed to the experimental ether anesthesia. Dr. Morton, the anesthetist, arrived 10 minutes late for the surgery, and Dr. Warren, the surgeon, was about to begin the surgery without anesthesia when he arrived. The operation with ether lasted 30 minutes (Ackerknecht, 1968; Marks, 1973).

General anesthesia was followed 40 years later by the use of local anesthesia. Howard Atwood Kelly, a recognized leader in gynecology, pioneered the use of cocaine for local anesthesia in 1881 and devised many new operations and instruments, including the Kelly clamp. Cocaine was first used in ophthalmology in 1884; conduction anesthesia was used in 1885; and infiltration anesthesia was used in 1894 (Ackerknecht, 1968; Marks, 1973).

As one would expect, anesthesia enhanced surgery as a treatment modality. American Civil War data promoted knowledge about fractures, gunshot wounds, amputations, excisions, fever, diarrhea, and dysentery. Good sterile technique was still lacking, however, because surgeons often donned waistcoats at the beginning of the day and hung them on a peg at night, to be worn the next day (Marks, 1973). Nurses continued to work alongside the surgeon, using equally poor sterile technique.

Surgical techniques continued to advance with the development of artery clamps, the development of an operating cystoscope, and the first clinical trial of electrocautery. Sterilization was achieved by boiling or autoclaving, and instruments were immersed in carbolic acid solution until needed. Caps and gowns were worn but no masks (Marks, 1973) (Figs. 1–1 and 1–2). Surgeons cleaned their hands, then immersed them in bichloride of mercury solution. In 1890, rubber gloves were introduced, but some surgeons feared they would reduce manual dexterity and delicacy of touch and did not use them. In 1889, a nurse in charge of the operating room complained of dermatitis from mercuric chloride. Because she was an "unusually efficient woman," a prominent surgeon, W. S. Halsted, took a cast of her hands and requested that the Goodyear Rubber Company make two pairs of thin rubber gloves as an experiment. Halsted wrote in *Surgical Papers*.

In the winter of 1889–1890—I cannot recall the month—the nurse in charge of my operating room complained that the solution of mercuric chloride produced a dermatitis of her arms and hands. As she was an unusually efficient woman, I gave the matter my consideration and one day in New York requested the Goodyear Rubber Company to make as an experiment two pair of thin rubber gloves with gauntlets. On trial these proved to be so satisfactory that additional gloves were ordered. In the autumn, on my return to town, the assistant who passed the instruments and threaded the needles was also provided with rubber gloves to wear at the operations (Halsted, 1952).

Even after wearing gloves became universally acceptable, this surgeon continued to remove his gloves to palpate the common bile duct (Marks, 1973). Surgery enjoyed a rise in prestige in the late 1880s because of technical and aseptic advances, although mortality rates for amputation were still 40%.

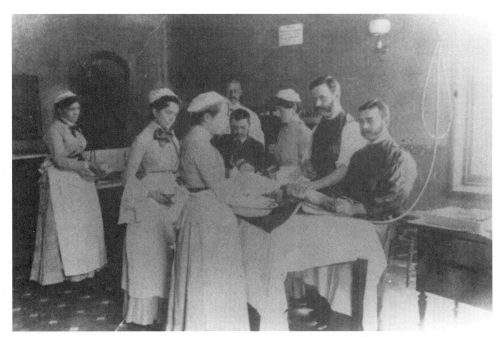

FIGURE 1-1. Mount Sinai Operating Room, circa 1890. The Archives of the Mount Sinai Medical Center.

Ethylene oxide was first described as a sterilant in 1859; the therapeutic effect of ultraviolet wavelengths was observed in 1895; and heat sterilization by boiling, steam, or hot oven was introduced in 1885. Schimmelbusch, an associate of von Bergmann in Berlin, sterilized white gowns and wore them over rubber aprons and street clothes. The Arnold pressure cooker was used to demonstrate steam sterilization, and the Wilmont Castle Company began manufacturing sterilizers in 1890. The American Sterilizer Company made its first tempera-

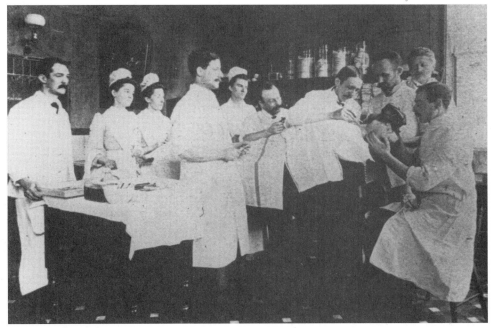

FIGURE 1-2. Mount Sinai Operating Room, circa 1900. The Archives of the Mount Sinai Medical Center.

ture-regulated pressure steam sterilizer in 1933 (Clemons, 1977; Altemeier, 1984).

Arpad Gerster provided the first English textbook, *The Rules of Aseptic and Antiseptic Surgery*, in 1888. A quote by Gerster taken from Clemons (1977, p. 20) reads:

> Whenever anyone engaged in an operation touches a not disinfected object, handles a chair, opens a window or door, helps the anesthetizer during a patient's vomiting spell, or scratches his face, or wipes his nose, it is absolutely necessary that his hands be scrubbed and disinfected anew. Instruments dropped on the floor should be left untouched. Raw assistants and especially nurses—male or female, trained or untrained—should be earnestly instructed beforehand and *constantly watched.*

PROGRESS IN NURSING

As surgery advanced as a science, so did the profession of nursing. In 1836 in Germany, Patrotor Fliedner and his wife Friederike instituted a 3-year course, consisting of bedside and classroom experience, to train deaconesses who would be nurses. Florence Nightingale studied with the Fliedners and with the Sisters of Charity in Paris. During the Crimean War, in 1854, Florence Nightingale became lady-in-chief, and her nurses worked in two fully-occupied hospitals under some very poor sanitary conditions. Army nursing under Nightingale's supervision advanced to a health service. While serving in the Crimean War, she developed and carried out nursing services, planned other services, and collected hospital statistics. She became aware of the need for nursing education and determined that nursing should be viewed as a health vocation independent of but closely allied with medicine.

Nightingale, as superintendent of Harley Street Clinic in London, took in 38 women and trained them as nurses. The initial 38 women Nightingale trained in nursing grew to a corps of 125. The Nightingale School of Nursing opened at St. Thomas' Hospital in London in 1860. She carefully selected young women for a 3- to 4-year course of study with a prescribed course of instruction and supervision on the wards (Jensen, 1955).

Nightingale's influence spanned the ocean, and soon schools of nursing were established in the United States. Mother Seton founded St. Joseph's Sisterhood in 1809. The Sisters of Mercy were established in 1843. By 1845, the Episcopal Sisterhood was established, and in 1858 the Episcopal sisters established and staffed St. Luke's Hospital in New York. In 1849, the Kaiserwerth deaconess order provided care to hospitalized patients (Jamieson, 1959).

In the United States before the Civil War, every large city had almshouses and infirmaries for the poor and sick. Some voluntary hospitals existed but the quality of care was poor. Often nursing was done by hospital inmates themselves, and no special training was provided. In 1839, Dr. Joseph Warrington organized the Nurse Society in Philadelphia and published *The Nurse's Guide for Infant and Mother Care*. In 1859, Drs. Elizabeth and Emily Blackwell planned to open a training school in New York, but the Civil War intervened. The first voluntary nursing group, organized by Dr. Elizabeth Blackwell, was the Women's Central Association for Relief intended to train supervisors and chief nurses.

Before the advent of the Nightingale training system in U.S. nursing schools, Linda Richards became the first trained nurse in America, graduating from the School of New England Hospital for Women and Children in 1873. Three schools based on the Nightingale system were then established in New York (Fig. 1–3). New Haven and Boston physicians provided most lectures, and nursing students learned by trial and error in a modified apprenticeship format (Jensen, 1955).

Professionalization of nurses began with the establishment of training schools for nursing. When early physicians were faced with the prospect of some women becoming trained nurses, some were opposed because, "they objected

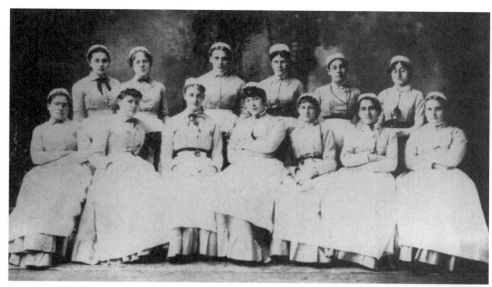

FIGURE 1-3. Mount Sinai School of Nursing Graduating Class 1881. The Archives of the Mount Sinai Medical Center.

that educated nurses would not do as they were told—a remarkable comment on the status anxieties of the 19th-century physicians" (Starr, 1982).

When the Civil War broke out, Lincoln called for volunteers to provide nursing services, for there were no trained nurses. President Lincoln established the U. S. Sanitary Commission in 1861 to secure healthier conditions in military camps and hospitals and to coordinate a nursing program with the Army. Dorothea Dix was commissioned as Superintendent of the U. S. Army Nurses on June 10, 1861. Her problem was the number of women already in the field and the others who wanted to join. She was concerned with their roles and found they varied from post to post. Some who joined lacked skills and were less meritorious and stole supplies (Jamieson, 1959). Dix demanded qualifications. Applicants had to be over 30 years of age, plain looking, wearing black or brown dresses and no bows, curls, jewelry, or hoop skirts. The Red Cross Society was founded in 1866. The work in Civil War hospitals was conducted by women and marked the beginning of public work by women (Flanagan, 1976). In October 1863, nurses were placed under the direction of medical officers. Clara Barton heard of men dying because they could not get to hospitals, so she personally took supplies to the front line and set up first aid stations (Jamieson, 1959). Six hundred women provided nursing care during the Civil War; however, after the war, few continued in the nursing profession. The Civil War brought an end to another era in nursing (Jamieson, 1959).

EMERGENCE OF OR NURSING TRAINING/EDUCATIONAL STANDARDS

In 1888, Isabel Hampton Robb became affiliated with Cook County Hospital to learn how to care for private patients. Robb wrote an important textbook in 1893, *Nursing: Its Principles and Practices in the Hospital and Home.* An excerpt reads:

To ensure thoroughness, one nurse should be given responsibility of the care of the operating room, a task which is sufficient to occupy her whole time. Pupils work under her direction and observance and in that way get their training . . . [because] the technique of the operating room has come to have such an important bearing on the outcome of surgical operations.

Because of the prevalence of new techniques and their impact on nursing care in the operating room, Robb recommended 2 months of orderly clinical operating room experience for nursing students (Clemons, 1977). During this period, nursing uniforms were developed, nurses strove to establish registration as legal distinction, and for the first time professional standards included graduation in addition to good character and good health.

In 1875, Johns Hopkins University opened. Isabelle Adams Hampton was superintendent of nurses and the principal of the Johns Hopkins Training School. The courses included elementary principles of asepsis and antiseptic surgery. The Johns Hopkins school planned and set precedents for nursing in the operating room. Still, during the Spanish American War of 1898, no provision for nursing services existed (Jamieson, 1959).

Johns Hopkins Hospital opened on May 7, 1889, with each division headed by a graduate head nurse on each ward. A surgical nurse, Carolyn Hampton (no relation to Isabelle) had been selected to be head nurse for the ward and the operating room on the day of opening, thus beginning clinical specialization in operating room nursing. Operating room nursing and surgical specialization for physicians began at the same time and place (Clemons, 1977; Lee, 1976). After surgical gloves were manufactured, Hampton was the only one to wear gloves for a long time in the operating room. She is credited with being the first operating room nurse of our modern time. It appears that the second operating room nurse, Nora Anthony, who was a classmate of Adelaide Nutting, was employed at Presbyterian Hospital in New York in 1892. Many other hospitals followed suit, adding nurses in charge of the operating room (Clemons, 1977).

Clemons cited *Asepsis for the Nurse*, published in 1889, which stated that the operating room nurse should have the following:

A level head and keen eyes, ever watchful for all that may be required, a mind not easily irritated or confused, combined with the facility of keeping out of the way and still being of the greatest help. . . . Thoroughness, speed and gentleness especially fit the surgical nurse.

The world's first operating room suite was developed by Gustav Neuber in 1884–1885. It contained five operating rooms and was built in Kiel, Germany. Neuber also introduced the surgical cap to cover hair (Clemons, 1977).

Massachusetts General Hospital Training School records note that female patients were taken to the operating theater without the presence of a nurse. Bellevue Hospital admitted nurses to the operating room when it was determined that boisterous medical students could be controlled by the presence of a nurse, and an 1877 Bellevue student prospectus promised that nursing students could expect to assist at operations. The advent of meticulous surgery, inflicting minimal trauma and providing good homeostasis, championed by Halsted, finally changed the role of the operating room nurse from taking care of sponges to assisting the surgeon.

During the late 19th century, student nurses were instructed to take baths before all procedures, to carbolize their hands and arms, and to cover cuts and abrasions with collodion. The scrub attire progressed from a black coat with buttons to white clothing. Robb, in *Aseptic Surgical Technique* (1894), advocated a complete surgical costume made of twilled muslin and sterilized before wearing. A 1905 guide advocated that nurses wear calico dresses without an aseptic gown over it.

In 1893, realizing the need to unite, the first international gathering of nurses was convened at the Chicago World's Fair in June 1893. On display at the World's Fair was an operating room with autoclave and rubber gloves. The nurses' conference, planned by Isabel Hampton Robb, Adelaide Nutting, and Lavinia Dock, focused on control of nursing training, registration of nurses, and formation of a national organization. Robb advocated an 8-hour workday and better nursing education. She published an outline detailing the content of 2-year programs, and by 1900, she was advocating 3-year programs and investigating the addition of nursing to college programs.

TWENTIETH CENTURY

Between 1910 and 1912, there were many advances in preventive medicine. Large-scale vaccination began to prevent disease, and antibiotics introduced in the second quarter of the 20th century reduced mortality. Methods for controlling the OR environment were improved as a consequence of the aerospace program, which led to the use of space suits for some operating surgeons and laminar airflow systems in the OR. Most instruments of the 1990s are made from stainless steel, titanium, and vitallium (Ackerknecht, 1968; Marks, 1973).

Education of operating room nurses was common in 1900. By 1909, hospitals numbered over 4000, and schools of nursing in hospitals proliferated to keep up with the demand for nurses. A 1917 survey noted that hospitals were dealing mostly with surgical patients. The National League for Nursing Education in 1917 published *Standards Curriculum Guide with Emphasis on Surgical Experience*. At the turn of the century, the specialty of nursing was established. In 1905, operating room nursing interventions included the prevention of infection, promotion of comfort, physical safety of patients, monitoring of patient condition, resuscitation, and psychologic support. In 1903, formal operating room experience was a requirement for nurse licensure (Clemons, 1977).

OR TEXTS

In 1902, the first operating room nursing textbook, *A Nurse's Guide for the Operating Room*, was published by Dr. Nicholas Senn. After World War I, the methods of sterilization included boiling, autoclaving, formaldehyde fuming, and immersion in 5% carbolic acid and cold bichloride solution in a 1 : 5000 ratio for 2 hours. Autoclaves accommodated different types and sizes of materials with different chambers for the varying needs of pressure and vacuum. Amy Armour Smith, author of the 1916 text *The Operating Room: A Primer for Pupil Nurses*, stated that the cap and mask should be put on first, that damp linen is unsterile, and that wrapped packages should not come in contact with the body. She also noted the need to autoclave scrub brushes, boil instruments after the operation, and patch linen holes. The book illustrated linen fan folds, elbow-operated soap dispensers, disinfection of the faucet each morning, and three separate mops on the floor for soap, water, and carbolic acid solution. She cautioned against leaning over the sterile field and wearing street shoes in the operating room.

Nursing textbooks of the 1920s describe how to turn the home into a surgical setting by removing the furniture, applying carbolic acid to surfaces, cleaning the wallpaper, covering the floor, fumigating the air, finding a sturdy table, and hanging sheets over the doors.

Between 1920 and 1940, most of the care in hospitals was provided by students, some of whom were listed as circulators. The Great Depression resulted in a decrease in the number of patients in the hospital and therefore the number of nurses employed (Groah, 1990). By the late 1940s, nurses engaged in collective bargaining through the ANA. Skin cleansing involved two processes, the first with soap and the second with chemical disinfectant. The scrub solution used by the team in preparing for surgery was based on surgeon preference. After scrubbing for 7 minutes, the hands and arms were rinsed with chloride of lime and soda, potassium permanganate, or iodine. When Edythe Alexander published *Operating Room Technique* in 1943, however, she advocated scrubbing the hands with soap and rinsing without the addition of the chemical rinse. In threading suture, Alexander advised that the short end should always be 4 inches long and the needle threaded inside out, placing the short end outside the curve of the needle.

World War II increased the demand for physicians and nurses. Military corpsmen returned from Army duty to assume roles as operating room technicians. In 1945, discussing the roles of operating room nurses, M. Crawford wrote:

> The nurse who is the immediate assistant to the surgeon is often called the "scrub" or "sterile" nurse. She first scrubs her hands and arms the required length of time, puts on sterile gown and gloves, and handles only sterile material,

and the circulating nurse is:

> In charge of the operating room, taking care of the needs of the room assigned to her. It is her responsibility to watch the aseptic technic of her team.

Crawford went on to note the qualities of a good operating room nurse:

> A surgery nurse must have many good qualities; but first of all, she must be most conscientious of sterile technic used, for the supervising nurse or surgeon is usually not present to watch the setting up of a case. Speed and efficiency are of no avail if a surgical wound breaks down due to an infection received in the operating room. The nurse must be enthusiastic about surgery or else is not able to continue in this type of nursing long, as it is physically as well as mentally tiring. Her disposition, patience, and control must be good; for under the strain of operation, conflicting orders are often given, specially to scrub nurses. Every move must mean something or much energy and time is wasted; therefore, a surgery nurse must have some knowledge of procedures, drapes, instruments, and sutures before being allowed to scrub on a case.

Crawford also noted that sterile rubber gloves were used in procedures except some eye procedures, such as cataract operations. She also advised that sterile cotton gloves were sometimes placed over sterile rubber gloves, particularly on bone or breast procedures, where the tissue is fatty and difficult to dissect because of the slipperiness of the gloves. Gloves were prepared by washing and drying each side and testing them for holes, which was done by the graduate nurses. Gloves were then powdered, packaged, and sterilized. Crawford also suggested that nurses report to duty with a cap, wear only white slips under their uniform, keep shoes and laces clean, keep fingernails short, remove lipstick, and refrain from unnecessary conversation. She also described the cleanup after contaminated procedures (Crawford, 1945).

E. A. Prickett in 1955 wrote a text aimed at helping the OR supervisor. The text, published by the National League for Nursing, described levels of personnel, such as the operating room supervisor, head nurse, general duty nurse, instructor, and nonprofessional personnel including practical nurses, surgical technical aides, nursing aides, and orderlies. Confusion existed because there were no standard titles in the operating room; nurse was used after scrub, suture, instrument, and sponge; but no one knew what to call the nonprofessional personnel who were employed to assist in scrubbing and circulating. Prickett (1955) noted that nonprofessional personnel were needed

> In order to meet the greatly increased demands for operating room service, the numbers and categories of nonprofessional workers assisting the professional nurse in the operating room have grown considerably. Leaders of the nursing profession and of hospital administration are in general agreement that nonprofessional workers can be used safely, effectively and economically for special assignments without compromising the quality of care given patients in the operating room.

OR NURSING EDUCATION

During the typical 6-month training program, the student learned how to scrub and prepare solutions, syringes, and needles, and became familiar with anesthesia and transfusions. The circulating nurse during surgery was responsible for tying the sterile gowns, connecting suction tubing, if used, changing the glove water when necessary, mopping the floor, and keeping the operating room clean and in order at all times. As instruments were thrown into the sink, the circulating nurse washed them and placed them in the small boiler. The soaked sponges were placed in the sponge pail, the square packs washed and hung over the side of the sink until the end of the operation — when the count was verified by the sterile nurse. The gloves were washed, and soiled basins were scoured and wrapped to be ready for sterilization immediately after the operation (St. Mary's Hospital, 1937).

In 1962, in *Logic of Operating Room Nursing*, J. Willingham described the surgical team as the anesthesiologist, surgeon, first assistant, second assistant, suture nurse who could be a nurse or a technician, and a circulating nurse who was preferably a registered nurse. Safety was emphasized, especially preventing infections and preventing explosions. To prevent explosions, Willingham recommended cotton clothing, conductive shoes, not smoking in the operating suite, testing floors and furniture for conductivity, insuring that the patient was conductive, taking care when disposing of used ether cans, avoiding the use of plastics, and making sure that the humidity was at least 55%. In describing the need for a surgical conscience regarding technique Willingham (1962) advised the nurse:

You have a very responsible position. Every set-up a doctor uses is prepared by a nurse. A good part of the doctor's success and the patient's well-being is in your hands. Remember this obligation. Only you can answer the question, 'Did I use good surgical technique while preparing and executing this procedure?' Everyone connected in the procedure is sure you did. Have you betrayed these people and yourself?

Anna M. O'Neill described an 8-week training course for operating room nursing, which included ethics, tours, preparation of the room, surgical technique, anesthesia, and instrumentation and solution preparation (Fig. 1-4). She described an operating room suite as needing an absence of the sun's glare, preferably with northern light, frosted glass or glass bricks for the windows, an abundance of fresh air free from dust and admitted without a draft, closed doors and a temperature of 80°F and a humidity of 45% to 60%. She also described the procedure for scrubbing and an open-gloving technique. The daily routine in the operating room included making sponges, attending end of shift conferences, and working from 7 AM to 7 PM.

A septic operating room was one in which a contaminated case had occurred, and she advised that septic cases be done in rooms that were connected to a sterilizer that could be isolated from the rest of the operating room (Fig. 1-5). Operating room attire was described as white surgical scrubs, caps of the turban style, white shoes with leather soles and heels, and cotton underwear. Masks

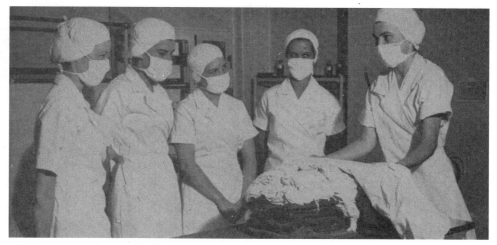

FIGURE 1-4. Teaching Methods of Sterilization. (Reprinted with permission from Davis & Geck, Danbury, CT.)

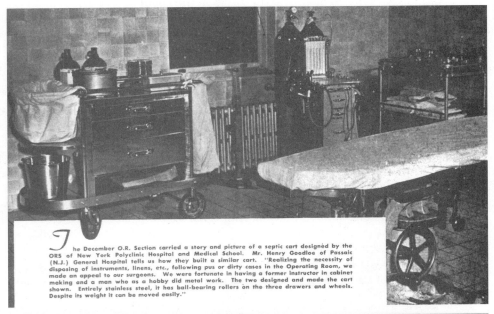

The December O.R. Section carried a story and picture of a septic cart designed by the ORS of New York Polyclinic Hospital and Medical School. Mr. Henry Goodloe of Passaic (N.J.) General Hospital tells us how they built a similar cart. "Realizing the necessity of disposing of instruments, linens, etc., following pus or dirty cases in the Operating Room, we made an appeal to our surgeons. We were fortunate in having a former instructor in cabinet making and a man who as a hobby did metal work. The two designed and made the cart shown. Entirely stainless steel, it has ball-bearing rollers on the three drawers and wheels. Despite its weight it can be moved easily."

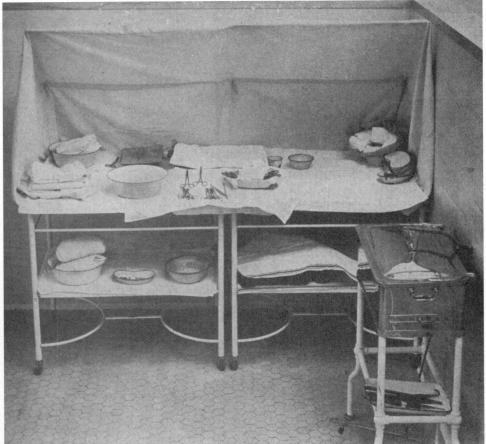

FIGURE 1–5. A Typical OR Suite of the 20th Century. (Top, Septic Cart, 1950, Hospital Topics. (Reprinted with permission of the Helen Dwight Reid Educational Foundation. Published by Heldref Publications, 1319 Eighteenth St., N.W., Washington, D.C. 20036-1802. Copyright © 1950.) Bottom, St. Mary's Hospital Sterile Setup, © 1937, W.B. Saunders Co., Philadelphia.)

were made of several layers of 8 X 5 gauze, thin muslin, or flannel. An extra piece of cloth was attached to the scrub gown in the front. It was open at the sides and served as a muff for the surgeon to keep his hands covered while waiting for the operation to begin (O'Neill, 1945). The role of the OR nurse at this time can best be described by this quote:

> If any surgeon is ever so unfortunate as to make a wrong diagnosis or error in judgment, it is the nurses' duty not to gossip or presume to criticize in any way. Most hospital staffs have surgeons of ability and good morale, so it is a privilege to give them a hearty cooperation, remembering that we are only pegs in the big operating system.

The average nurse's salary in 1955 was $246.58 per month, and the operating room nurses' time was spent in the following way: activities during surgery, 24.2%; personal and standby, 19.0% (personal and standby time included the time spent waiting for the surgeon, the patient, or others); care and preparation of supplies, equipment, environment, 15.2%; collateral duties in OB, ER, and administration, 13.6%; conference and consulting, 11.9%; preparation of the operating room and patient, 9.4%; recordkeeping, 4.2%; and postsurgery activities, 2.4% (Stewart, 1955). Stewart and Needham (1955) recommended that educators examine the daily activities of the OR nurse in order to plan educational programs.

EVALUATION OF THE ASSISTIVE PERSONNEL ROLE

When the American Hospital Association published *Surgical Technical Aides, Instructor's Manual* in 1954, the definition of the OR aide was as follows:

> Surgical technical aide is a selected lay person who by means of a well planned and well organized course of instruction is prepared to function intelligently under the direct and continuous supervision of qualified professional nurses within hospital areas intimately concerned with the principles and practices of surgical asepsis.

The suggested functions of the surgical technical aide included assisting with general nursing activities of the department under supervision; assisting with case preparation and maintenance of sterile and nonsterile supplies; general housekeeping duties and clerical work; taking messages; running errands; and transporting patients. He or she could act as circulating and scrub assistants during operative procedures, under supervision. The guide described phases of care as preoperative care, care during the operative procedure, and postoperative care. It also mentioned the need for research for operating room supervisors and staff nurses (AHA, 1954).

The issue of the use of technicians has been hotly debated from the beginning. AORN published a *Statement Relating to Non-professional Technical Assistants in the Operating Room* (AORN, 1966). It reads:

> The Association of Operating Room Nurses—due to the shortage of professional nurses—recognizes the need for non-professional assistance in the operating room.
>
> The Association acknowledges the fact that selected non-professional people can provide this assistance under the supervision of registered professional nurses, provided that they have been given proper training in established educational programs.
>
> The Association also acknowledges its responsibility to help establish sound educational programs for the purpose of training such non-professional operating room assistants. Therefore, a manual of instruction incorporating performance standards will be prepared for use as a guide in the setting up and carrying out of a comprehensive program of training.

A teaching guide for technicians was prepared by a committee appointed by the AORN Board of Directors.

The Board of Governors of the American College of Surgeons (ACS) was concerned with the shortage of operating room nurses. A committee was appointed to study the issue and propose a 6-month course outline of training for operating room technicians. AORN was at the forefront of the discussion. The operating room technician was defined as "a licensed practical nurse or a lay person who has been taught how to assist surgeons, anesthesiologists, and registered professional nurses in the care of patients in the operating room." The primary role of the technician was as a sterile instrument handler. He or she was also responsible for prepping patients, transporting, stocking, instrument assembly, specimen care, sponge counting, sterilization, positioning, and aiding the circulating nurse. "The Operating Room Technician works under the direct supervision of a registered professional nurse at all times, except for diagnostic procedures for which the direct supervision of the nurse may not be required" (Burns, 1967 p. 2).

By 1969, the Association of Operating Room Nurses had defined the practice of nursing in the OR as professional (Table 1–1). In an editorial (Rockwell, 1963) the future of the registered nurse in the operating room was challenged:

> What will our future be? Where are we going and where have we been? For those who believe in the professional role of the operating room nurse, in spite of what's behind and of the present wavering situation, there is a far greater challenge ahead, it's up to us to explain our being as well as accepting the responsibility to defend our position. We need united ranks and the will to accept the challenge. We must convince the world we operating room nurses are here because we are needed, and we are here . . . to stay!

Practical nurses were assigned to evening and night duty to assist professional nurses in their work and to eliminate the need to call in the nursing team from home. They circulated in emergency operations, set up intravenous lines, and scrubbed on surgical procedures. They also covered the emergency room but were not allowed to be in charge (Bell, 1952).

AORN has been consistently concerned with maintaining the role of the registered nurse in the operating room. Until June 1974, the Medicare conditions of participation required that the registered nurse circulate on all surgical cases. In 1974, the Department of Health and Human Services (HHS) published a notice in the *Federal Register* that it intended to change the conditions for participation to allow technicians to circulate. In 1977, HHS drafted a working paper that allowed operating room technicians to perform scrub duties or assist in circulating duties under the direct supervision of the registered nurse. However, in 1980, HHS published proposed changes in the *Federal Register* to allow registered nurses, licensed practical nurses, and surgical technologists to circulate. In 1983, HHS reversed its 1980 opinion and determined that only qualified registered nurses could circulate, allowing technicians to assist under the direct supervision of a

TABLE 1–1. A DEFINITION OF PROFESSIONAL NURSING IN THE OPERATING ROOM

Professional Nursing in the operating room is the identification of the physiological, psychological and sociological needs of the patient and the implementation of an individualized program of nursing care that coordinates the nursing actions, based on a knowledge of the natural and behavioral sciences, in order to restore, or maintain, the health and welfare of the patient before, during, and after surgical intervention.

CLINICAL PRACTICE OF PROFESSIONAL OPERATING ROOM NURSING

The objective of the clinical practice of Professional Operating Room Nursing is to provide a standard of excellence in the care of the patient before, during, and after surgical intervention.
This objective is achieved by:

1. Identification of the physiological, psychological and sociological needs of each individual patient;

2. Development and implementation of an individualized plan of nursing care that meets the identified needs of the patient;

3. Coordination of the individualized plan, with other members of the health team, to promote continuity of nursing care for each patient;

4. Application of the principles of asepsis and technical knowledge in making sound nursing judgements to ensure a safe environment for the welfare of the patient;

5. Provision for direction of other professional, and allied technical personnel, in implementation of the program of nursing care of the patient by teaching, supervising, and evaluating personnel performance;

6. Initiation of, or assistance with, research projects designed to develop a body of scientific knowledge relative to the care, and coordination of components of Professional Operating Room Nursing.

From Association of Operating Room Nurses. (1969). A definition of professional nursing in the operating room. *AORN Journal 10* (5), 48. Reprinted by permission.

registered nurse. The 1986 final regulations published in the *Federal Register* omitted the reference to direct supervision and allowed technicians to circulate when a registered nurse is immediately available.

The role of the registered nurse in the operating room was being challenged. Many schools of nursing, moving from hospital to university-based centers, were eliminating the education related to operating room nursing. Operating room nurses of that era tried to keep OR education included as a part of the curriculum, but most nursing educators failed to see the benefit of teaching aseptic technique to student nurses, and the education was eliminated from the programs. Jahraus (1955) described OR experience at the collegiate level:

> We urge nurses who complete our basic collegiate program to seek further experience and advanced education in their chosen field, since they are prepared for only first level positions in hospitals and in public health nursing agencies.

In a debate related to the professionalism of operating room nursing published in the *American Journal of Nursing* in 1965, Ginsberg said "every time anyone inquires about septic case technique, I explode a bomb by saying there isn't any. All cases are septic." She continued by saying, "There is no place in the operating room for a 'technical nurse.' There is a place for technical competence, but the need is for a professional nurse." The article described OR supervisors as clinical specialists and technicians as assistants to the professional nurse.

In 1973, a resolution reaffirming the role of the registered nurse in the operating room was approved by the AORN House of Delegates. By 1975, as a result of the issues related to the technician as the circulator, the House of Delegates passed a statement on the need for the circulator to be a registered professional nurse. By 1976, a task force was formed to define the role of the registered nurse in the OR. This resulted in the formation of the Project 25 Task Force appointed by the Board of Directors. At the 25th House of Delegates in 1978, the *Statement on the Perioperative Role* was adopted, officially expanding the role of the registered nurse in the OR to include the pre-, intra-, and postoperative periods of the patient's surgical experience. The statement was revised and the scope of perioperative nursing practice enlarged in 1984–85 and again in 1988 and 1994 (see Table 1–2).

Issues for Development

With the advent of health care reform, perioperative nursing practitioners must identify and validate the role of the registered professional nurse in the operating room. Although the profession has prided itself on its technical skills for several years, the time has come to examine the enhanced professional role of the perioperative nurse. Perioperative nurses must conduct studies that validate the outcomes of professional nursing care.

As the future overtakes nursing, perioperative nurses must be certain about the level of education necessary to compete in the marketplace of health care. The perioperative nurse of the future must be prepared minimally at the baccalaureate level. Graduate programs in nursing must begin to prepare perioperative clinical specialists and nurse practitioners who will provide comprehensive care to surgical patients regardless of the clinical setting and the operative procedure to be performed.

Finally, it is the responsibility of each perioperative practitioner to delegate effectively to unlicensed assistive personnel. Perioperative nurses must name what they do in ways that can be understood and reimbursed. AORN is accomplishing this through current work on the development of data elements for perioperative nursing. By identifying those interventions that perioperative nurses perform for patients, regardless of setting, the perioperative nurse will begin to

TABLE 1–2. SCOPE OF PERIOPERATIVE NURSING PRACTICE

Perioperative nursing practice begins with the prospect of an operative or other invasive procedure and is completed by evaluating the extent to which the recipient's needs have been met. Perioperative nurses interact with both the patient and/or the patient's significant other throughout the continuum of patient care. Perioperative nursing practice takes place in the patient's environment and includes, but is not limited to, surgical suites, ambulatory surgery settings, clinics, physicians' offices, communities, and homes.

The management of the recipient's needs, both unique and predictable, may be through direct or indirect interventions. These interventions are planned to assist the recipient in meeting the projected outcomes in an efficient and appropriate manner. Perioperative nursing care is implemented by registered nurses who strive to assist the patient to meet projected outcomes by functioning in various roles—clinical practitioner, manager, educator, and researcher.

Perioperative nursing varies and may include, but is not limited to,

- peer education and patient/family teaching,
- support and reassurance,
- advocacy,
- control of the environment,
- efficient provision of resources,
- maintenance of asepsis,
- monitoring physiologic and psychologic status,
- management of aggregate patient needs,
- supervision of ancillary personnel,
- perioperative exploration and validation of current and future practices,
- integration and coordination of care across settings and among disciplines, and
- collaboration and consultation.

These activities are based on using the problem-solving approach in practice, management, education and research.

The reason for the existence of perioperative nursing practice is the care of persons undergoing operative and other invasive procedures. Perioperative nursing services are extended to a variety of other groups to enhance the care ultimately provided to the patient. These groups include hospitals, clinics, schools and colleges of nursing, physicians, other nurses, insurers, and medical device and pharmaceutical manufacturers.

From Association of Operating Room Nurses. (1994). Scope of perioperative nursing practice. *AORN Journal*, *59*(1), 85. Reprinted by permission.

identify those interventions that have a direct impact on patient outcomes. This sentinel work by the Association will provide a basis on which to conduct outcome studies and validate the need for the registered nurse in perioperative patient care.

REFERENCES

Ackerknecht, E. H. (1968). *A Short History of Medicine*. Revised ed. New York: Ronald Press.

Alexander, E. A. (1953). Order out of chaos in the O.R. *American Journal of Nursing, 53*(3), 294–295.

Alexander, E. A. (1943). *Operating Room Technique*. St. Louis: C. V. Mosby.

Altemeier, W. A., Burke, J. F., Pruitt, B. A., Sandusky, W. R. (1984). *Manual on Control of Infection in Surgical Patients*. 2nd ed. Philadelphia: J. B. Lippincott.

American Hospital Association. (1954). *Surgical Technical Aides, Instructor's Manual*. Chicago: AHA.

American Journal of Nursing. (1984). *Pages from Nursing History*. New York: Author.

American Journal of Nursing. (1965). Operating room nursing: Is it professional nursing? *American Journal of Nursing, 65*(8), 58–63.

Association of Operating Room Nurses. (1994). Scope of perioperative nursing practice. *AORN Journal, 59*(1), 85.

Association of Operating Room Nurses. (1969). A definition of professional nursing in the operating room. *AORN Journal, 10*(5), 48.

Association of Operating Room Nurses. (1966). Statement relating to non-professional technical assistants in the operating room. *AORN Journal, 4*(1), 85.

Bell, H. S. (1952). Practical nurses in the operating room. *American Journal of Nursing, 52*(5), 581–582.

Burns, M. A., Lundahl, H. M., Rockwell, V. T., Redgate, J. M. (1967). *Teaching the Operating Room Technician*. New York: Association of Operating Room Nurses. (p. 2).

Clemons, B. (1976). Lister's day in America. *AORN Journal, 24*(1), 43–51.

Clemons, B. (1977). *Operating Room Nursing and Other Beginnings*. Phoenix: Author.

Crawford, M. (1945). *A Manual of Operating Room Technique*. Los Angeles: Hospital of the Good Samaritan. (p. 12).

Flanagan, L. (1976). *One strong voice: the story of the American Nurses Association.* Kansas City, Missouri: American Nurses Association.

Ginsberg, F., Brunner, L. S., Cantlin, V. L. (1966). *A Manual of Operating Room Technology.* Philadelphia, J. B. Lippincott Company.

Griffin, G. J., Griffin, J. K. (1973). *History and Trends of Professional Nursing.* 6th ed. St. Louis: C. V. Mosby.

Groah, L. K. (1990). *Operating Room Nursing: Perioperative Practice.* 2nd ed. Norwalk, Connecticut: Appleton and Lange.

Halsted, W. S. (1952). *Surgical Papers.* 2nd ed. Baltimore: The Johns Hopkins Press. (p. 38).

Jahraus, C. C. (1955). Clinical experience in the operating room. *American Journal of Nursing, 55*(1), 79–81.

Jamieson, E. M., Sewall, M. F., Gjertson, L. S. (1959). *Trends in Nursing History: Their Social, International, and Ethical Relationships.* 5th ed. Philadelphia: W. B. Saunders.

Jensen, D. (1955). *History and Trends of Professional Nursing.* 3rd ed. St. Louis: C. V. Mosby.

Lee, R. M. (1976). Early operating room nursing. *AORN Journal, 24*(1), 37–41.

Marks, G., Beatty, W. K. (1973). *The Story of Medicine in America.* New York: Charles Scribner's Sons.

National League for Nursing Education. (1917). *Standards Curriculum Guide with Emphasis on Surgical Experience.* New York: Author.

O'Neill, A. M. (1945). *Operating Room Technique* (reprint). Philadelphia: F. A. Davis.

Prickett, E. A. (1955). *The Operating Room Supervisor at Work.* New York: National League for Nursing Education.

Robb, H. (1894). *Aseptic Surgical Technique.* Philadelphia: J. B. Lippincott.

Rockwell, V. T. (1963). Editorial. *AORN Journal, 1*(1), 10.

Senn, N. (1902). *A Nurse's Guide for the Operating Room.* Chicago: Keener.

Smith, A. R. (1916). *The Operating Room: A Primer for Pupil Nurses.* Philadelphia: W. B. Saunders.

St. Mary's Hospital. (1937). *The Operating Room Instructions for Nurses and Assistants.* 3rd ed. Philadelphia: W. B. Saunders.

Starr, P. (1982). *The Social Transformation of American Medicine.* New York: Basic Books. (p. 155).

Stewart, D. S., Needham, C. (1955). Operating room nurses' functions are studied. *American Journal of Nursing, 55*(11), 1347–1349.

Willingham, J. (1962). *Logic of Operating Room Nursing.* New York: Springer.

U.S. Dept. of Health and Human Services. (1986). Federal Register Medicare and Medicaid Programs; Conditions of participation for hospitals; final regulations 51(116)22009–22052.

Chapter Two

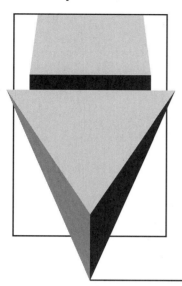

Professional Perioperative Nursing Development

Kathie G. Shea, RN, BSN, CNOR

Prerequisite Knowledge   Chapter contents will correlate with AORN positions, standards, and recommended practices. These standards may be considered a prerequisite prior to beginning the chapter or a refresher upon completion of the chapter.

Mission and philosophy

Competency statements in perioperative nursing

Standards of administrative practice

Standards of perioperative clinical practice

Standards of perioperative professional practice

Quality improvement standards for perioperative nursing

Patient outcomes: Standards of perioperative care

Recommended practices for perioperative nursing

Chapter Outline

Professional Development
  Professional organization membership
  Specialty certification

Perioperative Nursing Standards
  Definition
  Purpose
  Scope
  Categories

Recommended Practices for Perioperative Nursing
  Definition/purpose
  Basis
  Development
  Structure

Perioperative Nursing Roles
  Role definitions
  Responsibilities

Unlicensed Assistive Personnel
  Role definition
  Trends in utilization
  Nursing's role and responsibilities

Personal Values
  Values clarification
  Professional codes
  Ethical dilemmas

Learning Objectives

1. Identify resources for professional development.

2. Relate the concepts of perioperative nursing practice to professional nursing.

3. Interpret the importance of recommended practices to the perioperative nurse.

4. Compare and contrast perioperative nursing roles.

5. Analyze the relationship between the perioperative nurse and unlicensed assistive personnel.

6. Assess personal values in light of perioperative ethical dilemmas.

One does not graduate from a nursing program with the competency necessary to practice perioperative nursing. It takes time and effort to acquire the knowledge, skill, and ability that will enable the nurse to competently practice in the perioperative milieu. Thus, the new graduate will need to seek avenues for professional development.

Professional Nursing Organization Membership

One avenue for professional development is membership in a professional nursing organization. Membership can be of great value to the novice as well as the experienced nurse. There are many reasons to join a professional nursing organization.

These organizations provide current information to their members on a wide variety of clinical, managerial, research, and legislative topics. The nurse who remains informed on these topics has the opportunity to improve practice and is better equipped to anticipate and deal with the myriad changes taking place in the health care arena. Current information also allows the nurse to be proactive rather than reactive in regard to legislation impacting nursing practice.

Professional organizations facilitate group problem solving and exchange of ideas. Problems can be shared and resolution found through meetings of the organization and through journals and newsletters published by the organization. In addition, meetings of the organization can provide an opportunity for nurses to relate experiences and ideas that help in their practice setting. Professional organizations provide nurses with a voice in local and national decision making that shapes their future. Many large organizations, such as the American Nurses Association, hire lobbyists who monitor legislation related to nursing and health care and make legislators aware of nursing's position on various issues.

Membership in a specialty nursing organization, such as the Association of Operating Room Nurses, helps develop an increased awareness of perioperative nursing—its scope, factors that have an impact on practice, current research, and legislation. Exposure to current research and knowledge, awareness of trends in nursing, and access to legislative decision making provide nurses with tools to deliver quality patient care.

The Association of Operating Room Nurses

The Association of Operating Room Nurses (AORN) is an excellent resource for professional development of perioperative nurses. From its inception in 1949, AORN's mission has been to enhance professionalism, promote standards of perioperative nursing, and provide a forum for the interaction and exchange of ideas (AORN, 1993a). As a result of this mission, AORN has defined perioperative nursing and developed tools to identify the role and scope of the perioperative nurse. Among these tools are a model of care, nursing standards, recommended practices, and competency statements, which identify the fundamental knowledge and skills necessary to fulfill the role of a registered nurse in the perioperative setting.

PHILOSOPHY

AORN's philosophy, based on fundamental beliefs regarding nursing, serves to delineate perioperative practice as one in which the nurse, working in collaboration with other health care professionals, identifies and meets the needs of patients having surgical, therapeutic, or diagnostic intervention. Rapid changes in our society require that the perioperative nurse be responsive and adaptable. These changes bring about the necessity for perioperative nurses to be well-educated, skilled practitioners who continue the learning process throughout their careers.

ORGANIZATIONAL STRUCTURE

AORN is a specialty nursing organization of nurses throughout the United States and around the world. Members are organized into local geographic chapters following guidelines set forth by AORN.

Local chapters allow members input to the national organization and allow for collaboration and networking. Figure 2–1 shows the AORN organizational chart. Chapter members serving as delegates make up the House of Delegates and represent their chapter in official business, which is brought before the House annually by the national Board of Directors. The Board of Directors is elected annually by the House of Delegates. It is this Board that governs the organization.

AORN has several national committees whose functions are to carry out tasks assigned by the Board and provide information to assist the Board in decision-making processes. National committee membership is open to all active members by annual appointment of the president-elect with approval of the Board of Directors.

The Board is also assisted in accomplishing the work of the association by the AORN headquarters staff. Located in Denver, Colorado, AORN headquarters is divided into three service centers and two support divisions.

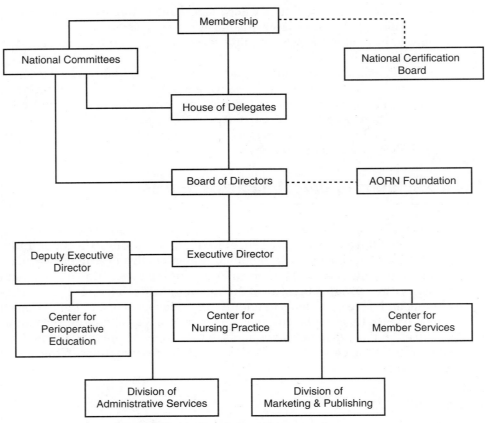

FIGURE 2-1. AORN Organizational Structure.

The Center for Perioperative Education develops and presents continuing education programs for perioperative nurses. This center also assists individual chapters with developing educational activities for their local area.

The Center for Nursing Practice focuses on consultation, specialized practice resources, standards, and recommended practices for perioperative nurses. An average of 700 telephone consultations a month are conducted by this busy center.

The Center for Member Services serves individual members and chapters in a variety of ways including chapter relations activities, member recruitment and retention programs, and customer service (e.g., liability and disability insurance, travel benefits, and credit cards).

Administrative Services is one of two support divisions within the AORN headquarters structure. It handles accounting, meeting services, information systems, and facilities management. The other support division, Marketing and Publishing, is responsible for production of the *AORN Journal*, advertising sales, marketing, and exhibit sales (*AORN Journal*, 1993a).

Although they are not part of the direct organizational structure of AORN, the National Certification Board: Perioperative Nursing Inc. (NCB:PNI) and the AORN Foundation have indirect connections with it. The National Certification Board conducts a voluntary certification and recertification program for registered nurses practicing in the perioperative setting. The AORN Foundation was formed to provide resources to support the mission of AORN related to research and educational pursuits of AORN members.

BENEFITS

The AORN offers perioperative nurses many professional development tools including educational offerings, publications, and other resources. AORN conducts several regional workshops and symposia throughout the nation each year. Topics, determined by identified member needs, are presented by experts in the field and offer participants the most current information on a wide variety of topics. The AORN Congress, which occurs annually, brings perioperative nurses together for a week of education, networking, and organizational decision making. Biannually the World Conference of Operating Room Nurses is held. It is here that perioperative nurses from around the world share knowledge and address common concerns of their practice. For those unable to attend educational meetings, AORN offers continuing education home study courses and videotapes.

Publications are another professional development tool offered by AORN. The *AORN Journal*, published monthly, is the premier publication for perioperative nurses. In-depth articles feature the latest in technologic advances, nursing theory, patient care, and surgical intervention. Clinical and legal topics are addressed in a question and answer format in each issue. Subscribers are also kept informed about legislation and other issues that have an impact on perioperative nursing. Specific AORN publications focus on perioperative nursing standards, recommended practices, ethics, and quality improvement, to name a few.

Other resources offered by AORN include information management software, consultation services, their library, and access to literature searches.

Certification

Certification in one's specialty can be viewed as evidence of professional development. Certification builds upon licensure in that it identifies specific knowledge that is above and beyond that of entry level for competent functioning in a nursing specialty (Allen, 1992). The NCB:PNI is the national certifying body for perioperative nursing. The NCB:PNI defines certification as "the documented validation of the professional achievement of identified standards of practice by an individual registered nurse providing care for patients before, during, and after surgery" (NCB:PNI, 1993).

OBJECTIVES/PURPOSES

The objectives of the certification program as stated by NCB:PNI are
- To recognize the individual nurse who is proficient in practice
- To strengthen conscious use of theory in planning and implementing patient care
- To enhance professional growth through continued learning

Certification objectives provide accountability for nursing practice, enhanced quality of care, recognition for the nurse who has demonstrated professional achievement, and personal satisfaction for the individual perioperative nurse.

ELIGIBILITY

Certification in perioperative nursing (CNOR) is available to experienced perioperative nurses who pass a written examination developed by their colleagues. Content of the examination is based on knowledge and skills related to perioperative nursing. Because some content is experiential, only registered nurses with

---

CONTROVERSY BOX

Certification

The issue of certification is not without controversy. Many believe certification demonstrates competence in nursing practice (Perry, 1989), while others see it as important in improving patient care skills and self-image (Faherty, 1991). Those who criticize certification believe that basing competency on a written test does not verify competency in actual nursing practice (del Bueno, 1988). A study of perioperative nurses in Texas revealed that performance in the clinical setting is a better indicator of quality care than certification, but that preparing for certification improves perioperative nursing ability (Allen, 1992). Regardless of the controversy surrounding certification, perioperative nurses are motivated to seek certification as fulfillment of a personal goal and as validation of their professional achievement (Allen, 1992).

---

a minimum of 2 full years of practice in perioperative nursing are eligible to take the examination.

Perioperative Nursing Standards

Nursing standards are important for professional development because they define responsibilities for a professional nurse practicing in the perioperative setting. Novice and experienced nurses alike need to be familiar with the standards in order to understand their scope of practice and accountability to the institution, to those they work with, to the public, and most importantly to those they care for.

The AORN *Standards of Nursing Practice* were developed in 1975 by AORN using the American Nurses Association (ANA) *Standards of Clinical Nursing Practice* as a guide. The revised *Standards of Perioperative Nursing Practice*, published in 1981, are approved by the ANA Division of Medical-Surgical Practice and the AORN Board of Directors.

DEFINITION

AORN defines standards as "authoritative statements that describe the responsibilities for which nursing practitioners are accountable" (AORN, 1993). Standards reflect the values and priorities of the nursing profession and define the professional's responsibilities. The standards developed by AORN focus specifically on the individual experiencing surgical intervention. They apply to all registered nurses engaged in perioperative practice regardless of the setting. The nurse is responsible for meeting the standards unless prevented from doing so by working conditions or lack of resources.

PURPOSE

Standards help to measure the quality of nursing care for surgical patients and can easily be adapted for use in quality assessment and improvement activities by comparing the standards with the nursing care provided in the practice setting. Standards reflect the definition, purpose, and framework for the perioperative setting, making them useful for developing policies and procedures. Standards are also a means to direct and evaluate professional nursing practice and can form the basis for job descriptions and performance appraisals.

CATEGORIES

The *Standards of Perioperative Nursing* are divided into three functional categories: structure, process, and outcome (Fig. 2–2).

- *Structure* standards focus on administrative practice.
- *Process* standards focus on clinical practice, professional performance, and quality improvement.
- *Outcome* standards focus on patient outcomes of perioperative care.

The *Standards of Perioperative Administrative Practice* are structure standards designed to guide nurses in administrative roles by providing a framework for the organization and administration of the perioperative setting. They also form the basis on which administrative nurses can evaluate their practice.

The process standards are composed of three separate standards:

- *Standards of Perioperative Clinical Practice*
- *Standards of Perioperative Professional Performance*
- *Quality Improvement Standards for Perioperative Nursing*

The *Standards of Perioperative Clinical Practice* describe a competent level of care provided by the nurse. These standards use the nursing process as a foundation for describing the nurse's responsibilities.

The *Standards of Professional Performance* describe a competent level of behavior for the nurse. Examples of professional behavior identified in these standards include activities related to providing quality care, performance appraisal, education, collegiality, ethics, collaboration, research, and use of resources.

Quality Improvement Standards for Perioperative Nursing serve as a guide to assist perioperative nurses in the assessment and improvement of quality patient care. The quality improvement standards are based on the Joint Commission on Accreditation of Healthcare Organizations criteria for patient care assessment and its standards for quality assessment and improvement.

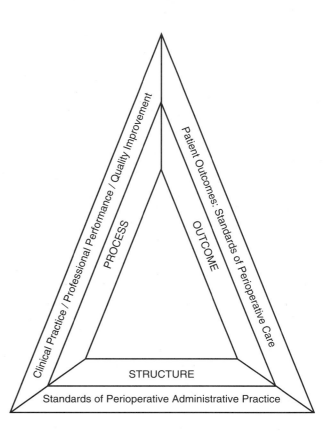

FIGURE 2–2. Perioperative Nursing Standards.

Patient Outcomes: Standards of Perioperative Care are outcome standards that describe the basic level of care a patient can expect to receive. Identified patient outcomes are observable or measurable responses to perioperative nursing intervention. Outcome standards assist the nurse in planning, implementing, and evaluating care. They may also be used to establish a data base to support existing practice or provide rationale for a change in practice.

Recommended Practices for Perioperative Nursing

Recommended practices are technically focused documents designed to assist nurses in their daily practice. Recommended practices are guidelines that represent an optimal level of practice. They focus on a wide variety of technical and professional perioperative nursing practices. They describe what procedures the nurse should follow in an ideal situation. All recommended practices are based on principles of microbiology, research, scientific literature review, and opinions of experts in the field.

AORN recognizes that perioperative nursing is practiced in a variety of settings and under many different conditions. These factors may influence the degree to which the recommended practices can be met. Therefore, it is important to emphasize that recommended practices represent an *optimal* level of practice and that compliance with the recommended practices is *voluntary*. They are not mandates, which must be followed, but rather guidelines to assist in delivering safe care that is of high quality.

PROCESS FOR DEVELOPMENT, REVIEW, AND REVISION

Recommended practices are reviewed and revised by the AORN Recommended Practices Committee. This multidisciplinary committee is composed of AORN members and representatives from the American College of Surgeons, the Centers for Disease Control and Prevention, the American Society of Infection Control Practitioners, the American Society of Anesthesiologists, and the American Society of Hospital Central Services Personnel. Recommended practices are examined at frequent intervals to insure that they reflect advances in technology and current research findings. Newly developed recommended practices and revisions to existing ones are published in the *AORN Journal* as drafts. AORN members and others are given the opportunity to comment on these drafts. Following the comment period, the Recommended Practices Committee completes a final review/revision based on the comments received. A final draft is sent to the AORN Board of Directors for approval. The approved recommended practice is then printed in the *AORN Journal*.

STRUCTURE/FORMAT

All recommended practices follow the same format — an introduction, a purpose statement, and a description of the recommended practice, followed by one or more interpretive statements with rationale provided for each interpretive statement. A reference list accompanies all recommended practices, providing resources for further study. The following outline is an example of one recommended practice related to monitoring the patient receiving intravenous conscious sedation.

Recommended Practices for Monitoring the Patient Receiving Intravenous Conscious Sedation

PURPOSE

These recommended practices provide guidelines for the registered nurse monitoring the patient receiving IV conscious sedation. The selection of patients managed in this way should be determined by established criteria developed through an interdisciplinary approach within the practice setting. The type of monitoring to be used, the medications that may be given, and the interventions that may be taken must be within the defined scope of nursing practice.

Certain patients are not candidates for IV conscious sedation with monitoring by the registered nurse. These patients may require more extensive and intensive monitoring and sedation, as provided by anesthesia personnel, and should be identified in consultation with anesthesiologists, nurses, certified registered nurse anesthetists, surgeons, and other physicians. It is not the intent of these recommended practices to address situations that require the services of the anesthesia department.

The patient care and monitoring outlined in these recommended practices may be exceeded at any time. Their intent is to encourage high-quality patient care; however, implementation of these recommended practices cannot guarantee a specific patient outcome. These recommended practices are subject to revision as warranted by the evolution of practice and technology.

RECOMMENDED PRACTICE I

The nurse should know the goals and objectives of IV conscious sedation.

Interpretive Statement 1

The primary goal of IV conscious sedation is to allay patient fear and anxiety regarding the planned procedure.

Rationale

Adequate preprocedure preparation and verbal reassurance from nursing personnel facilitate the effects of IV conscious sedation and may allow for a decrease in the dosage of opioids, benzodiazepines, and sedatives used.

Interpretive Statement 2

Objectives for the patient receiving IV conscious sedation include

- alteration of mood
- maintenance of consciousness
- maintenance of ability to cooperate
- elevation of pain threshold
- minimal variation of vital signs
- lessened degree of amnesia
- a rapid, safe return to ambulation

Rationale

Intravenous conscious sedation produces a condition where the patient exhibits a depressed level of consciousness but retains the ability to independently and continuously maintain a patent airway and respond appropriately to verbal commands or physical stimulation. Misunderstanding of the objectives of IV conscious sedation may jeopardize the quality of care.

From *AORN Standards and Recommended Practices.* Denver, Association of Operating Room Nurses, Inc., 1993.

Perioperative Nursing Practice

INTRODUCTION

Perioperative nursing practice has changed significantly in the past 25 years primarily owing to advancing technology and changes in the health care delivery system. Traditionally the operating room nurse was accountable for the care of patients only in the surgical suite. This role was expanded in 1978 to include nursing activities performed before and after surgery as well. The patient's surgical experience was divided into three distinct phases:

- preoperative
- intraoperative
- postoperative

Nursing responsibilities were identified for each phase. Currently the registered nurse who performs nursing activities in these three phases of the patient's surgical experience is defined as a perioperative nurse.

The scope of perioperative nursing practice is quite broad under the existing definition. The nurse's responsibilities may begin in the physician's office when the decision for surgical intervention is made, continue through the surgical procedure, and end with an evaluation in the patient's home. However, the emphasis for most perioperative nurses continues to be the intraoperative phase with responsibility for preoperative assessment just preceding surgical intervention and postoperative evaluation shortly after the surgical procedure concludes.

Perioperative nursing practice may take place in a variety of settings— hospitals, freestanding ambulatory treatment centers, clinics, or physician's offices. It is important to remember that the focal point of perioperative nursing practice is the individual undergoing surgical, therapeutic, or diagnostic intervention rather than where that intervention takes place.

Perioperative nursing practice does not exist in a vacuum. Perioperative nurses are part of a team of health care professionals who collaboratively work together to provide continuous quality care to all surgical patients. Collaborative teamwork presumes that the role and responsibilities of each member of the team are important. Collaborative teamwork also acknowledges and appropriately utilizes the knowledge and skills of all members of the team. Studies have shown that the results of collaborative practice are better patient care, increased job satisfaction, reduced cost, and reduced length of patient stay (Giordano, 1993). Barriers to collaboration include sex role stereotypes and differences in education, practice focus, and jurisdiction. Because collaboration has a direct impact on positive patient outcomes, barriers must be identified and resolved. Collegiality is slowly emerging between the nurse and physician. Perioperative nurses can take the lead in fostering its development by maintaining a current perioperative nursing knowledge base and exhibiting professional behavior.

The broad definition and scope of perioperative nursing allows the professional a variety of roles in which to practice. These roles include

- scrub person
- circulator
- manager
- researcher
- educator
- registered nurse first assistant (RNFA)

The perioperative nurse may assume many of these roles in the course of a single day depending upon the specific facility or patient population served.

The AORN *Standards of Perioperative Nursing* serve as the basis for delineating responsibilities of perioperative roles. A detailed characterization of these responsibilities is found in the AORN *Competency Model* (AORN, 1992) and the job analysis developed by the NCB:PNI. The *Competency Model* consists of 18 competency statements, which are believed to be "essential in providing an understanding of the fundamental knowledge and skills necessary to fulfill the functions/activities of a registered nurse in the practice setting." Each statement is accompanied by measurable criteria, which can gauge achievement of the competency statement, and examples of how achievement may be documented. A *Job Analysis and Test Specifications* describes 21 basic perioperative nursing responsibilities. Knowledge and skills required for proficiency in carrying out each responsibility are listed. The learner is encouraged to read the AORN *Competency Model* and the NCB:PNI *Job Analysis* for an in-depth look at the responsibilities that are generally described in this text. Developing an awareness of the roles of the nurse in the perioperative setting allows the nurse to coordinate patient care activities and develop a concept of the teamwork necessary to provide care.

SCRUB PERSON

The scrub person may be a registered nurse, licensed vocational/practical nurse, or surgical technologist. If the scrub person role is assumed by a registered nurse whose actions are based on the nursing process, that individual is practicing nursing. Activities of the scrub role are seen as an integral part of perioperative nursing practice. A surgical technologist who assumes the role of the scrub person is "doing so as a delegated technical function and under the direction of a perioperative nurse" (*AORN Journal*, 1988).

Qualifications for the scrub role include knowledge of aseptic technique, instruments, and equipment; anatomy and physiology; and surgical procedures. This knowledge assists the scrub person in anticipating needs of the scrub team.

Responsibilities of the scrub person are usually confined to the intraoperative phase of the patient's surgical experience. This individual may also be involved in gathering supplies and equipment for the operative procedure or assisting the circulator. The scrub person performs a hand scrub; dons a sterile gown and gloves; sets up and maintains the sterile field; hands supplies and instruments to the surgeon and assistants; keeps an accurate count of sponges, sharps, and instruments; and monitors aseptic technique.

CIRCULATOR

The circulating nurse or circulator is a registered nurse who, using the nursing process, assists the patient to meet individual needs. The circulating nurse, in collaboration with other members of the health care team, assesses the health status of the patient, develops an individualized plan of care, implements the plan, and continuously evaluates progress of the plan toward identified outcomes.

Responsibilities of the circulating nurse span all three phases of the surgical experience (Fig. 2–3). Preoperatively, the circulator collects data and identifies patient needs, which are used to develop the plan of care. For example, upon assessing the patient preoperatively, the nurse finds that the patient is 92 years old and severely under normal weight. The nurse develops a plan of care that includes particular attention to padding bony prominences. The nurse may obtain extra aids during this preoperative phase to ensure that no nerve injury results.

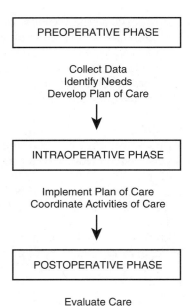

PREOPERATIVE PHASE

Collect Data
Identify Needs
Develop Plan of Care

↓

INTRAOPERATIVE PHASE

Implement Plan of Care
Coordinate Activities of Care

↓

POSTOPERATIVE PHASE

Evaluate Care
Communicate Information

FIGURE 2-3. Circulating Nurse Responsibilities.

Intraoperatively, the circulating nurse implements the plan of care and coordinates activities that serve to ensure that safe, efficient, quality care is delivered. In the case of the aging emaciated patient, the patient may be positioned while awake to solicit feedback as to comfort level. In this particular case, the nurse would apply additional padding to anticipated pressure areas depending on the position in which the patient was placed. Other activities during the intraoperative phase include providing emotional support to the patient, family, and significant other; serving as the patient's advocate; anticipating and meeting the needs of the anesthesiologist and scrub team; monitoring and controlling the operating room environment; documenting nursing care; monitoring blood loss; and completing the sponge, sharps, and instrument counts.

In the postoperative phase, the circulator evaluates the nursing care that has been provided. In the underweight patient, the nurse would carefully check all pressure areas and bony prominences for skin integrity and signs of redness. In the postoperative phase, the nurse also insures continuity of nursing activities by communicating pertinent information regarding the patient, including any unique needs, to the post-anesthesia care unit (PACU) nurses. Any redness or skin breakdown would be documented on the nurse's notes and verbally communicated to the PACU nurses.

MANAGER

The perioperative nurse manager is the individual who coordinates the activities that are related to the nursing care of surgical patients. The size and complexity of the organization in which the nurse manager practices will determine the areas of responsibility and position title. The nurse manager may administer and supervise activities only in the surgical suite or may be responsible for additional nursing units that care for the patient preoperatively and postoperatively. In some facilities, nurse managers are also responsible for areas such as central processing, which provide support services to the surgical suite.

The AORN *Standards of Perioperative Administrative Practice* state that the nurse manager "is responsible for the interpretation, direction, and evaluation of nursing practice and the coordination of operating room services through the use of clinical, management, and leadership skills" (AORN, 1993b). This includes activities related to patient care, human resources, and organizational management.

Given the description of the role and responsibilities of nurse manager, *every* perioperative nurse is a manager in daily practice. For example, although the nurse may not be managing 12 operating rooms, he/she is managing the one assigned. And, although the nurse may not be evaluating overall departmental nursing care, he/she is evaluating care and supervising others providing care. The nurse may not be responsible for the departmental budget but is responsible for managing the judicious use of supplies. Management, in one form or another, is applicable to all perioperative nurses.

RESEARCHER

Nursing is a science based on research and knowledge from biologic, physiologic, behavioral, and social disciplines. The knowledge gained from research forms the basis of nursing practice and demonstrates a relationship between nursing interventions and patient outcomes. Perioperative nurses use research findings in their practice. In the past, perioperative nursing has taken research from outside its specialized practice and incorporated it into the specialty. As more perioperative nurses seek advanced degrees, there has been an increase in the amount of research related specifically to perioperative nursing.

Not all perioperative nurses conduct formal research, but all perioperative nurses can use research to demonstrate the relationship between the nursing care provided and patient outcomes. Perioperative nurses may involve themselves in research by identifying clinical problems, participating in collecting data for research studies, reading research to determine how it might apply to practice, sharing research with others, participating on a research committee, or using information gained from research to initiate change in the practice setting.

EDUCATOR

The perioperative educator is a nurse who provides staff development for operating room personnel. Large facilities may have the luxury of a designated, full-time educator, whereas smaller facilities rely on nurses in the department to accomplish staff development activities.

Staff development is composed of three areas:

- orientation
- in-service training
- continuing education

The nurse educator is responsible for formal orientation of new employees as well as orientation of current employees who are assuming new roles within the operating room setting. During orientation, the educator introduces the employee to the philosophy, goals, policies, procedures, role expectations, physical facilities, and special services of the unit. The educator assesses the employee's knowledge and skill level and assists in planning an individualized clinical orientation. The educator then works with the nurse manager and perioperative preceptors to coordinate the clinical orientation.

The nurse educator is also responsible for developing, planning, coordinating, and implementing in-service and continuing education programs and activities. The first step for the educator in accomplishing these tasks is to conduct an assessment of the staff, which serves to identify learning needs and to determine priorities for programs. These identified needs are then addressed by two categories of programs: those that assist employees in performing their assigned functions (in-service) and those that build on previous experience to enhance practice (continuing education).

In many facilities the nurse educator works with an education committee of nurses, technologists, and ancillary personnel. The committee provides input and feedback on programs and may assist the educator in planning and implementing learning activities.

The perioperative nurse educator may be involved in teaching patients, physicians, students, and other groups of nurses within the facility. The role of the nurse educator is not the exclusive domain of one individual. All perioperative nurses have the opportunity to participate in teaching patients, families, colleagues, and students, and all perioperative nurses orient their patients to the surgical environment in the course of providing care.

REGISTERED NURSE FIRST ASSISTANT

The registered nurse first assistant (RNFA) is an emerging perioperative role that is gaining acceptance as a way to serve the public's health care needs in a cost-effective manner. It is an expanded role in which the perioperative nurse works under the direct supervision of the surgeon as a first assistant during surgery. To assume this role, the experienced perioperative nurse must obtain additional education and training. Registered nurse first assistants must also be credentialed by the facility in which they intend to practice.

The RNFA may perform the following functions as first assistant during the surgical procedure:

- handling tissue
- providing exposure
- suturing
- providing hemostasis

These functions are independent of the scrub nurse role. The RNFA does not concurrently function as the scrub person.

In 1993, the NCB:PNI offered the first certification examination for RNFAs. To be eligible for certification, the RNFA must be certified as an operating room nurse (CNOR) and have completed a minimum of 2000 hours of practice as a registered nurse first assistant. Content for the certification examination is based on the knowledge and skills outlined in a job analysis similar to the one developed for certifying perioperative nurses.

Unlicensed Assistive Personnel

A fundamental component of every health care system is the delivery of nursing care. The provision of care involves the nurse, assisted by numerous individuals with different knowledge levels and capabilities. These assistive personnel work with the nurse in the provision of quality patient care.

ROLE DEFINITION

The American Nurses Association (ANA) has defined unlicensed assistive personnel as "individuals who are trained to function in an assistive role to the registered professional nurse in the provision of patient/client care activities as delegated by and under the supervision of the registered professional nurse" (ANA, 1992b).

In the perioperative setting, the term "unlicensed assistive personnel" applies to such job titles as nurses aides, patient care aides, orderlies, nursing attendants, anesthesia technicians, and surgical technicians. These individuals are not authorized to perform activities that have been defined as nursing acts by individual state nurse practice acts, but they may assist in providing some direct patient care.

TRENDS IN UTILIZATION

Over the past decade there has been a dramatic increase in the utilization of unlicensed assistive personnel. This has occurred in response to health care reform brought about by public concern regarding the increasing resources allocated to health care and the inability of the health care system to use resources to deliver services in a cost-effective and efficient manner.

During the early 1980s there was a general decrease in unlicensed assistive personnel and an increase in registered nurses in hospitals. The severe illnesses of patients in the acute care setting had risen, and sophisticated technology was at an all-time high. By the end of the decade, however, the utilization of unlicensed assistive personnel had changed owing to changes in a variety of factors, including economics, health care delivery systems, patient populations, and opportunities for allied health careers (ANA, 1992b).

By 1991, a survey revealed that over 80% of hospital registered nurses and 98% of long-term care registered nurses were working with unlicensed assistive personnel (Bergman, 1991). The Bureau of Labor Statistics predicts that by the year 2005, nursing assistant positions will increase by 45% and home health aides by 138% (U.S. Bureau of Labor Statistics, 1993).

In 1989, the North Dakota Nurses Association (NDNA) reported 109 assistive personnel job descriptions in just 37 institutions within their state alone (NDNA, 1989). Roles that in the past have been clearly defined by education, training, and responsibility are becoming a collection of titles with hazy expectations. This, coupled with the rapid growth in the numbers of unlicensed assistive personnel, has caused confusion and concern for registered nurses.

THE NURSING PROFESSION'S ROLE

The role of nursing with regard to unlicensed assistive personnel is based on the fundamental principle that the nursing profession is directly accountable for its practice to the public; therefore, it is the nursing profession that must define and supervise the education, training, and utilization of any unlicensed assistants involved in providing direct nursing care.

The development of education standards, roles, and activities for unlicensed assistive personnel is currently being addressed by a variety of professional organizations including the American Nurses Association, National Council of State Boards for Nursing, Tri-Council for Nursing, and American Hospital Association. These organizations are working collaboratively to provide a common basis for standardization of this category of health care worker. Training and orientation of unlicensed assistive personnel is accomplished in individual practice settings following institutional policies and guidelines that flow from the education standards being developed. Competencies must also be created to assist the nurse in utilizing and evaluating unlicensed assistive personnel.

When utilizing unlicensed assistive personnel, nurses must adhere to the professional standards of nursing practice and the definitions of nursing in their state nurse practice act, as well as the specific rules of various regulatory bodies. These clearly delineate the scope of professional practice and how it may be applied to a variety of practice settings and staff compositions. The nurse must be clear as to what constitutes professional nursing care and what activities or tasks may be appropriately performed by unlicensed assistive personnel in the delivery of patient care. The nurse must also be reasonably assured that the assistant can function in a safe and effective manner based on education, training, orientation, and documented competencies.

Management of unlicensed assistive personnel falls into two broad categories — supervision and delegation. Both categories carry accountability for the registered nurse.

Supervision is "the active process of directing, guiding, and influencing the outcome of an individual's performance of an activity" (American Nurses Association, 1992b). Supervision may be *on-site* where the nurse is physically present or immediately available while the activity is being performed, or *off-site* where the nurse is not physically present but provides direction through written or verbal communication or both. Having an orderly assist in the transfer of a patient from the gurney to the operative bed is an example of on-site supervision in the perioperative setting.

When supervising unlicensed assistive personnel, the nurse must insure that there are criteria in place to determine that expectations for activities have been met. Written policies should describe what measures can be taken by the nurse to stop an inappropriate act or to regain control of an activity.

Delegation is the second management activity. Delegation is "the transfer of responsibility for the performance of an activity from one individual to another while retaining accountability for the outcome" (American Nurses Association, 1992b). When delegating, the nurse uses professional judgment to decide which nursing activities may be delegated, to whom, and under what circumstances.

State laws may vary somewhat in specific interpretation, but it is generally agreed that the registered nurse is legally responsible for activities that are delegated to unlicensed assistive personnel. The nurse and the assistant share *responsibility* for the correct performance of the task, but it is the registered nurse who is *accountable* for the performance of the assistant.

In deciding what nursing activities should be delegated to an assistant, the nurse must take into account the following:

- the condition of the patient
- the capabilities of the assistant
- the complexity of the nursing task
- the amount of supervision the nurse will be able to provide
- the available staff assigned to accomplish the unit workload (American Nurses Association, 1992b)

Certain nursing activities should *not* be delegated. These activities include the processes (assessment, diagnosis, planning, and evaluation) that require specialized knowledge, judgment, and skill. Unlicensed assistive personnel may be delegated to perform activities that are components of the nursing process, such as data collection during assessment, but it is the nurse who must analyze the data, using professional nursing knowledge, to formulate the nursing diagnoses and individual plan of care for the patient.

NURSING RESPONSIBILITIES

Unlicensed assistive personnel provide important contributions in the provision of nursing care. They can support nurses by performing certain activities so that nurses will have more time to concentrate on nursing care. The growing number and utilization of these health care workers have brought added responsibility to the registered nurse. The nurse has the fundamental responsibility to be familiar with nursing standards, the state nurse practice act, and any other regulation that is applicable to nursing practice. This knowledge enables the nurse to develop a clear understanding of what constitutes professional practice and to employ this understanding to ensure that the public will receive safe and effective nursing care.

Each perioperative nurse who interacts with unlicensed assistive personnel is also responsible for

- remaining current on the emerging roles and utilization of unlicensed assistive personnel
- providing training and orientation
- ensuring that appropriate policies and documented competencies are in place
- acquiring knowledge and skill in supervising and delegating activities for unlicensed assistive personnel

Personal Values

Values are social principles that are accepted by an individual. They are the worth placed on an object, idea, or action. Values are not something one thinks about every day and are often taken for granted. For these reasons, each of us may not realize that a given set of values is maintained or that decisions are based on these values. Values become important when something goes wrong or when a situation arises in which the nurse must choose between values. The process of values clarification is an important activity in developing professionally. If values are clarified, the nurse will be better prepared to deal with the ethical dilemmas in the perioperative setting.

VALUES CLARIFICATION

Values clarification is a process whereby each nurse identifies the values that have personal significance. Once identified, the nurse examines personal beliefs based on the truth, beauty, or worth of the value.

The purpose of values clarification is to examine one's life in an effort to foster the making of choices and facilitate decision making (Davis, 1991). Values clarification is a first step to be taken in order to deal with the ethical dilemmas encountered as perioperative nurses. When faced with selecting certain values, the following basic principles apply.

- *Intrinsic values are favored over extrinsic values.* Something is intrinsically valuable when it is good in itself, when it is valued for its own sake and not for what it has the ability to lead to. Most of the things used in daily life have extrinsic value; they are a means to attain other things. Intrinsic and extrinsic values are not always mutually exclusive, however. Knowledge is an example of this. Knowledge, in and of itself, is good, but it may also lead to other goals, such as recognition by peers or increased respect by colleagues.
- *Values that are productive and fairly permanent are favored over those that are less productive and not as permanent.* For example, some individuals believe that social or religious values tend to provide more permanent satisfaction than material objects.
- *Values should be selected on the basis of self-chosen ends or ideals.* Values should be based on personal beliefs not on the expectations of others or the demands of society.
- *Given two positive values, the nurse should select the most positive of the two.* When choosing between two negative values, select the less negative of the two. Take for example, the nurse who is assigned to circulate for an emergency operative procedure. The patient's life is seriously threatened by massive hemorrhaging, and time is of the essence. Should the nurse choose to *disregard* the facility's policy of counting sponges on all cases (a negative value) or take time to count and *possibly place the patient in further jeopardy* (another negative value)? In this case, the less negative of the two values would be to begin the procedure without a sponge count.

ETHICS

Ethics is the study of values in human conduct. It is an investigation of the principles of morality, of right and wrong conduct, or of good and evil as they correlate to human conduct (McCloskey, 1990). Ethics is based on theories, principles, and rules that are used in the process of making ethical decisions.

Ethical theories were developed to explain and provide a general basis for making decisions when principles or rules conflicted with one another. There are two fundamental types of theories — teleological and deontological. Teleological theories endeavor to justify moral principles in terms of the overall goal or purpose of the human experience. The outcome or consequence of the decision is what is most important. In contrast, deontological theories are concerned with the action involved in making the decision. Proponents of deontological theories believe that it is not the consequences of an act that make it right or wrong, but the moral intention of the person making the decision.

Ethical principles are derived from one or both of the theories described. Principles serve as a guide to action. They are presumptions about what is good or right. Principles are universal truths that can generally be applied to a situation. Some examples of ethical principles are autonomy, beneficence, utility, and paternalism. *Autonomy* recognizes the individual's independence in making choices and carrying out actions based on these choices. *Beneficence* dictates that people ought to do good and avoid doing harm. The Hippocratic oath is based on the principle of beneficence. When the nurse weighs the benefit of doing good against the harm that might result, he/she is using the principle of *utility*. The principle of *paternalism* states that restricting a person's rights is justified if the individual's actions would result in serious harm or fail to produce a positive benefit. The decision to withhold negative test results from a patient is paternalistic.

Ethical rules flow from principles. Rules identify specific actions that should or should not be taken because they are either right or wrong. Professional rules are the result of responsibilities as registered nurses. They are manifested in professional codes of ethics, which reflect expectations of our society. Confidentiality is an example of an ethical rule that comes from the principle of autonomy. Patient advocacy is another rule that springs from the beneficence principle.

PROFESSIONAL CODES

Professional codes, as stated previously, are rules and principles by which the profession regulates its members and demonstrates its accountability to society (Bandman, 1990). The American Nurses Association's *Code for Nurses* is an example. This code, originally adopted in 1950 and revised periodically, consists of eleven statements that guide the nurse in conduct and relationships in the provision of nursing care. Each of the eleven statements is accompanied by an interpretation of the statement. The ANA describes the *Code for Nurses* as a characterization of nursing conscience and philosophy rather than a series of rules placed upon the nurse. The code itself does not insure the integrity of the nurse unless the nurse is committed to the code.

In 1993, AORN's Special Committee on Ethics developed a proposed statement that adapts the *Code for Nurses* to the perioperative setting (*AORN Journal*, 1993b). This document lists each statement in the ANA code and applies the statement specifically to perioperative nursing practice. The AORN statement also identifies examples of perioperative behaviors that reflect each statement.

The ANA's *Code for Nurses* is the primary guide for nursing, but other professional codes may have an impact on our practice as well. Among these are the International Council of Nurses' *Code for Nurses: Ethical Concepts Applied to Nursing*, the American Hospital Association's *Patient's Bill of Rights* and *Nuremberg Code*.

ETHICAL DECISION MAKING

Making an ethical decision refers to determining what is the morally right thing to do in a given situation. The nurse who is faced with an ethical problem can apply the problem to a model, such as the Husted ethical decision-making model (Husted, 1991) or can apply a decision-making process to assist in resolution. The decision-making process consists of three steps:

- identifying the problem
- collecting data
- exploring options

To identify the problem, the nurse must be able to clearly and objectively describe the situation and the circumstances surrounding the situation. If in doubt, the nurse should collaborate with colleagues or other health care professionals in order to validate the problem.

Once the problem has been identified, information must be collected. This information takes into consideration the individuals involved and most importantly, what the patient wants. If the patient is unable to communicate, the nurse is responsible to ascertain what the patient would want given the situation. This information may be obtained from the patient's family or friends.

Options are based on the information obtained. The nurse explores each option from a personal and professional viewpoint by answering the following questions:

- What actions are required?
- What are the possible and probable outcomes of the actions?
- What is the intention or purpose of the actions?
- What are the alternatives to this option?

There are no ready-made solutions to ethical problems. Most are frustrating and difficult to deal with. Using the universal principles of ethics, nurses must choose the courses of action that best reflect their judgment.

ETHICAL DILEMMAS

An ethical dilemma is a choice between equally undesirable alternatives. Throughout its history nursing has faced such dilemmas. However, current health care economics, recent technologies, and an increasingly complex society have produced dilemmas that were previously nonexistent.

What follows is a presentation of three perioperative situations involving nursing dilemmas — abortion, organ harvesting and transplant surgery, and intraoperative suspension of do-not-resuscitate (DNR) orders. The purpose of this presentation is not to provide answers but to furnish information and present issues and ethical positions for consideration. Using the principles of values clarification and ethics, the nurse can work toward personal resolution of the dilemmas presented.

ABORTION

In 1973, based on the cases of *Roe v. Wade* (410 U.S. 113) and *Doe v. Bolton* (410 U.S. 179), the U.S. Supreme Court established the right of every woman to have an abortion legally. The foundation of the Court's decision was the constitutional right to privacy. Currently, abortion is legal in the United States. However, in 1977, the Supreme Court ruled in favor of two cases that affect the implementation of the *Roe v. Wade* (1973) decision. In *Beal v. Doe* (U.S.L.W. 4787) and *Maher v. Roe* (U.S.L.W. 4787), the Court ruled that states were not required to spend Medicaid funds for elective, nontherapeutic abortion. In this decision the Court said that the state could not prevent abortions, but that it did not have to help poor women obtain abortions as a remedy for social and economic ills (Segers,

1977). Following this decision, Congress immediately banned the use of federal funds for abortions, with some exceptions. As it now stands, "one social class, the poor, is singled out for the restriction of the fundamental right to abortion because of the inability to pay" (Bandman, 1990).

The ethical dilemmas in abortion surround three separate rights:

- the rights of the fetus
- the rights and obligations of the mother
- the rights and obligations of society (Davis, 1991)

The notion that a fetus is a person can be neither proved nor disproved to everyone's satisfaction. The lawyer who presented *Roe v. Wade* (1973) before the Supreme Court argued that although the Constitution uses the word "person," there was no assurance that this word had prenatal application. From this, the lawyer concluded that the unborn fetus is not a person. The counterargument is that the fetus had the potential to become a person and therefore had the same right to life as any other person. Those who believe that the fetus is a human being from the moment of conception must accord it all human rights, including the right to life. In the case of abortion, the dilemma arises over a conflict between the right of the fetus to life and the right of the mother to her life and to determine what is allowed to happen in and to her body. Some believe that individuals do not have a right to control their fate when other individuals share it. Opposing this position are those who say that no one has the right to continued dependence upon another person's bodily processes when it is against the other person's will. The circumstances in which a pregnancy occurred (rape, failed contraception, voluntary) and the condition of the fetus (deformed, healthy) are two factors that add to the complexity of this issue.

A society will determine its abortion policy. If the policy is very restrictive, some argue the results would be that a number of women would be threatened by continuation of the pregnancy, that the new child would place greater psychologic and economic burdens on the family, and that more children would be born who were mentally and physically challenged. There are others who argue that if a liberal abortion policy is accepted it would have grave consequences on other values in our society, such as a diminished respect for life. They believe that perhaps a liberal abortion policy would lead to other policies affecting the elderly, the mentally challenged, and the mentally ill. Davis (1991) sums up the issue regarding abortion and the rights of society by asking if there are benefits to the society that override the benefits to the prospective mother. A balance needs to be established concerning the rights and obligations of the society as a whole against the rights and obligations of an individual member of the society. This question, like many others surrounding abortion, remains unanswered.

ORGAN PROCUREMENT AND TRANSPLANT SURGERY

Transplant surgery has been characterized as a modern miracle and a medical triumph. However, it has also created ethical dilemmas for health care providers, families of donors, and society in general. Two such dilemmas concern:

- determination of death
- allocation of organs

Advanced technology has contributed to the ethical dilemma surrounding death. Traditionally, death has been determined by absence of a pulse and respiration, but current medical technology can sustain these functions indefinitely. Patients who would have died 10 years ago are now being successfully resuscitated and maintained on life support systems. When severe brain damage occurs, individuals lapse into an unresponsive state from which they will never recover. The result is that the patient is deprived of death with dignity, and the family is subjected to emotional and economic stress (Allan, 1989). In such cases, death may be established using brain death criteria developed by the Harvard Medical School (Journal of the American Medical Association, 1968). The physician must make the diagnosis of brain death based on these criteria, realizing that "no absolute test or procedure exists to verify their conclusions" (Kawamoto, 1992). Thus, the decision to declare the patient legally dead must be based on ethical decision making to reflect what is in the best interest of the patient.

The patient who has been declared brain dead and arrives in the operating room for organ retrieval may not *appear* dead. The IVs are running, the heart rate is displayed on the monitor, and the patient is warm to the touch. The patient may look like any other critically ill patient who comes to surgery. It can be emotionally upsetting for the perioperative nurse to assist with organ procurement realizing that the patient outcome is physical death rather than recovery. Assistance must be provided for the nurse to express feelings and resolve conflicts surrounding participation in the procedure.

The number of transplants performed in this country in 1990 was 15,165. The number of organ donors was 4,357. By 1992, the number of people on the waiting list for organs had risen to 24,791 (Martinelli, 1993). This discrepancy between the number of available organs and demand for these organs produces a dilemma in which a decision must be made regarding who receives them.

The government has helped to alleviate the supply versus demand problem by passing legislation that makes it easier to donate organs and by providing funds for kidney transplants. In 1984, Congress passed the *National Organ Transplant Act.* This law prohibits the selling of organs or the withholding of them from patients who are poor. Additionally, the law prevents families from requesting that organs be given to a person of a particular race, creed, sex, or color (Smith, 1992). It is hoped that this law will assist in increasing the number of donors.

Medicine has also assisted in resolving the supply versus demand dilemma in a variety of ways including use of living-related donor transplants where the organ recipient is related to the living donor; "domino" transplants where the organ recipient also becomes an organ donor; segmental transplants where only a portion of the organ is donated or where a single organ can be divided among more than one donor; immunosuppressive medications; and tissue typing to insure the best match between organ and recipient.

The current system for organ sharing in this country is coordinated by the United Network for Organ Sharing (UNOS). This organization maintains a national registry for potential transplant recipients. Recipients are selected for an organ on the basis of several factors including blood and tissue type and urgency of need.

Will medical science develop a method for unequivocally determining death? Will the supply of organs ever exceed the demand? Or, will artificial organs be developed, making organ allocation a moot point? Perhaps, but determination of death and allocation of organs are only two ethical problems surrounding this issue. A more basic starting point for your deliberation of organ donation and transplantation might be to examine the terms "life" and "death" and determine what they mean to you as an individual and a professional.

INTRAOPERATIVE SUSPENSION OF DO-NOT-RESUSCITATE (DNR) ORDERS

"Patients have the right to participate in decisions made about their care, including the right to refuse treatment, even if those decisions result in death" (Reeder, 1993). The decision not to resuscitate the patient who has suffered cardiac arrest is reached consensually by the patient and the physician. When the patient is incompetent, the decision is made by a family member or court-appointed conservator and the physician. The decision must be agreed upon by all parties involved. This decision should be reached only after the patient or family member or conservator, depending on the circumstance, has been fully informed of the patient's condition and prognosis. The physician documents the decision in the patient record and writes the DNR order. This order is reviewed at frequent intervals in the event that the patient's condition improves. Frequently, this order is suspended when the patient undergoes surgery. Why?

The practice of suspending DNR orders intraoperatively has its historical basis in events that occurred during World War II where countless numbers of people were killed with "terminal anesthesia." These acts were later outlawed in the Nuremberg and Geneva conventions. In response to this, a new rule of medical practice evolved in the United States whereby surgeons and anesthesiologists would not allow a patient to die while under anesthesia even if the patient had previously authorized DNR orders (Vaux, 1992). History is not the only contributing factor to the tradition of suspension of DNR orders during surgery. Medical ethics, which weigh heavily on the principle of beneficence or do no harm, create conflict within the physician. Being prohibited from resuscitating patients intraoperatively may also cause feelings of failure and fear of condemnation by colleagues. And, in today's litigious society, there is a fear of prosecution for negligence (Martin, 1991).

The conflict between the patient's autonomy and the medical profession's beneficence gives rise to the ethical dilemma. Contrary to abortion and organ transplant dilemmas, the legal system has provided little toward resolving the issue of suspension of DNR orders. Patients have the legal right to refuse resuscitation; however, there is no case law or statutory law that specifically addresses suspension of this right intraoperatively (Murphy, 1993). A survey of practicing anesthesiologists found that 60% of them automatically suspended DNR orders when the patient arrived in surgery. Almost 50% of the time this was done without the patient's knowledge (Clemency, 1993). If patients are resuscitated against their wishes, they could sue under the theory of negligence, battery, or "wrongful life," but this has never been reported. "To date, courts have been reluctant to hold nurses or physicians liable when they act to maintain life — even when it is done against a patient and a family's wishes" (Murphy, 1993).

Various approaches have been put forth to resolve the issue. For example, DNR orders could simply be disregarded during surgery. However, this approach denies patients the right to participate in decisions affecting their health and violates the *Patient Self-Determination Act of 1991*.

On the other end of the spectrum might be enforcing a policy whereby all patients who enter surgery would be resuscitated regardless of pre-existing DNR orders. This approach would satisfy the beneficence principle for the health care team but would also put their needs before those of the patient.

A third approach to resolving this dilemma is "required consideration" as described by Cohen (1991). Prior to surgery, the physician and patient discuss the DNR orders in light of the risks and benefits of anesthesia care during the upcoming operative procedure. The patient may then decide to continue with the DNR order or temporarily suspend it. This approach allows the patient to participate in decisions that affect his/her care.

In an effort to assist nurses, the American Nurses Association (ANA) has published a list of specific recommendations to resolve some of the ethical dilemmas surrounding DNR orders. According to this position statement, the patient's choices and values are given priority over those of health care providers. The statement also suggests that if the nurse's personal belief or moral integrity is compromised by the professional responsibility to carry out a DNR order, the care of the patient should be relinquished to another nurse (American Nurses Association, 1992a).

The perioperative nurse who has been assigned to care for the patient with a DNR order must validate information regarding the continuation or suspension of the order intraoperatively. If this validation is not possible and the need arises to resuscitate the patient intraoperatively, the nurse, under law, should participate in the resuscitation as directed by the physician.

The Nurse's Responsibilities

The brief introduction to values clarification, ethics, and ethical dilemmas provided in this chapter is merely a starting point for perioperative nurses. The nurse's responsibilities as a professional are to

- become informed through literature and discussion
- give consideration to situations one may be involved in
- clarify values and formulate ethical/moral positions
- arrive at a balance between individual values and professional obligations to the patient

Issues for Future Development

What does the future hold for nursing in general and perioperative nursing specifically? No one knows. But one thing is certain, the delivery of health care in this nation is on the brink of what could be sweeping changes. The U.S. Congress is currently considering the concept of access to health care for all. If health care is made available to everyone in America, the impact on nursing will be significant.

Advanced practice nursing roles will probably be increasingly utilized under health care reform. In the future, nurse practitioners staffing clinics might serve as the individual's sole entry into the health care system. These nurses would be responsible for initial assessment of all individuals and referral for treatment as indicated. The current scope of the advanced practice nurse would increase and new roles would be created.

Along with the increased dependence on nurses in advanced practice, expanded roles, such as the RNFA, would become the norm rather than the exception. Perhaps cost reimbursement for services performed by these nurses would also become the standard.

Nurses practicing today have an uncertain but exciting future. The perioperative nurse must be prepared for the changes that will come and be positioned to direct those changes in ways that benefit nursing and society. How can the nurse best accomplish this?

- By staying informed on proposed changes
- By guiding those changes through participation in professional nursing organizations
- By acquiring new knowledge, skills, and abilities, which will provide versatility in future nursing roles

REFERENCES

A definition of irreversible coma: report of the ad hoc committee of the Harvard Medical School to examine the definition of brain death. (1968). *JAMA (205)*, 337–340.

Allan, D. (1989). Brain death. *Nursing Times, 85*(35), 30–32.

Allen, D. E., Girard, N. J. (1992). Attitudes toward certification. *AORN Journal, 55*(3), 817–829.

American Nurses Association. (1992a). *ANA Position Statement: Do-Not-Resuscitate (DNR) Orders.* Washington, DC: ANA.

American Nurses Association. (1992b). *Registered Professional Nurses and Unlicensed Assistive Personnel.* Washington, DC: ANA.

AORN moves to new headquarters, changes to meet members' needs. (1993a). *AORN Journal, 57*(2), 382–410.

AORN Special Committee on Ethics. (1993b). ANA Code for nurses with interpretive statements—explications for perioperative nursing. *AORN Journal, 58*(2), 369–388.

Association of Operating Room Nurses. (1992). *Competency Model.* Denver, CO: AORN.

Association of Operating Room Nurses. (1993a). *Standards and recommended practices.* Denver, CO: AORN.

Association of Operating Room Nurses. (1993b). *Standards of perioperative administrative practice.* Denver, CO: AORN.

Bandman, E.L., Bandman, B. (1990). *Nursing ethics through the life span.* 2nd ed. Norwalk, CT: Prentice Hall.

Beal v. Doe, U.S.L.W. 4787 (1977).

Bergman, E. (1991). Nurse extenders now found in 97% of hospitals. *American Journal of Nursing, 91*(9), 88, 90.

Clemency, M.V., Thompson, N.J. (1993). Do not resuscitate (DNR) orders and the anesthesiologist: a survey. *Anesthesia and Analgesia, 76*(2), 396.

Cohen, C.B., Cohen, P.J. (1991). Do-not-resuscitate orders in the operating room. *The New England Journal of Medicine, 325*(26), 1879–1882.

Davis, A.J., Aroskar, M.A. (1991). *Ethical dilemmas and nursing practice.* 3rd ed. Norwalk, CT: Prentice Hall.

del Bueno, D. (1988). The promise and the reality of certification. *IMAGE: Journal of Nursing Scholarship, 20*(4), 208–211.

Doe v. Bolton, 410 U.S. 179 (1993).

Faherty, B. (1991). Why bother getting certified? *Home Healthcare Nurse, 9*(4), 29–31.

Giordano, B.P. (1993). Symposium on the operating room environment. *AORN Journal, 55*(2), 840.

House adopts resolution on the role of scrub person. (1988). *AORN Journal, 47*(5), 1118.

Husted, G.L., Husted, J.H. (1991). *Ethical decision making in nursing.* St. Louis: Mosby-Year Book.

Kawamoto, K.L. (1992). Organ procurement in the operating room. *AORN Journal, 55*(6), 1541–1546.

Maher v. Roe, U.S.L.W. 4787 (1977).

Martin, R.L., Soifer, B.E., Stevens, W.C. (1991). Ethical issues in anesthesia: Management of the do-not-resuscitate patient. *Anesthesia and Analgesia, 73*(2), 221–225.

Martinelli, A.M. (1993). Organ donation. *AORN Journal, 58*(2), 236–251.

McCloskey, J.C., Grance, H.K., eds. (1990). *Current issues in nursing.* St. Louis: C.V. Mosby.

Murphy, E.K. (1993). Do-not-resuscitate orders in the OR. *AORN Journal, 58*(2), 399–401.

National Certification Board: Perioperative Nursing, Inc. (1993). *Certification and recertification guide.* Denver, CO: NCB:PNI.

North Dakota Nurses Association, Congress on Education and Professional Nursing Practice. (1989). *Study of unlicensed personnel who provide assistance to the nurse.* Bismarck, ND: NDNA.

Pearson, L.J. (1993). 1992–93 update: how each state stands on legislative issues affecting advanced nursing practice. *Nurse Practitioner, 18*(1), 23–38.

Perry, L. (1989). Nursing societies promote certification. *Modern Healthcare, 19*(41), 50.

Reeder, J.M. (1993). Do-not-resuscitate orders in the operating room. *AORN Journal, 57*(4), 947–951.

Roe v. Wade, 410 U.S. 113 (1973).

Segers, M.C. (1977). Abortion and the Supreme Court: some more equal than others. *The Hastings Center Report, 7*(4), 5.

Smith, K.A. (1992). Demystifying organ procurement. *AORN Journal, 55*(6), 1530–1540.

U.S. Bureau of Labor Statistics. (1993). Monthly Labor Review, Vol. 116, Number 11.

Vaux, K.L. (1992). *Death ethics.* Philadelphia: Trinity Press International.

SUGGESTED READING

American Nurses Association. (1992). *Registered professional nurses and unlicensed assistive personnel.* Washington, DC: ANA.

AORN Special Committee on Ethics. (1993). ANA code for nurses with interpretive statements—explications for perioperative nursing. *AORN Journal, 58*(2), 369–388.

Association of Operating Room Nurses. (1991). *Perioperative nursing process.* Denver, CO: AORN.

Association of Operating Room Nurses. (1992). *Competency model.* Denver, CO: AORN.

Association of Operating Room Nurses. (1993). *Standards and recommended practices.* Denver, CO: AORN.

Bandman, E.L., Bandman, B. (1990). *Nursing ethics through the life span.* 2nd ed. Norwalk, CT: Prentice Hall.

Davis, A.J., Aroskar, M.A. (1991). *Ethical dilemmas and nursing practice.* 3rd ed. Norwalk, CT: Prentice Hall.

Dougherty, C.J., Edwards, B.J., Haddah, A.M. (1990). *Ethical dilemmas in perioperative nursing.* Denver, CO: AORN.

Groah, L.K. (1990). *Operating room nursing: Perioperative practice.* 2nd ed. Norwalk, CT: Appleton & Lange.

Husted, G.L., Husted, J.H. (1991). *Ethical decision making in nursing.* St. Louis: Mosby-Year Book.

McCloskey, J.C., Grance, H.K., eds. (1990). *Current issues in nursing.* St. Louis: C.V. Mosby.

National Certification Board: Perioperative Nursing, Inc. (1992). *A job analysis and test specifications.* Denver, CO: NCB:PNI.

Rothrock, J.C. (1990). *Perioperative nursing care planning.* St. Louis: C.V. Mosby.

Spry, C. (1988). *Essentials of perioperative nursing: A self-learning guide.* Rockville, MD: Aspen Publishers, Inc.

Practice Scenario 1
Professional Development

by Donna Benotti, RN, CNOR

SCENARIO

Anna Rodriguez, RN and Donna Smith, RN are assigned to scrub and circulate for a 0900 gastrostomy on William Jones, a 79-year-old emaciated male. Since his hospitalization 3 days ago, he has managed to remove his intravenous line and nasogastric tube several times. Consequently, he has been restrained in his room and on the stretcher during transport to the operating room. His medical diagnosis is chronic alcoholism and chronic brain syndrome. He is noncommunicative. Mr. Jones appears to acknowledge Donna Smith's presence with a half glance in her direction. He does not respond to the anesthesiologist or to his questions. Mr. Jones is supported on the stretcher in a semi-Fowler's position with several pillows. Further examination reveals that Mr. Jones has contractures of the hips and knees.

PERIOPERATIVE INTERPRETATION

Using what you have just learned in this chapter, as an experienced perioperative nurse you would consider the following in the care of this patient.

1. Assessment:
   - Based upon the preoperative assessment, Donna Smith identifies that the surgical consent is not signed. Does the patient have the necessary mental capacity to make the surgical decision for or against the proposed surgical procedure?
   - How severe are the contractures of the patient's hips and knees? Will they allow him to be positioned supine on the operating room bed?
   - If the patient has repeatedly discontinued his intravenous lines, what is his current nutritional and fluid/electrolyte status?
   - Does Mr. Jones understand the questions and instructions given to him or is he simply ignoring the health care personnel? Is his refusal to communicate a desire to "end it all?"
   - Examine personal dilemma regarding the patient's surgery. The gastrostomy tube will provide life-sustaining nutrition according to the principle of beneficence versus the patient's right to self-determination (possibly not to have the surgery at all) according to the principle of autonomy.

NURSING DIAGNOSIS

Alterations in thought processes related to chronic brain syndrome

Impaired verbal communication related to unknown cause

Fluid volume deficit and possible electrolyte imbalance related to inadequate fluid intake

Impaired physical mobility related to contractures of lower extremities

Potential for impaired skin integrity related to emaciated state

2. Planning:
   - Call the patient's nursing unit to check on Mr. Jones' behavior on the unit and his willingness to communicate with the nursing staff.
   - Review the operating room's policy manual to ascertain the options for obtaining surgical consent, court-appointed guardian, two-surgeon, co-validation of need for surgery, and so forth.
   - Communicate with the surgeon regarding the lack of a signed surgical consent. Consult with the OR charge nurse and discuss hospital approved options with the surgeon. Suggest the possibility of cancellation/delay until a court-appointed guardian is identified.
   - Procure additional personnel and pillows and gel mattress pad for positioning Mr. Jones on the operating room bed.
   - Review the patient's skin turgor and laboratory results to assess fluid and possible electrolyte imbalances.
   - Plan on remaining with the patient once the restraints have been removed to prevent the patient from doing injury to himself until he is anesthetized.

3. Implementation:
   - Consultation with the surgeon has determined that the patient has diminished mental capacity and is medically judged unable to give informed surgical consent. The surgeon states that he has thoroughly discussed the situation and need for a gastrostomy tube with the referring physician since Mr. Jones has no known relatives. Both physicians have documented their findings and plan in the medical record according to the hospital's policy.
   - Once the appropriate surgical consent has been obtained, transport the patient into the operating room. Communicate to Mr. Jones, in spite of his lack of response, all interventions and activities prior to their initiation.
   - Place the gel mattress pad on the operating room bed prior to the positioning of the patient. Using additional personnel, move the patient to the bed. Place pillows under the patient to support the patient's contractures of the hips and knees.
   - Document on the intraoperative record the lack of the signed consent preoperatively and the actions taken to secure surgical consent. Also record the positioning aids and techniques used.
4. Evaluation:
   - Convey to the nurse in the post-anesthesia care unit the patient's lack of verbal communication, fluid and electrolyte status, and prior history of alcoholism and chronic brain syndrome.
   - Evaluate the patient's dependent skin areas for any areas of redness or impaired integrity.

Practice Scenario 2
Professional Development

by Doris A. Porter, RN, BSN, MS, CNOR

SCENARIO

Cathy Butler, RN and Bea Davis, RN are assigned to scrub and circulate (respectively) on a patient having a therapeutic abortion. Cathy accepts the assignment and proceeds to prepare the OR. Bea has not received this type of assignment before nor is she eager to participate in the procedure. She does not want to let her team members down.

Bea considers many issues which include

- She has a right to determine her personal values and decide how deeply she is committed to them.
- Her personal beliefs can differ from her therapeutic responsibilities to the patient.
- To give psychologic support to the patient, she must respect differing values and beliefs.
- Care must be delivered in a nonjudgmental manner.
- She must check on the rules and regulations of the institution regarding the staff participation in therapeutic abortion.
- Her responsibility to herself includes minimizing her emotional turmoil (guilt, anxiety, agitation, feelings of powerlessness).
- Her options are to circulate for the scheduled case, request another assignment, or transfer the patient's care to another equally qualified nurse.

Donna Ross is a 36-year-old divorced female who has been admitted to the same day surgery unit for a suction curettage procedure. The patient is 5 feet 9 inches tall and weighs 172 pounds. Her obstetric history includes five prior pregnancies. She has a daughter 4 years old and a son 2 years old. Her current pregnancy is of 9 weeks duration. She has experienced three incomplete abortions for which dilatation and curettage were performed. Ms. Ross answers questions quietly and appears weepy. She has hypertension associated with pregnancy. She underwent right shoulder rotator cuff repair 18 months previously.

Bea Davis decides to participate in the procedure.

PERIOPERATIVE INTERPRETATION

Using what you have just learned in this chapter, as an experienced perioperative nurse you would consider the following in the care of this patient.

1. Assessment:
   - Based upon the nursing preoperative assessment of this patient and knowledge of the planned surgical procedure, the patient will be placed in lithotomy position.
   - The patient's height and weight require special care when placing the patient in and out of lithotomy position.
   - The patient's history of hypertension during pregnancy must be considered as it has an impact on position and anesthesia.
   - The history of right rotator cuff repair poses a problem for positioning of the right arm so as to limit extension.
   - The mannerisms of the patient in answering questions suggest anxiety and apprehension.

NURSING DIAGNOSIS

High risk for skin damage related to pooling of prep solution.

High risk for hemodynamic changes related to history of hypertension and postural change.

High risk for injury related to prior shoulder surgery and surgical positioning.

Anxiety related to the surgical procedure and outcome.

2. Planning:
   - Inform the surgeon, anesthesiologist, and other members of the surgical team of history of hypertension and prior orthopedic surgery.
   - Secure positioning aids to protect bony prominences from nerve and soft-tissue injuries.
   - Provide drip towels to collect prep solution used to prevent the patient from lying in excess solution.

- Position the awake patient to assess for comfort in the surgical position.
- Procure all needed supplies prior to bringing the patient into the OR room so the nurse can stay with the patient during induction to offer physical and emotional support.

3. Implementation:
- With another person, place the awake patient in lithotomy position. Protect the patient's privacy during positioning.
- Place padding under right shoulder with arms aligned on arm board at 45-degree angle.
- Place padding on all body parts where pressure points are located.
- Assess the patient's comfort and make adjustments as necessary. Check the patient's peripheral pulses prior to and after positioning the patient.
- Place drip towels under the patient's buttock prior to the surgical prep and remove after the prep is completed.

- Return the patient's legs to the supine position slowly with another person at the completion of the procedure.

4. Evaluation:
- Assess the patient's skin integrity for breaks, marks, or bruises.
- Ask the patient, when awake, if she has any discomfort in her shoulder, back, hips, or arms.
- Evaluate the patient's peripheral pulses to evaluate circulation after the surgical position.
- Convey to the nurse in the post-anesthesia care unit the patient's hypertension status, prior shoulder injury, and identified need for emotional support.
- Document in the nursing record the patient's position, positioning aids and prep solutions used, nursing activities, and achievement of outcomes.

Chapter Three

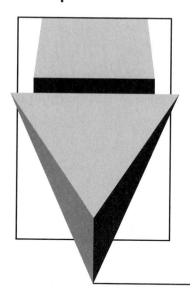

Asepsis: Protecting the Patient, Personnel, and Environment

Leana Revell, RN, MSN, CNOR

Prerequisite Knowledge   Prior to beginning this chapter, the learner should review concepts of microbiology and infection theory.

Chapter content correlates with several AORN recommended practices. These recommended practices may be referred to as a prerequisite, or upon completion of the chapter as a refresher.

Recommended practices for aseptic technique

Recommended practices for surgical attire

Recommended practices for protective barrier materials for gowns and drapes

Recommended practices for surgical hand scrub

Recommended practices for laser safety in the practice setting

Recommended practices for selection and use of packaging systems

Recommended practices for reducing radiologic exposure in the practice setting

Recommended practices for sanitation in the surgical practice setting

Recommended practices for sponge, sharp, and instrument counts

Recommended practices for traffic patterns in the surgical suite

Recommended practices for universal precautions in the perioperative practice setting

Learning Objectives

1. Define asepsis.

2. Discuss traffic patterns for the surgical suite.
3. Describe proper surgical attire for designated areas of the surgical suite.

4. Discuss sanitation practices appropriate for the surgical suite.

5. Define the meaning of surgical conscience.

6. Discuss the procedure of a surgical scrub.
7. Describe the sterile application of gown and gloves.
8. Identify the principles of surgical draping.

Infection Control in Surgical Settings

Today's operating room or surgical suite is quite different from its predecessor of 100 years ago, yet the main principles of asepsis and infection control within the surgical environment remain as significant today as they were in the past. Without care and concern about infection, the success of every surgical procedure would be in great jeopardy. Each nurse, scrub person, and housekeeper, and all ancillary personnel within the surgical environment must develop a strong surgical conscience. A surgical conscience dictates an awareness of and a strict adherence to cleanliness, aseptic principles, and sterile technique. Adherence to aseptic practices, which control infection, provides protection not only for the patient but also for the surgical personnel who work within the environment.

Asepsis by definition means absence of pathologic organisms. However, it is impossible to exclude all microorganisms from the environment. Asepsis in the surgical setting refers to the efforts made by the surgical team to prevent the transmission of microorganisms to patients and personnel. Aseptic technique includes those practices that prevent the patient and staff from acquiring an infection. These may include nonsterile activities, such as washing hands, or sterile activities, such as donning surgical gloves, which require a more complex knowledge base and stringent application of sterile technique.

The concepts of asepsis apply to delivery of patient care during the entire perioperative experience. It is the role of all direct and indirect caregivers in these settings to control situations that promote the spread of infection to a compromised patient and to minimize the spread of infection to themselves and to future patients. The control of infection can be achieved by aseptic practices, appropriate sterilization and disinfection, prophylactic antibiotics, and vaccination where necessary (Tait, 1993).

Some of the aseptic practices performed in the surgical setting are mandated by regulations. Others come from years of ritual practice or from scientifically validated studies which direct the development of regulations. Recommendations for practice can come from many sources such as the Centers for Disease Control and Prevention (CDC), Association of Operating Room Nurses (AORN), Association for the Advancement of Medical Instrumentation (AAMI), Joint Commission for Accreditation of Healthcare Organizations (JCAHO), and Occupational Safety and Health Administration (OSHA). Recommendations from these regulatory bodies are incorporated into daily activities to maintain infection control and optimum patient care.

MICROBIOLOGIC CONSIDERATIONS

A variety of microorganisms can be found in hospitals and surgical settings, including gram-positive bacteria (Streptococcus, Staphylococcus), gram-negative bacteria (Pseudomonas, Escherichia coli, Mycobacterium tuberculosis), fungal growth (Candida albicans, Aspergillus), and viral organisms (herpesvirus, hepatitis virus, human immunodeficiency virus). Contamination and possible infection from microbes during surgical procedures are controlled through the use of disinfection and sterilization processes.

Disinfection kills disease-causing organisms but not spores. Several types of disinfectant or germicidal agents are available to kill these microorganisms. High-level disinfectants destroy all vegetative bacteria, fungi, and viruses but not necessarily bacterial spores. Intermediate-level disinfectants destroy vegetative bacteria, including Mycobacterium tuberculosis, most fungi, and most viruses, but not bacterial spores. Low-level disinfection will destroy most vegetative bacteria, fungi, and some viruses but not Mycobacterium tuberculosis or bacterial spores (Young, 1990).

Sterilization renders an object free of all organisms, including bacterial spores and viruses. In the surgical setting, sterile areas or fields are established to insure that patients have minimal exposure to harmful microbes that can cause infection. Other factors that may contribute to the development of infection in the surgical setting include the patient's susceptibility, the type of invasive procedure performed, and the presence of antibiotic resistant bacteria.

Patient Considerations

The surgical setting is an area where invasive procedures are performed upon patients. Invasive procedures vary in complexity and may range from excisions of a superficial mass or endoscopic observations to major surgical interventions, such as thoracotomies. Since surgical procedures are invasive, they transgress normal body protective barriers. As the patient's normal body barriers, such as skin or mucous membranes, are broken or compromised, the patient becomes vulnerable to acquisition of an infection. There is increasing evidence that anesthetic agents administered during the invasive procedure may further alter the patient's immune response (Tait, 1993). Without the application of aseptic practices, which are directed at interrupting infectious cycles, the patient may develop a hospital-acquired infection.

Approximately 5% of all patients entering hospitals acquire some type of microbial infection that was not present upon admission. These are termed hospital-acquired or nosocomial infections. Nosocomial infection rates vary depending upon the type of procedure and the general health of the patient. Overall infection rates do not reflect the quality of care but are indicators to be monitored and investigated if increases are noted.

The more critically ill and compromised the patient, the higher the probability of the patient's acquiring a nosocomial infection and becoming infective to others. Patients may harbor unusual, antibiotic-resistant virulent microorganisms. In addition, patients may have compromised immune systems and may be unable to resist minimal microbial exposure. Factors predisposing a surgical patient to infection include age; burns; obesity; diabetes; smoking history; pre-existing infection; poor nutritional status, such as is found in alcoholic or drug-addicted patients; and immunocompromised conditions, resulting from chemotherapy, radiotherapy, or AIDS.

Personnel Considerations

From the health care worker's perspective, the issue of infection control is more complex. The protection of the health care worker, as well as the patient, is now necessary since it is not possible to identify which patients may be hazardous. In the past, patients were considered as "contaminated" when a known infection, such as hepatitis, was identified, and the procedures were designated as "dirty cases." Stringent aseptic techniques were used, such as fogging a room with disinfectant and closing the room for 24 hours after treating a contaminated patient. During the 1970s, this practice changed to incorporate the principles of confine and contain to decrease microbial contamination (Rothrock, 1991).

It is no longer possible to screen patients for communicable diseases. Furthermore, the antibodies of a newly acquired exposure may not be detected. These factors necessitate stringent infection control measures, called universal precautions, on all patients. With universal precautions, all patients are treated as if contaminated. These practices provide a maximum level of protection for patients and personnel at all times. Routine aseptic techniques and universal precautions are practiced whether or not an infection or communicable disease is suspected. In the surgical setting, personnel are exposed to infectious material, and other body fluids routinely. Exposed health care workers are required to take protective measures and wear additional protective attire to decrease their potential for infection.

Within the health care facility, the primary culprit for infection of health care personnel is not human immunodeficiency virus (HIV), but the hepatitis B virus (HBV) (Giordano, 1993). Nearly 8,700 health care workers become infected with HBV annually, and of these 200 die each year. The CDC recommend that all operating room personnel, as well as others coming into contact with blood and other body fluids, be vaccinated to prevent HBV infections (Lisanti, 1992).

Universal Precautions

Universal precautions provide an infection control approach that states that all human blood and other potentially infectious materials are to be treated as if known to be infected with HIV, HBV, or other bloodborne pathogens (Bruning, 1993). The Occupational Safety and Health Administration (OSHA) presumes that all patients and personnel represent a potential source of infection. In order to protect health care personnel as well as patients from infection, OSHA requires that certain precautions be universally applied when dealing with body substances such as blood, semen, saliva, unfixed tissue and organs, pleural fluid, pericardial fluid, peritoneal fluid, synovial fluid, vaginal secretions, cerebrospinal fluid, and amniotic fluid. Handling substances such as feces, urine, tears, breast milk, and vomitus requires nursing judgment. If blood is present, it is considered contaminated. All body fluids are considered to be potentially contaminated and may infect an individual through broken skin or mucous membranes. Universal precautions are an integral part of all procedures in the surgical setting. Principles of universal precautions include the use of personal protective barriers, handwashing, and care in the use and disposal of needles and other sharp instruments. These topics are discussed individually, but the concept of universal precautions applies in each situation.

TRAFFIC PATTERNS

Within surgical settings there are real and/or conceptual geographic divisions, or areas, which are designated as restricted, semirestricted, or unrestricted. The purpose of these zones is to control contamination through the establishment of traffic patterns and designations of specific surgical attire for each area. The closer to the sterile field, the greater the need for control of contamination, and the more restrictive the dress and activities. Where architectural design permits, clean and contaminated items are moved using separate traffic patterns. Soiled materials are isolated from clean and sterile supplies to prevent cross-contamination. Ideally, separate traffic patterns will prevent contact between clean and contaminated equipment, but environmental design may limit the implementation of this practice.

The unrestricted area includes the area that interfaces with public access to the surgical suite. Areas that may be classified as unrestricted may include dressing areas, patient-holding areas, and adjoining offices. An unrestricted area usually includes a control center, which monitors patients, family, and personnel, and equipment entering the surgical suite. Street clothes are permitted in the unrestricted area. Equipment that enters the unrestricted area and needs to be taken to the semirestricted and restricted areas will require special handling or preparation in this area. If an external cover is not in place, articles are wiped down with a disinfectant solution prior to movement into semirestricted and restricted areas. Supplies are removed from external shipping containers or covers in the unrestricted areas to prevent dust, debris, and insects from entering controlled areas.

Semirestricted areas are frequently separated from unrestricted areas by closed doors or markers that indicate that traffic is limited to authorized personnel and patients. Semirestricted areas include clean and sterile storage areas, work areas for processing equipment, peripheral support areas, and corridors to restricted areas. Patients entering this area should wear clean gowns and a hair covering and have clean linens on the stretcher or bed. Personnel in semirestricted areas wear scrub attire including head coverings.

The restricted area is where surgical procedures are performed and unwrapped supplies are sterilized. It includes the operating room, clean core, and scrub sink areas. Surgical attire, head coverings or hoods, and masks are required in this area at all times, even if the area is not in use. Although all personnel are required to wear masks in this area, patients do not wear masks.

SURGICAL ATTIRE

Patient Attire

Physical barriers to infection impede the movement of microbes from the human body to the atmosphere. Clean gowns, linens, and hair coverings are worn to contain debris and dead cells shed by the patient. Hair coverings are applied after the patient is checked for metal hairpins or clips, which might function as a ground during electrosurgical cautery or cause unwanted pressure points during positioning. A clean gown and hair covering must be in place from the time the patient enters the semirestricted area. Although not considered surgical attire for patients, warm blankets or thermal coverings should be available. These decrease the potential for hypothermia in the cool environment of the surgical suite.

Personnel Attire

One of the most obvious visual designations of the surgical setting is the apparel of the staff. Surgical scrub suits, masks, and hair coverings are required by all personnel (Fig. 3–1). Warmup jackets and shoe covers are also appropriate attire for the surgical suite. These items may be disposable or reusable and provide barriers that interfere with the passage of microorganisms. Dressing rooms are located in the unrestricted area and allow personnel to change into scrub attire prior to entering the semirestricted and restricted areas.

Head and facial hair are gross contaminants and sources of bacteria. Hats or hoods which *completely* cover the hair, sideburns, and beards should be worn to decrease the spread of microbes. The hair covering should be single use and disposable, or if reusable, should be laundered after each use. The head covering is placed over the hair prior to putting on scrub attire to confine as much contamination as possible. Hair should not be combed while wearing scrub attire.

Surgical attire worn in the surgical environment consists of either a one-piece coverall or a two-piece scrub suit. The two-piece scrub suit must fit the body snugly. Loose-fitting shirts are tucked into the pants to prevent the shirt from touching sterile areas and to reduce fallout of skin debris. A tunic top that fits snugly may be worn on the outside of the pants. Disposable or freshly laundered scrub suits should be worn. Individuals should not launder their own clothing at home. Scrub attire should be laundered in the facility laundry, which provides hospital-grade detergent germicides for removal of blood and body

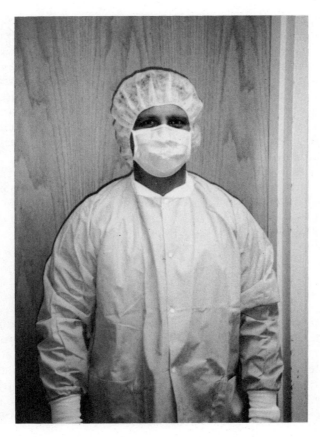

FIGURE 3–1. Surgical Attire

COVER GOWNS

Scrub Attire

Current AORN Recommended Practices (AORN, 1993) state that if it is necessary to leave the surgical suite, scrub attire should be covered completely with a cover gown that closes in the back. Upon return to the surgical suite, the disposable cover gown should be discarded, or if reusable, placed in the laundry. The value and cost-effectiveness of cover gowns in reducing contamination has not been well established (Patterson, 1991). Alternatives to the cover gown include donning fresh scrubs upon return to the surgical suite, wearing a lab coat over scrubs, or requiring no coverage of scrubs.

fluids. The use of the hospital laundry facilities also prevents possible contamination of the home environment of the health care worker with hospital-acquired microorganisms. Scrub attire should be changed anytime it becomes wet or visibly soiled and should be worn only within the surgical suite. When personnel leave the surgical suite, it should be removed and placed in the laundry or discarded if disposable.

Warmup jackets with long sleeves are worn by unsterile team members over the scrub suit. These jackets serve two purposes. They decrease the shed of bacteria from uncovered forearms and keep the unscrubbed person warmer in the cooler temperature of the operating room. Warmup jackets should be kept buttoned or snapped and should be changed if visibly soiled or wet. Warmup jackets are removed when it is necessary to scrub.

Masks are worn at all times in the restricted area where sterile supplies will be opened, in clean cores, and at scrub sinks. Masks with face shields or masks and protective eyewear are required whenever any splashes, spray, or aerosol of blood or other potentially infectious materials may be generated. Masks can be found in various shapes with a variety of different features. Special masks may be required for higher particle filtering of microbes, such as during laser surgery.

Masks are effective only if worn properly. Masks decrease the passage of air and bacterial particles from the wearer into the environment. It is not uncommon to see masks poorly fitted, placed below the nose, or wet with blood or body fluids. Masks should be comfortable and cover both the nose and mouth completely. The fit should assure that there is no tenting at the sides of the mouth that would allow dispersion or entry of microbes. A small pliable metal strip at the nose area should promote a close fit. Masks should be changed frequently and anytime they become wet. When removing the mask, handle it only by the strings and promptly discard it into the waste receptacle. A mask should never be

MASKS

Masks and Patient Infection Rates

Research suggests that masks may not significantly decrease patient infection rates. In foreign countries, it is not uncommon for surgical procedures to be performed by scrubbed personnel who do not wear masks. Some experts state that masks should be required only for scrubbed personnel working directly over the surgical wound. Others advocate that masks are needed only if the health care worker has a cold. Other sources state that a plastic face shield alone is sufficient in providing protection for patient and health care worker (Mathias, 1993).

allowed to hang or dangle around the neck, nor should it be folded and placed in a pocket for later use. Masks should be either on or off.

Fingernails should be short, clean, and free of chipped polish, artificial nails, and bonding materials (AORN, 1993). Artificial nails have been shown to harbor microorganisms, particularly fungal growths. Jewelry, including necklaces, earrings, watches, and rings should be removed or confined within the scrub attire. These articles prevent effective handwashing, harbor organisms in crevices, and have the potential of falling into wounds. Makeup should be minimal, because it can flake and fall into open wounds or sterile fields.

Comfortable supportive shoes should be worn. Cloth shoes, such as tennis shoes and sandals, provide no protection against spilled fluids or dropped instruments and should not be worn. Clogs and shoes without enclosed heels and/or toes are not recommended for daily wear. Shoes must be cleanable. Disposable shoe covers may be worn over shoes for protection but should be changed whenever torn, wet, or soiled. Fluid-resistant shoe covers should be worn when contact with blood or body fluids is unavoidable or excessive, such as during joint replacement surgery.

Special Attire Situations

Personal Protective Attire

Personal protective equipment is specialized clothing or barriers that prevent the passage of microorganisms from the patient to the health care worker, or from the health care worker to the patient. It does not include general work clothing such as scrub suits unless they are specifically designed to provide protection against a hazard (Bruning, 1993). Barriers include fluid-resistant gowns, aprons, gloves, masks, shoe covers, and eyewear or face shields. These protective barriers should be liberally used by all personnel (Fig. 3–2). Personnel should never assume that just because they are not close to the sterile field that they are not at risk of being splattered by blood or irrigation fluids (Hubbard, 1992).

Although not required for all surgical procedures, disposable fluid-resistant shoe covers protect personnel from spills and splashes of blood and body fluids. Shoe covers should be changed whenever torn, wet, or contaminated by blood or other potentially infectious materials. Protective shoe covers are available in various heights from ankle to above the knee. The fluidproof shoe cover may be required in procedures where an abundance of fluids or potentially infected fluid will be contacted, such as orthopedic or urologic procedures.

Plastic aprons may not usually be thought of as a fluid barrier, but they can prevent fabric scrub clothes from becoming wet in specific procedures. Aprons can be worn under permeable reusable sterile gowns. Fluid-resistant aprons are worn when there are copious irrigations (such as in cytoscopy) or when contact with fluids is possible (emptying suction canisters, cleaning instruments). Fluid-

---

SHOE COVERS

Shoe Covers for Routine Surgery

Shoe covers are not required for routine surgical attire. They are worn predominantly to keep contamination off shoes. If shoes are able to be decontaminated after contact with body fluids, covers are not required. If contact with body fluids is anticipated, shoe covers are worn as personal protective attire. Some experts consider shoe covers costly and unnecessary.

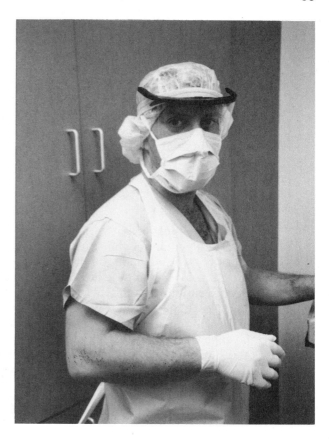

FIGURE 3-2. Personal Protective Attire

resistant gowns should be worn whenever blood or other potentially infectious material could splash, spatter, or spray the health care worker.

Gloves should be worn when contact with blood and body fluids may occur, such as in starting intravenous infusions, intubation, or dressing application. Gloves should be worn when handling blood, drainage, secretions, tissue specimens, or items contaminated with blood or body fluids. Gloves should be changed between patient contacts or after contact with contaminated items when the task is completed. Gloves may be sterile for invasive procedures or nonsterile for all other activities that do not require sterile techniques. General purpose utility gloves are worn for sanitation purposes, then decontaminated and reused. Reusable utility gloves should be inspected prior to use for cracks, punctures, or evidence of deterioration.

Handwashing is the single most important means of infection control and should be practiced frequently. Even if gloves have been worn, impeccable handwashing should be accomplished before entry into the restricted area and after every direct contact with patients or items in contact with blood, body fluids, or excreta.

Eye protection, along with a surgical mask, is worn to protect the health care worker from contamination caused by splashing, spraying, and spattering. Eyewear is appropriate for cleaning personnel who are emptying suction canisters or hazardous wastes as well as for those individuals who have the potential of being spattered by blood, body fluids, and tissues at the surgical field. Prescription glasses are not considered protective eyewear. Protective eyewear includes perspective glasses with side shields, which provide a formfitting barrier for the eye; goggles; and face shields, which protect the entire facial area. Antifog goggles can be worn over prescription glasses. Protective eyewear or face shields that become contaminated should be discarded or decontaminated promptly according to the manufacturer's recommendations.

To provide *complete* isolation and face protection for sterile surgical team members, a helmet-type device may be worn on the head. The helmet is used selectively, such as in orthopedic procedures, where a high-speed drill may tend to splatter or aerosolize fluid and tissue. This helmet usually requires a venting system for circulation and filtration of air to the surgical team member. During the gowning process, the helmet is covered with a fitted drape, which contains a clear plastic face shield to protect staff from exposure to blood, tissue, and body fluids. A surgical mask is not necessary when a disposable face shield and helmet are worn.

Laser Surgery

When entering procedures where a laser is in use, special glasses and masks must be worn by all personnel and conscious patients. Laser glasses should be appropriate for the laser wavelength and optical density that is in use. These glasses may vary in color and should contour to the face with side shields to insure no contact between the laser beam and the eye. Without these laser glasses, permanent damage can occur to the cornea or retina of the eye. Masks for laser procedures have a higher filtration than other masks for removal of particles that have become vaporized with the laser beam. The plume of laser smoke is considered a potential hazard owing to viable viral microorganisms that are found in laser smoke. Without the appropriate mask, these potentially harmful vaporized cells may be inhaled into the lungs of the health care team members. Even though mechanical smoke evacuator systems decrease the amount of laser plume, special laser masks should be worn during laser procedures.

Radiologic Procedures

Personnel and patients exposed to ionizing radiation during fluoroscopy or surgical procedures require special protective devices (Fig. 3–3). Radiation monitor badges are required for personnel who are in frequent proximity to radiation sources. This radiation monitor badge is worn outside of lead aprons at the neckline. Portable radiographc shielding partitions may be brought into the room for additional protection. Leaded glasses may be used to protect eyes, and leaded gloves reduce the exposure to hands. Body shields, such as aprons or collars, are used to cover areas, such as gonads or the thyroid, that are at risk for high radiation dosage. Leaded thyroid collars should be provided for patients and anesthesia personnel when x-ray films are made of the upper extremities, trunk, and head. Leaded shields are used to cover the patient's pelvis and gonads while doing x-ray examinations of the hips and upper legs. Leaded aprons and collars should be visually inspected for cracks prior to use and should be stored flat or hanging to maintain structural integrity. Structural integrity of leaded shields should be routinely inspected by radiographic methods to insure safety for patient and staff.

Environmental Control

TEMPERATURE AND HUMIDITY

Since temperature and humidity have the potential for increasing or inhibiting bacterial growth, the control of the surgical environment is monitored and regulated. The temperature is maintained at 70°F to 75°F with a humidity of 50% to 60% (Bartley, 1993). These temperature and humidity ranges are helpful for the

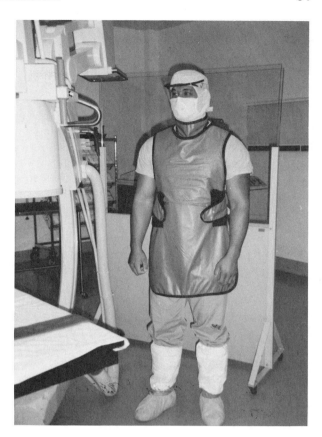

FIGURE 3–3. Radiologic Protective Devices

reduction of bacterial counts and static electricity, and for the comfort of the sterile-attired surgical staff. These lower room temperatures may cause extremely adverse effects to the patient. Patents whose thermoregulation abilities are compromised, such as the elderly, malnourished, or neonate, require careful monitoring and additional nursing interventions in the surgical environment, such as warming blankets, thermal body drapes, or warmed solutions.

AIR EXCHANGES

In an attempt to minimize the potential for infection, health care facilities and surgical settings are designed with air handling systems that comply with local, state, and national regulations. These regulations dictate the number of air changes per minute; whether the air must be fresh or can be recirculated; whether special circuits are required for air that is grossly contaminated; or whether special handling devices, such as an anesthetic gas exhaust, are necessary. Ventilation systems are designed to provide positive pressures within the operating room and to lower the pressure within adjoining corridors. This positive pressure decreases the mixing of the operating room air and the corridor air, thereby decreasing contamination and bacterial counts.

Air currents are a significant source of contamination within surgical settings. Bacteria are shed by patients and personnel within the operating room from skin and airborne droplets. These organisms have the ability to travel on dust particles and air currents. Greater amounts of airborne contamination can be expected with increased movement of people and supplies. As the number of people present in the room increases, the amount of activity in the room increases, potential for bacterial shedding increases, and potential for contamination from air turbulence also increases.

Several aseptic practices decrease airborne contamination. The number of individuals within the operating room is controlled to minimize traffic and potential sources of bacteria (Ritter, 1988). Dust is minimized through stringent housekeeping practices throughout the day. Surgical drapes are never fanned, as this action would increase air currents. Contaminated liquids, such as blood or pus, have the ability to dry and become airborne particles. Therefore, soiled sponges, instruments, or laundry are placed in impervious containers to decrease potential airborne contamination. Room doors remain closed to decrease air currents except when patients, personnel, or equipment must move. Regular maintenance of the air handling systems, exchange of filters, and cleaning of vents are essential to reduce the number of airborne bacteria.

A high-flow, unidirectional ventilation system, called laminar airflow, may be found in the surgical setting. The purpose of the laminar airflow is to provide the cleanest air possible with minimal air turbulence. This is an ultraventilation system where essentially bacteria-free air is introduced through a perforated end wall or ceiling. The air is circulated over the patient from a filtered air outlet, and then returned through a receiving air inlet. The airflow within the room is unidirectional over the working area and the patient. Care must be taken to have only sterile items at the air outlet and within the working area. Clean equipment and contaminated items are placed at the air inlet in the working area.

Ultraviolet lights may be found in some operating rooms. These are utilized to destroy airborne and surface microorganisms that are rapidly affected by ultraviolet radiation. The ultraviolet lights are inexpensive and easy to install but do have some disadvantages. The effectiveness of the ultraviolet lights can be affected by dust on the light tubes and by distance. The ultraviolet radiation may be hazardous to both patient and personnel when used continuously and requires protective glasses, hoods, and gowns to avoid conjunctivitis, skin erythema, and corneal burns (Wenzel, 1993). In some operating rooms, ultraviolet lights are turned on only when patients and personnel are not in the rooms.

OPERATING ROOM SANITATION

A surgical environment that insures cleanliness and minimal bacterial growth is essential to the well-being of patients and personnel. Unless properly cleaned and disinfected, the surgical area can become heavily contaminated by microbes. Consistent implementation of sanitation procedures is required for all cases, since all patients are considered potentially contaminated. Good housekeeping techniques within the surgical setting should reduce microbial flora by approximately 90% (Atkinson, 1992).

The supplies and equipment used in sanitation procedures include lint-free cleaning cloths, detergent germicidal solutions, WetVac system or clean mops, floor scrubber, gloves, and carts for linen and trash disposal. Prompt disinfection of furniture, equipment, and floors, and disposal of waste and laundry should be accomplished so that debris does not dry and become an airborne contaminant.

AIR CURRENTS IN THE SURGICAL SETTING

Laminar Airflow

Experts disagree that unidirectional airflow is the most effective and efficient system for reducing airborne contamination. Proponents of laminar airflow identify it as an optimal, cost-effective mechanism for reducing contamination. Other experts believe that prophylactic antibiotics and standard aseptic technique are equally, or more effective, than laminar airflow in reducing wound infection (Laufman, 1990).

In all cleaning procedures, friction increases the removal of debris. All individuals who carry out these sanitation duties should wear protective attire, such as gloves, masks, and eyewear. Additionally, shoe covers and gowns should be donned if heavy contamination is present.

Preliminary Cleaning

The room should be inspected for soiled areas that may have been missed during previous cleanup. It is the responsibility of the perioperative nurse to establish that the room is clean prior to the opening of any sterile supplies. Before the first scheduled procedure, all horizontal surfaces within the room are damp-dusted with a lint-free cloth containing a hospital-grade germicide. The surgical bed, overhead lights, room furniture, and room equipment should be carefully damp-dusted. Equipment from other areas, such as electrosurgical units (ESU), gas tanks, x-ray machines, supply carts, and any pieces that come from a storage area, should be damp-dusted prior to being brought into the room.

Interim Cleaning

During the surgical procedures, contamination should be confined and contained as much as possible. Most contamination occurs within the immediate vicinity of the surgical field. If gross contamination occurs and is difficult to confine, such as might be the case in a large trauma case, sterile and nonsterile personnel should wear gowns, goggles, gloves, shoe covers, aprons, and other appropriate personal protective equipment.

Accidental spills of blood and body fluids should be promptly cleaned with a disposable cloth that is saturated with a germicide solution (Fig. 3–4). Disposable gloves are worn when handling contaminated items. Nonsterile instruments

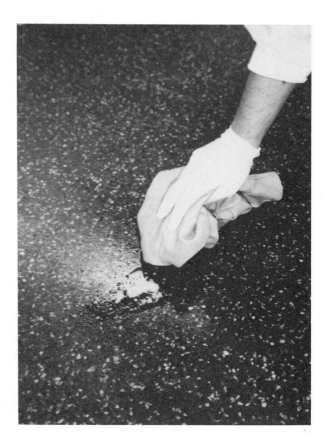

FIGURE 3–4. Interim Cleaning of Spills

may also be used to handle contaminated articles. If an instrument from the sterile field falls to the floor and becomes contaminated, it should be deposited in a pan of germicide if it is submersible. This will prevent drying of bioburden or debris, which could become additional airborne contamination. Nonsubmersible instruments are placed in an impervious container. Those instruments that are required to be immediately resterilized should be washed in germicide and rinsed prior to sterilization.

Confine all disposable items used during the procedure in impervious containers (Fig. 3–5). Trash and linens are placed in separate impervious containers, sealed, and removed to designated receiving areas. Trash bags must be leakproof, sealed, and of sufficient thickness to maintain their integrity as they are transported. Reusable anesthesia tubing, masks, and equipment are confined and transported for terminal cleaning. Items that are grossly contaminated with blood, tissue, or body fluids will require special handling as hazardous wastes.

Hazardous wastes may include grossly contaminated sponges, drapes, gowns, or fluids contained in suction tubing and canisters. Disposal of fluids in suction canisters is done according to hospital policy and local regulations. This may include emptying contents into a flushing hopper or addition of chemicals that cause solutions to become gelatinous or inactivated. Sharps, such as needles, syringes, knife blades, some electrocautery tips, and pins, are disposed of in special punctureproof receptacles (Fig. 3–6). OSHA regulations require that sharps containers be closable, puncture-resistant, leakproof, and labeled or color-coded. These containers should be readily available in each room. Small sterile sharps containers may be placed on the sterile back table for sharps disposal at the sterile field.

Specimens that are handed off the sterile field for examination are carefully placed in an impervious container. Exterior surfaces of specimen containers are

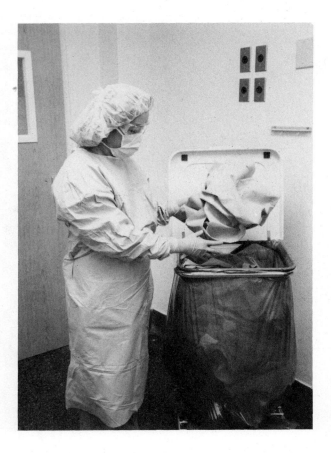

FIGURE 3–5. Disposal of Used Linens

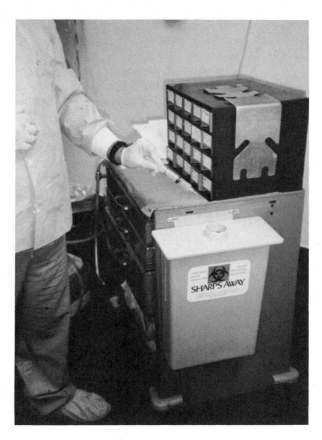

FIGURE 3-6. Disposal of Used Sharps

wiped with a disinfectant solution before being removed from the surgical room. Culture tubes or blood-filled syringes may be placed into impervious containers, such as plastic bags, for transport. Insure that documents submitted with specimens are free of contamination.

Gloves should be worn when handling items that are in contact with the patient. These items, although they may appear outwardly clean, are contaminated. Instruments that were not used during the surgical procedure are separated from instruments that were used (Rutala, 1990). Contaminated used instruments will require additional care, as follows:

- Irrigate suction tips to clear internal debris.
- Remove all visible bioburden from instruments.
- Open box-lock devices on instruments.
- Separate delicate instruments or those requiring special handling.
- Disassemble those instruments that can be reasonably handled without losing parts.

Sharp instruments are separated from other instruments in a small basin. Disposable sharps, such as knife blades, are deposited in appropriate puncture-proof containers. If a substerile area is adjacent to the surgical room and contains a washer-sterilizer, place opened instruments in a wire mesh tray for processing. Specialty instruments, such as endoscopes, drills, saws, and delicate instruments, are not processed in washer-sterilizers and require separate cleaning procedures. If the processing area is not adjacent to the surgical rooms, isolate and enclose contaminated instruments for transport in impervious containers, closed carts, or plastic bags.

Clean supplies, equipment, and activities should be distinctly separate from contaminated supplies, equipment, and activities. The separation of clean and contaminated items can be accomplished by traffic patterns when transporting items by different routes, by different time periods, or by space when enclosed in sealed containers/bags. Cross-contamination must be avoided in all sanitation activities.

Contaminated or used disposable items should be discarded according to local, state, and federal regulations. Contaminated linen is confined in a leak-proof laundry bag. Linen is handled as little as possible to prevent airborne contamination. Trash is separated into routine trash and hazardous waste and is placed into separate receptacles (McVeigh, 1993). Methods of handling and disposing of hazardous waste should comply with current OSHA and local regulations. Reusable items should be processed according to institutional policy. Equipment that will not be used in future cases is returned to the appropriate storage area after it is cleaned, restocked, and reassembled.

At the end of each procedure, after all trash, linen, instruments, and equipment have been removed, all horizontal surfaces should be cleaned with a detergent germicidal solution. Inspect the room walls for contamination and spot-clean as necessary. Cleaning should begin with ceiling items and proceed downward. Surgical lights that have been placed over the sterile field are carefully inspected for blood, wiped, and returned to the center of the room. Surfaces that have come into contact with the patient or patient secretions are thoroughly cleaned using mechanical friction. The surgical bed and mattress pad are wiped, paying particular attention to the sides of the bed and areas that may have contacted patient blood or other body fluid. Handles of cabinets and push plates of doors are cleaned. The floor is flooded with a detergent germicide, the wheels of the surgical bed are moved through the solution, and the immediate area is wet-vacuumed. If wet vacuums are not available, a clean mophead that is soaked in a fresh detergent germicide solution is used (Fig. 3–7). Mopheads are reprocessed or discarded after each case. Kick buckets, linen hamper frames, suction canis-

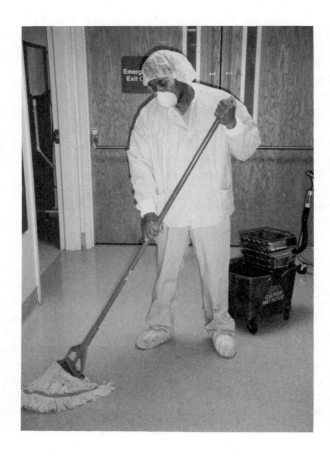

FIGURE 3–7. End-of-Procedure Cleaning

ters, and other waste receptacles are cleaned, and new liners are placed in them. The bed is made with fresh linens and the room is readied for the next procedure.

Terminal Cleaning

At the end of each day, all operating rooms, substerile areas, scrub sinks, scrub/utility areas, hallways, furniture, and equipment are terminally cleaned. Storage areas where sterile supplies are contained should be carefully cleaned, taking care not to contaminate packaging with cleaning fluids, which might splash. Furniture is wiped down and inspected. Casters on movable equipment should be inspected for suture material, which frequently accumulates around wheels. Operating rooms are cleaned by removing all portable items, flooding the floor with detergent germicide solution for 5 minutes and thoroughly scrubbing it with a floor scrubber. Floor baseboards are cleaned. The solution is removed with a wet vacuum or clean mophead. The room furniture is replaced; fresh trash liners, linen bags, suction canisters, and tubing are reapplied; and linen is placed on the bed. Anesthesia equipment and any other needed equipment are set up for the next day.

Scrub sink areas, which have been cleaned periodically during the day, are terminally cleaned at the end of the day. Reusable soap dispensers are disassembled, cleaned, and autoclaved, if possible, prior to being refilled with scrub solutions. Spray heads of faucets are removed, cleaned, and may be autoclaved. Walls around the scrub sinks are checked for cleanliness. Scrub brushes and supplies are restocked.

Corridors often become cluttered with equipment and supplies during the day. These items are returned to their appropriate storage areas after they have been stocked and wiped down. Corridors are thoroughly cleaned.

After performing OR sanitation, disassemble and clean the housekeeping equipment. Before storing the equipment, ensure that it is dry. This will decrease the growth of microbes.

Weekly/Monthly Cleaning

Periodic sanitation of the surgical suite is established in health care facility policies. These procedures specify a cleaning schedule for items that require routine, but not daily cleaning. Some of the items included in these policies are closets, cabinets, shelves, walls, ceilings, air conditioning equipment, return ventilation and heating grills, overhead lighting tracts, ducts, and filters. Equipment such as sterilizers, warming cabinets, refrigerators, and ice machines require routine scheduled cleaning. Lounges, offices, and locker rooms may be cleaned daily or weekly.

Aseptic Technique

SURGICAL CONSCIENCE

Professionalism in nursing requires that patient safety never be compromised. In the surgical setting, consistent incorporation of aseptic principles, perpetual attention to each detail in providing cleanliness or sterility, and constant monitoring of one's own actions in the surgical setting are the fundamentals of a surgical conscience. The significance of the surgical conscience is that it does not permit a nurse to excuse an error in technique, but rather leads to identifying an error, rectifying it, and moving on to other activities. The surgical conscience dictates that the nurse correct the error whether he/she is observed or unobserved. In daily practice this issue is critical, because sterility and strict aseptic technique are essential (Radke, 1993).

ESTABLISHING A STERILE FIELD

The required sterile supplies and equipment for the surgical procedure should be selected and brought to the room. The physician preference card is reviewed and items to be placed in the sterile field are separated from items for possible or later use. Rooms are arranged so that when opening a door, nonsterile personnel will not enter directly into the sterile field.

The sterile field includes all the furniture and equipment that will be covered with sterile drapes; the personnel, who are gowned and gloved; and the draped surgical area, where the procedure will take place. The sterile field should be prepared as close to the time of the procedure as possible. The longer the supplies are open, the greater the possibility of airborne contamination. Once the sterile field is established, it should be constantly monitored and maintained. If the sterile field is not monitored, it should be considered contaminated. If there is any doubt about the sterility of an item, it is considered contaminated (Gruendemann, 1990). Sterile tables should not be covered for later utilization, since it is impossible to uncover a table without contamination of sterile contents (Smith, 1992).

Sterile packages are placed on dry surfaces and handled with clean, dry hands. Certain guidelines will apply to sterile packaging in general. If a sterile package that is wrapped in permeable materials becomes wet or damp, it will become contaminated through a process of bacterial migration through a wicking action and should be discarded or resterilized. A dropped package may be considered contaminated. If an article is dropped on the floor, or other area of contamination, the packing may allow implosion of air into the contents, thereby contaminating the article. If the dropped article is wrapped in impervious materials and is dry and intact, the article may be opened and immediately transferred to the sterile field (Atkinson, 1992). Textiles should be treated with caution when they are dropped owing to their absorbency (Patterson, 1991). Dropped articles that are not used should not be returned to sterile storage.

The sterile field is frequently established by opening a table cover or drape pack over a back table (Fig. 3–8). The sterile drape pack or table cover is opened by placing hands under the protective cuff, opening the fanfolded drape completely, and allowing the excess and touched areas to fall below the table level. The sterile inside of the drape should cover the table and become a sterile area or field where other sterile supplies can be placed. The sterile wrappers from skin preparation sets, instrument sets, and basin sets can also be considered as smaller sterile fields.

Most articles are sterilized in a sequential wrap, peel packaging, or rigid containers. When opening packages, first check the external chemical indicator, package integrity, and expiration date. The nurse observes for punctures, tears, and areas where heat seals may have become broken or where linen or disposable wrappers have opened for any evidence of wetness. After the article is inspected, it may be opened. To open the sequential-wrap package (Fig. 3–9), open the first flap outward from the opener, then open the wrapper to either side, and finally open the final flap toward the opener. Ends of the wrapper are secured in the hand so that they do not dangle and inadvertently contaminate other articles. A second wrapper is found inside the first wrapper and is opened in the exact manner as the first. If internal indicators are visible, these are observed prior to delivering the contents to the sterile field.

Peel packages should be inspected for tears, punctures, or poor areas of heat sealing. The inner edge of the heat seal is considered to be the demarcation line for sterility. Peel-open packages should be pulled back to expose sterile contents.

PACKAGE WRAPPING

Single and Double Wrapping

Some items are single-wrapped, not double-wrapped. From a safety and function viewpoint, single wrapping is all that is required if the packages are stored in clean, dry conditions, with no damage to package integrity. Some experts advocate double wrapping for barrier protection and greater opportunity for sterility to be maintained. If several small items are contained in the wrapper, a second wrap will facilitate transfer of items to the sterile field.

Practice is required to assure sterility of items placed on the sterile field. Contents should be flipped from the package or lifted outward and not allowed to slide over or touch the areas of heat sealing. Articles can be flipped or lightly tossed onto the sterile field if they are small, not likely to roll off the sterile field, and will not penetrate the sterile surface.

Rigid container systems may also be utilized for maintaining sterile supplies. These containers should be inspected for exposure to sterilization processes and intact filters or valve systems per the manufacturer's recommendations. If the filter is found to be damaged, dislodged, or damp, the supplies within are contaminated. The tops of rigid container systems are removed for access to internal sterile supplies by the scrub person.

As the sterile field is being established, the following principles should be applied.

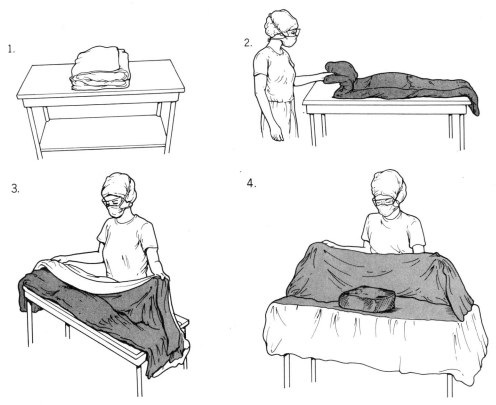

FIGURE 3-8. Establishing a Sterile Field (From Fairchild, S. *Perioperative Nursing.* © 1993. Boston: Jones and Bartlett Publishers. Reprinted by permission)

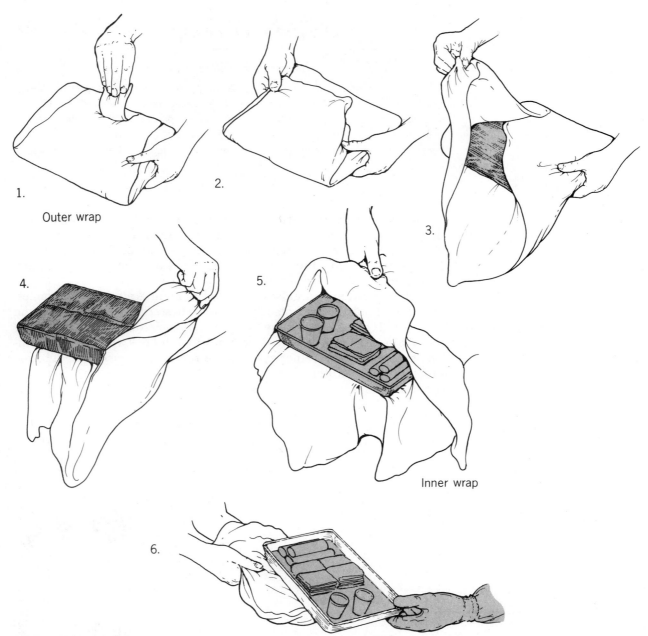

1.

Outer wrap

2.

3.

4.

5.

Inner wrap

6.

FIGURE 3–9. Opening Sterile Wrapped Supplies (From Fairchild, S. *Perioperative Nursing.* © 1993. Boston: Jones and Bartlett Publishers. Reprinted by permission)

1. *Movement and air currents around a sterile area are kept to a minimum to avoid contamination.* Talking is kept to a minimum.
2. *All items used within the sterile field must be sterile.* Only scrubbed personnel in sterile gown and gloves are allowed within the sterile field. The circulating nurse does not directly contact the sterile field. If an item is of unknown sterility, it is considered contaminated.
3. *All sterile supplies are inspected prior to being opened.* All items presented to the sterile field should be checked for proper packaging, processing, expiration date, contamination of evidence, seal integrity, package integrity, and external sterilization chemical indicator appearance.

4. *Items introduced onto the sterile field should be opened, dispensed, and transferred by methods that maintain sterility and integrity.*
5. *Tables are sterile only at and above the table level.* Any edges of drapes that overhang the table are not considered sterile.
6. *Wrappers are considered sterile to within 1 inch of edges.*
7. *Do not turn your back toward a sterile area.* Sterile and unsterile persons face the sterile area to maintain visibility.
8. *Do not reach over sterile areas.* Unscrubbed personnel should never lean or reach across a sterile field. Unscrubbed arms should not cross over the sterile field while transferring a sterile item. This practice decreases the potential of contamination from skin shedding.

Containers that will receive solutions are placed at the near edge of the sterile field or are held by the scrub person. Unsterile personnel, without reaching over sterile supplies, pour solutions in such a way that splashing or dripping is avoided (Fig. 3–10). The entire contents are poured at one time whenever possible. With multiple-use solution containers, pour a small amount of fluid over the lip of the solution container to remove any debris that may be near the opening before pouring contents into the sterile field.

Sterile items should be placed securely on the sterile field or should be presented to the scrubbed person. Additional supplies are provided to sterile team members by the circulating nurse after the initial sterile area has been established and scrubbed personnel are within the sterile field. Sharp, heavy, and difficult to handle or difficult to open articles should be opened on a separate surface or presented directly to a scrubbed person.

SURGICAL HAND SCRUB

It is impossible to sterilize personnel, but the skin of those who enter the sterile field should be rendered as clean as possible. Although surgical team members wear sterile gloves, the skin of their hands and forearms should be prepared to reduce the number of microorganisms in the event of glove tears. This is done with a surgical hand scrub. Any personal protective equipment, such as masks or

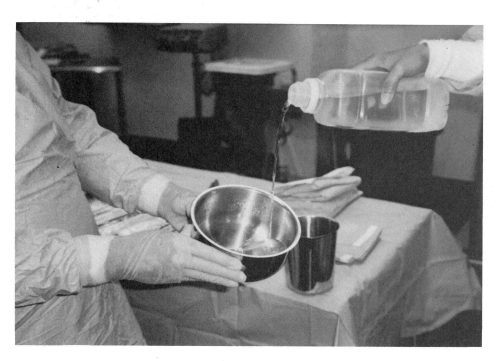

FIGURE 3–10. Pouring Sterile Solutions

goggles, required for the procedure should be donned prior to the scrub procedure. All jewelry should be removed from hands. Jewelry may be pinned to scrub suits or placed in lockers to assure that valuables are not lost. Cuticles, hands, and forearms should be free of open lesions and breaks in skin integrity. Individuals with weeping dermatitis or exudative lesions should not scrub, be involved in direct patient care, or handle medical devices in invasive procedures. Fingernails should be short and free of chipped polish, artificial nails, or bondings (Baumgardner, 1993).

There are a variety of antimicrobial solutions that are appropriate for surgical hand scrubbing (Table 3–1). The solution chosen should be approved by the Food and Drug Administration (FDA) and should inhibit the growth of bacteria and viruses on intact skin. Other qualities of a hand-scrub agent are that it should be nonirritating and fast-acting, have a residual effect, and should be an effective detergent. Chlorhexidine gluconate, iodophor, triclosan, and hexachlorophene solutions are among the most commonly found products (Leclair, 1990). If skin sensitivity is a problem, a liquid nonmedicated soap may be used followed by an application of alcohol-based hand cleanser. Personal preference and availability usually dictate the solution. Prefilled brushes may be impregnated with antimicrobial solutions, or the solutions may be dispensed at the scrub sink area and added to reusable or disposable brushes.

There are a variety of methods for the actual scrub. Each institution should have a written policy that specifies the facility's procedure. Several principles apply no matter what method is selected. The scrub begins with selection of water temperature, prewash, and nail-cleaning (Fig. 3–11). The hands are prewashed with the selected antimicrobial solution to remove gross dirt and skin oils. This preliminary prewash should include hands and forearms and should extend 2 inches above the elbows. Friction should be applied while washing. After the prewash of hands and arms, the undersides of individual fingernails are cleaned, and debris is removed from the nail cleaner using running water. Cuticles are lightly pushed back and any debris is removed from the cuticle area of each finger.

After this is completed, the fingers and hands are scrubbed (Fig. 3–12), followed by the arms up to 2 inches above the elbow. A standardized timed ana-

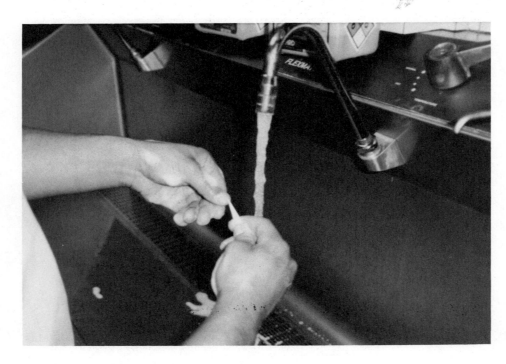

FIGURE 3–11. Nail Cleaning Process

TABLE 3-1. CHARACTERISTICS OF SIX TOPICAL ANTIMICROBIAL AGENTS

AGENT	MODE OF ACTION	RAPIDITY OF ACTION	RESIDUAL ACTIVITY	USUAL CONCEN- TRATION (%)	AFFECTED BY ORGANIC MATTER	SAFETY/ TOXICITY	ACTIVITY AGAINST					
							Gram-Positive Bacteria	Gram-Negative Bacteria	Mycobacterium Tuberculosis	Fungi	Viruses	
Alcohols	Denaturation of protein	Most rapid	None	70–92	No data	Drying, volatile	Excellent	Excellent	Good	Good	Good	
Chlorhexidine gluconate	Cell wall disruption	Intermediate	Excellent	4.2 in detergent base; 0.5 in alcohol	Minimal	Ototoxicity, keratitis	Excellent	Good	Poor	Fair	Good	
Hexachlorophene	Cell wall disruption	Slow to intermediate	Excellent	3 by prescription only	Minimal	Neurotox- icity	Excellent	Poor	Poor	Poor	Poor	
Iodine and iodophors	Oxidation/ substitution by free iodine	Intermediate	Minimal	10, 7.5, 2, 0.5	Yes	Absorption from skin with possible toxicity, skin irritation	Excellent	Good	Good	Good	Good	
Chloroxylenol	Cell wall disruption	Intermediate	Good	0.5–3.75	Minimal	More data needed	Good	Fair	Fair	Fair	Fair	
Triclosan	Cell wall disruption	Intermediate	Excellent	0.3–1	Minimal	More data needed	Good	Good except for Pseu- domonas	Fair	Poor	Unknown	

Adapted from Larson, E. (1988). APIC Guidelines for infection control practice, guideline for use of topical antimicrobial agents. *American Journal of Infection Control, 16*, 253–266.

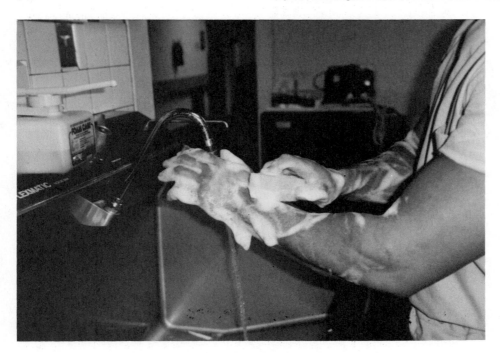

FIGURE 3-12. Surgical Hand Scrub

tomic scrub or a counted-stroke method should be followed for all surgical hand scrubs. The timed scrub method begins by scrubbing nails and hands a half minute for each hand, rinsing, then reapplying antimicrobial solutions. The hands are then rescrubbed, and the arms are scrubbed for 3 minutes. In the anatomic scrub method, the procedure recommends scrubbing the nails of each hand with 30 strokes, each finger with 20 strokes to each side of the finger, the back of the hand with 20 strokes, the palm surface of the hand with 20 strokes, and each third of the arm with 20 strokes.

During the entire procedure and during rinsing, the hands should always remain higher than the elbows so that contamination will be rinsed away from the hand area (Fig. 3-13). If the hand or arm comes in contact with faucet head, sink, scrub attire or other surface, the process should start again. The length of time for a surgical scrub is between 5 and 10 minutes. A vigorous 5-minute scrub with a reliable agent may be as effective as a 10-minute scrub done with less mechanical action (Atkinson, 1992). Subsequent scrubs during the day require the application of the same process for the same amount of time.

Upon completion of the surgical scrub, the nail cleaner, brush, or sponge should be discarded in the proper receptacle without lowering the arms or hands. Disposable items may be placed in the trash. Reusable brushes and nail cleaners require decontamination and sterilization before reuse. The hands and arms are rinsed making sure that the hands stay higher than the elbows, allowing water to drip off the elbow, not the fingertips. The excess water is allowed to drip over the scrub sink area, and the scrubbed person enters the operating room to begin application of gown and gloves.

GOWNING AND GLOVING

Sterile team members maintain contact with the sterile field by means of sterile gowns and gloves. The function of surgical gowning and gloving is to establish a barrier between sterile and nonsterile areas. This barrier should prevent the passage of microorganisms and should be nonabrasive, fire-retardant, and fluid-repellent. Gowns are available in different sizes and may be reusable or dispos-

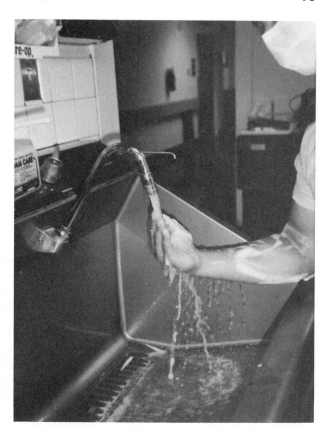

FIGURE 3–13. Surgical Hand Scrub Rinse Procedure

able. Gowns may be classified as fluid-resistant or fluidproof. The surgical gown should prevent fluids from contacting the skin and scrub clothing of the surgical team. Fluid-resistant gowns should be worn whenever the presence of blood or other body fluids is anticipated and whenever potential exists for clothing to become soaked with blood or other infectious materials. Although gowns are classified as fluid-resistant, the type of procedure, the length of procedure, and the type of fluid exposure may cause the gown to become soaked. In procedures where fluidproof gowns are needed, such as vascular surgery, the manufacturer provides reinforced gowns with protective films or membranes for additional protection. These gowns are costly and are not needed for all cases but should be available for selective procedures.

Gloves should be of appropriate size and may be hypoallergenic if skin sensitivity is a problem (Smith, 1993). Studies have shown that latex and vinyl gloves worn during delivery of patient care acquire microscopic holes. Gloves are protective but should not be thought of as a total barrier for personnel from all contamination (Jackson, 1992). Double gloving is frequently used to decrease the potential for infection (O'Neale, 1993) and may be recommended at specific facilities. In this situation, a second set of gloves, one-half size larger, is placed over the first set of gloves. Double gloving does not prevent puncture wounds but may reduce exposure to blood and other body fluids.

Gowning and gloving should take place in a sterile field other than the main instrument table. This practice avoids contamination from water dripping from forearms or hands. Grasp and open the towel completely, bending forward slightly so that the towel does not come into contact with the surgical scrub suit. Use one end of the towel to dry each finger and hand; use a rotating movement to dry up the arm toward the elbow. After one arm is dried, reverse the end of the towel and use the dry end for the other arm. After hands and arms have been thoroughly dried, the folded gown is lifted from the sterile packaging.

The gown is grasped at the neckline and allowed to unfold. The inside of the gown will come into contact with bare skin, but the outside surface of the gown should not be touched while unfolding. Hands are slipped into both armholes of the gown simultaneously, and the circulating nurse may assist in pulling the gown onto the scrubbed person. The arms are not extended through the cuff of the gown for purposes of closed gloving (Fig. 3–14). In closed gloving, the right glove is placed over the cuff area of the right sleeve. The thumb side of the glove will touch the sleeve of the gown and be held in place by the encased hand within the sleeve. The fingers of the glove will be pointing toward the elbow. The cuff of the glove is then pulled over the stockinette cuff of the gown, and the hand is gently inserted into the glove. The glove should completely cover the cuff of the gown. The skin of the scrub person should not come into contact with the exterior surface of the glove during this procedure. The second glove is applied in the same manner. Gloves are inspected for integrity, and glove powder is removed with a moistened towel or in a designated glove-rinsing basin (Fay, 1992). The circulating nurse ties or snaps the back of the gown at the neckline and waist. If a sterile back is on the gown, the nurse assists the scrubbed person in turning around.

The scrub person gowns and gloves self, then gowns and gloves the surgeon and assistants (Fig. 3–15). When gowning and gloving others, begin by providing an opened towel for drying the hands without actually touching the hand. Hold the neckline area and unfold the gown allowing it to open completely. Place a protective cuff of the gown over the gloves and hold the gown at the top of the sleeve area. Offer the inside of the gown to the person to be gowned. As the individual's arms are placed inside of the sleeves, release the gown and allow the individual to work their arms into the sleeves, extending their hands through the cuffs. Pick up the right glove and grasp it at the edges. Stretch the cuff open wide and point the thumb of the glove toward the midline of the individual putting the glove on. Firmly hold the glove as the individual places their hand into the glove. Repeat the process for the opposite hand and assist in turning those individuals with sterile-backed gowns.

Although the entire gown has been subject to sterilization, the surgical gown is considered sterile only in the front, even if the gown has a wraparound sterile-backed feature. Since the back of the gown cannot be continuously monitored for sterility, it is considered contaminated. Areas considered sterile are from the gloved hand up the sleeve to 2 inches above the elbow. The front of the gown is sterile from the level of the chest to the sterile table. Necklines, shoulders, under the arms, back and cuffed portions of the sleeves are moisture-collection and friction areas, which should be considered unsterile. Once gowned and gloved, the sterile team members may not lower their forearms below waist level. Scrubbed persons keep gloved hands in sight at all times. Scrubbed persons should keep arms and hands within the sterile area at all times. Hands are never folded under the armpits, because perspiration in the axillary region may cause contamination (Atkinson, 1992).

Scrubbed persons are aware of the height of the sterile field. Changing levels at the sterile field is avoided. The gown is considered sterile at the highest level of the table. If a scrubbed person must stand on a platform during the surgical procedure, the platform should be positioned at the beginning of the procedure. Scrubbed persons should sit for a surgical procedure only when the entire procedure is performed at this level, otherwise contamination from changing the levels of the gown and the sterile field may occur.

If gloves become contaminated during the procedure, the preferred method of changing gloves is for one member of the sterile team to glove the other. If this is not possible, the contaminated glove should be changed by an open-glove

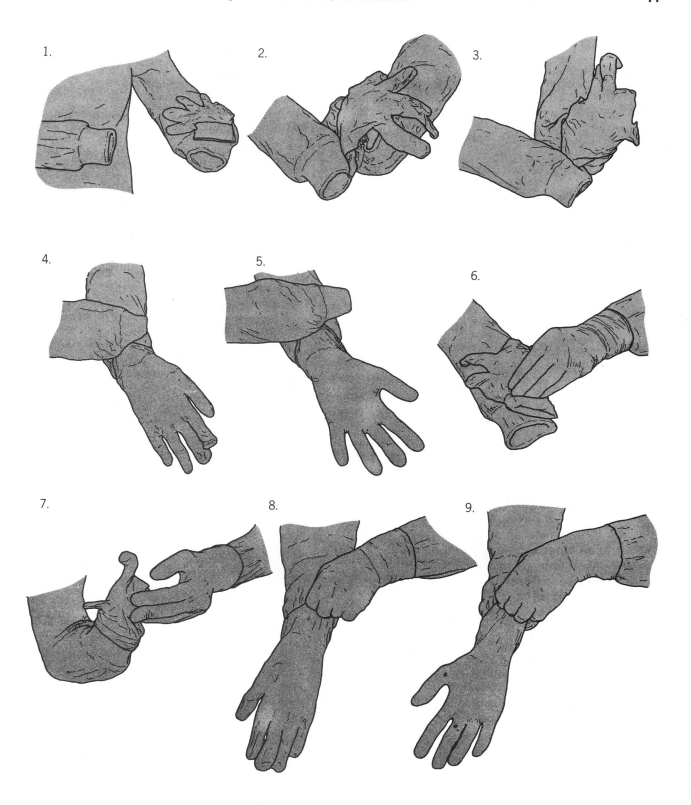

FIGURE 3–14. Closed Gloving Technique (From Fairchild, S. *Perioperative Nursing.* © 1993. Boston: Jones and Bartlett Publishers. Reprinted by permission)

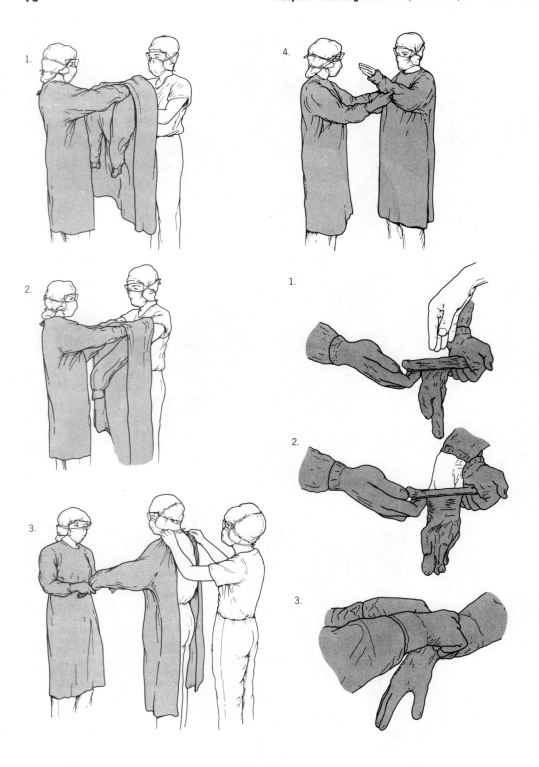

FIGURE 3–15. Gowning and Gloving Others (From Fairchild, S. *Perioperative Nursing.* © 1993. Boston: Jones and Bartlett Publishers. Reprinted by permission)

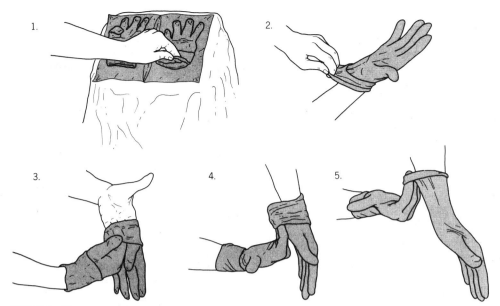

FIGURE 3-16. Open Gloving Technique (From Fairchild, S. *Perioperative Nursing.* © 1993. Boston: Jones and Bartlett Publishers. Reprinted by permission)

method (Fig. 3-16). The open-glove method is the same method taught for catheterization or other sterile procedures. In the surgical environment, the open-glove method adds a new dimension. The glove must be applied so that the sterile gown is not contaminated and the exterior of the glove and gown both remain sterile. If one glove becomes contaminated, the circulating nurse, wearing unsterile gloves, removes the contaminated glove from the scrubbed person. New sterile gloves are placed in the field for the scrubbed person. The scrub person uses the remaining sterile gloved hand to pick up the replacement glove, gliding the gloved hand under the cuff of the new glove. The ungloved hand is placed inside the new glove taking care that the bare hand does not touch the outside of the new glove during application. The cuff of the glove is pulled over the gown cuff for complete coverage.

At the end of the procedure, the gown is untied by unsterile personnel, pulled downward from the shoulders turning the sleeves inside out as it is pulled off the arms. The gown is folded inward upon itself to help confine contamination and then placed in the laundry if reusable or in the trash if disposable. Visibly contaminated gowns should be discarded in hazardous-waste receptacles. After the gown is disposed of, gloves are removed. Gloves are removed by pulling the gloves off inside out to confine gross contamination. Hands are washed after gloves are removed.

DRAPING

Sterile drapes are used to establish sterile fields. The drapes create barriers to transmission of microbes to and from nonsterile and sterile areas. Materials utilized for drapes are fluid-resistant, fire-resistant, lint-free, tear-resistant, nonglare, and nontoxic, and they should contour easily around patients and equipment.

Drapes may be reusable or disposable. Reusable drapes, such as woven cloth, will require processing, which may compromise the protective barrier after many uses. Reusable drapes are therefore monitored for the number of uses, are heat-seal patched to maintain integrity, and are laundered before each sterilization. This laundering rehydrates the strands of fabric and reduces the breakdown of fabric by heat sterilization. Disposable nonwoven drapes, often referred to as plastic or paper drapes, are single-use drapes. Both types of drapes, reusable and disposable, should prevent strikethrough. Strikethrough is soaking of moisture through layers, which renders an article unsterile.

There are numerous varieties of drapes available for surgical procedures. Some drapes, such as towels, half sheets, and full sheets have no precut opening or fenestration. Other drapes, such as laparotomy sheets, transverse laparotomy sheets, thyroid sheets, lithotomy drapes with leggings, extremity sheets, and split sheets, have an opening that corresponds with the incision to be made. Some draping packs, such as cardiovascular packs, orthopedic packs, head and neck packs, craniotomy packs, and laparoscopic packs, among others, come prepackaged and will contain several types of drapes in one package, which can be used for a particular type of procedure. These packages list drapes contained within and may be cost-effective when several types of drapes are needed for routine procedures.

A variety of other draping materials are available to create sterile fields. Stockinette may be used over extremities. Plastic cover drapes, especially designed for equipment such as laser, microscopes, or x-ray machines, are frequently used to create and maintain sterile fields. Plastic incise drapes, which cover the incision area, may be used prior to draping or after drapes are in place to prevent strikethrough of fluids and bacteria. Barrier drapes, which isolate around and not over the incision area, may be used, such as a U-drape or buttocks drape.

After the appropriate drapes have been selected for the case, they are arranged in order as needed on the back table. Basic principles to remember when applying drapes include the following:

1. *Do not fan drapes because this will increase air turbulence and potential for contamination.*
2. *Handle drapes as little as possible.* Hold material above waist level whenever handling. Stand back a safe distance from nonsterile items when draping to avoid contact with sterile gown.
3. *Establish an initial barrier with smaller drapes.* Small drape towels are placed around the proposed incision site. The larger drapes are then placed over these initial drapes as needed.
4. *Drape from operative site to periphery.* A sterile person first covers the near side of any unsterile surface with sterile drapes and will then cover the far side. The drapes then are applied from operative site to periphery. This helps to protect the sterility of gowned personnel.
5. *Gloved hands are protected by drapes during application of drapes.* A cuff of draping material covers the hand during placement of the drape.
6. *Do not remove drapes once they are in place.* Once placed in position, sterile drapes are never moved or shifted since this would compromise the sterility of the field.

Any part of the drape that drops below the table surface is considered unsterile. Only the top of a draped table is considered sterile; edges and sides of the drape extending below the table level are considered unsterile. Any object that falls below the level of the table is considered unsterile. All cables, cords, and tubings are secured to the sterile field using nonperforating devices so that the sterile barrier will not be compromised. Two common draping procedures for abdominal and lithotomy procedures are illustrated in Figures 3–17 and 3–18.

MAINTAINING A STERILE FIELD

Every team member continuously observes for events that may contaminate the sterile field and initiates corrective action when breaks in technique are noted.

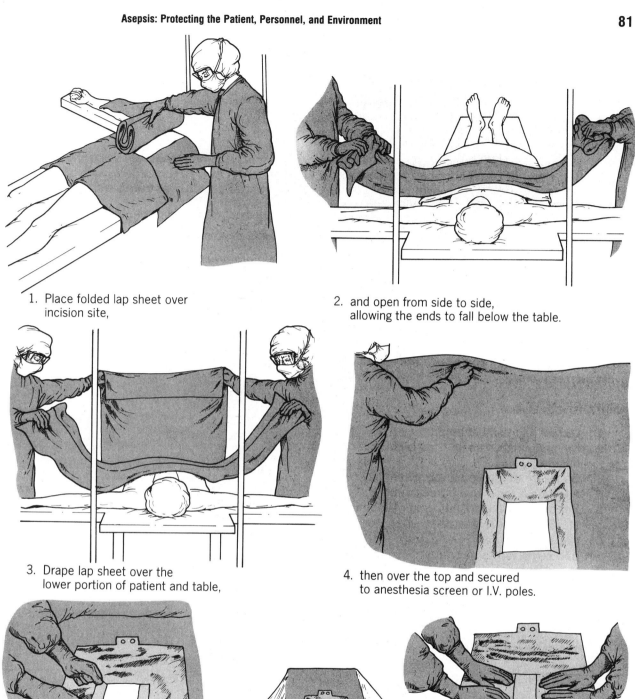

1. Place folded lap sheet over incision site,

2. and open from side to side, allowing the ends to fall below the table.

3. Drape lap sheet over the lower portion of patient and table,

4. then over the top and secured to anesthesia screen or I.V. poles.

5. Surgeon removes release paper from adhesive strips on both sides of fenestration,

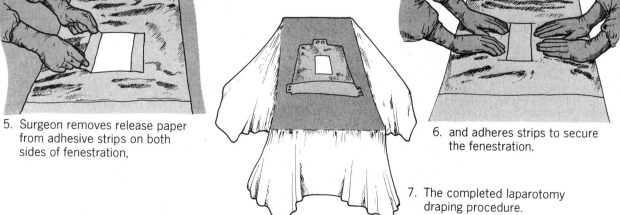

6. and adheres strips to secure the fenestration.

7. The completed laparotomy draping procedure.

FIGURE 3–17. Draping for Abdominal Surgery (laparotomy drape) (From Fairchild, S. *Perioperative Nursing.* © 1993. Boston: Jones and Bartlett Publishers. Reprinted by permission)

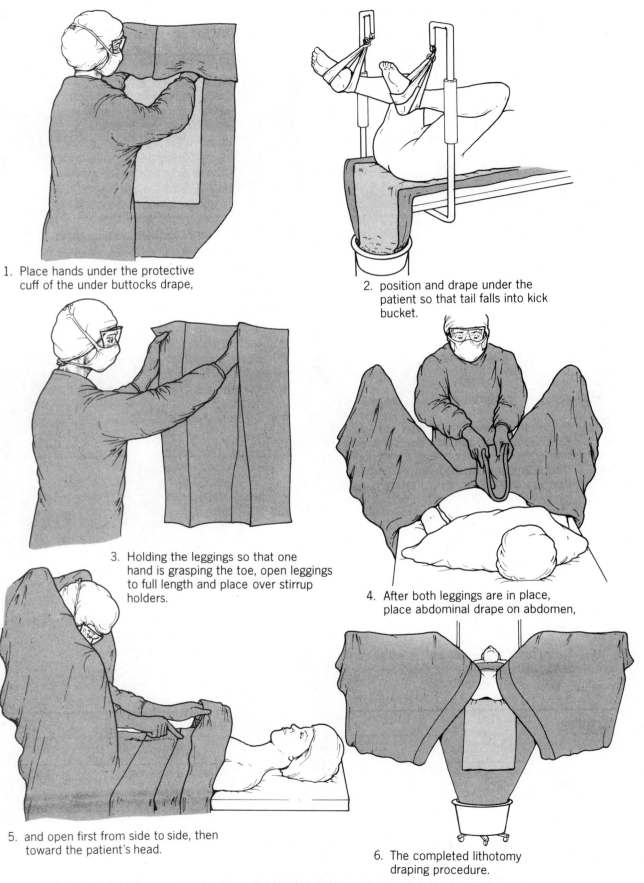

1. Place hands under the protective cuff of the under buttocks drape,

2. position and drape under the patient so that tail falls into kick bucket.

3. Holding the leggings so that one hand is grasping the toe, open leggings to full length and place over stirrup holders.

4. After both leggings are in place, place abdominal drape on abdomen,

5. and open first from side to side, then toward the patient's head.

6. The completed lithotomy draping procedure.

FIGURE 3-18. Draping for Lithotomy Position (From Fairchild, S. *Perioperative Nursing.* © 1993. Boston: Jones and Bartlett Publishers. Reprinted by permission)

Some measures will be ongoing throughout the procedures. Efforts that decrease air turbulence will help to maintain the sterile field. These include, but are not limited to, keeping doors closed except during transport of patients and equipment, not fanning sheets or drapes, keeping conversation to a minimum, and limiting the number of personnel who are allowed into the room.

Movement within and around a sterile field is kept to a minimum to avoid contamination of sterile items and personnel. All personnel moving within or around a sterile field should do so in a way that maintains the integrity of the sterile field. Unsterile personnel restrict their activity near sterile fields by maintaining a distance of at least 12 inches from the sterile field. Also they may not move between two sterile fields. Nonsterile equipment brought into and/or over the sterile field should be draped with a sterile material or covering. Examples may include microscopes, endoscopic equipment, x-ray equipment, or fluoroscopy equipment.

Sterile personnel always face the sterile field. They do not turn their backs to the sterile field, even though they have donned a sterile-backed gown at the beginning of the procedure. Since it is not possible to monitor contamination of the back of the gown at all times, the back of the gown is considered to be contaminated, and movement within the sterile field is done with this thought in mind. To avoid potential contamination, sterile-attired persons should move either back to back (contaminated to contaminated) or front to front (sterile to sterile) (Crow, 1990). If a scrubbed person needs to pass an unsterile object or person, a margin of 12 inches should be maintained and the scrubbed person should maintain the right of way. Sterile personnel do not walk around or go outside of the room. They remain at the sterile field.

A no-touch or hands-free technique may be chosen to pass instruments during the surgical procedure. This can help to prevent needle sticks during surgery (Fox, 1993). Loaded needle holders, knife blades, and other sharp instruments are placed in a neutral zone (on a Mayo tray or in an emesis basin) for the surgeon/scrub person to pick up rather than placed directly into the hand (Fig. 3–19). Needles are loaded on the holder and placed point down when storing them on the Mayo stand to avoid snagging gloves and hands. After needles are used they are placed directly into a needle counter device (Hubbard, 1992).

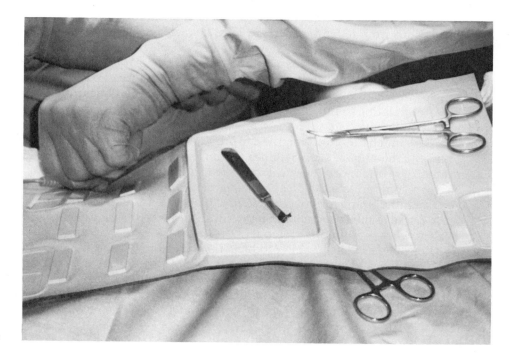

FIGURE 3–19. No-Touch Technique

Other preventive measures include applying or removing a disposable knife blade on a scalpel handle or placing a needle on a syringe with an instrument. Any sharp is always handled by personnel employing instruments, not the bare hand, and is isolated in a protective area, such as a needle counter or sharps pad, as soon after use as possible. Injection needles are not recapped except with re-capping safety devices (McPherson, 1992).

Gowns and gloves should be periodically inspected during the procedure for strikethrough, tears, and puncture sites, and should be replaced as needed. If a glove is torn or punctured, remove the contaminated needle, blade, or instrument from the sterile field immediately and change the glove. If skin is torn or punctured, apply pressure to encourage bleeding to clean the wound, and wash the area immediately with an antimicrobial solution. Repeat the incident immediately and follow the facility's procedure for biohazardous exposures.

Aseptic technique is a continuous process in the surgical environment, one that requires continuous monitoring, evaluating, and observing. The application of this technique in our daily practice provides better patient care by establishing and maintaining the sterile field and by preventing the spread of infection. Aseptic practices also ensure the safety and well-being of health care personnel. Consistent application of aseptic technique is an essential component of perioperative nursing practice.

Issues for Development

Standards for classifying gowns and surgical drapes that are labeled fluid-resistant and fluidproof should be established by regulating agencies. Current drape and gown material, although labeled fluid-resistant, may not be totally resistant to strikethrough. The ability to prevent strikethrough from bloodborne pathogens should be established for personal protective attire (Mathias, 1993).

Hazardous-waste disposal should be further defined with emphasis upon what measures provide maximum infection control for minimum cost. Some OR wastes have been found to be less contaminated than usual landfill contents (McVeigh, 1993). The costliness of disposal of hazardous waste and conflicting regulations from federal, state, and local agencies have led to some confusion. Some operating rooms place all disposable materials that have come into contact with the patient in hazardous-waste containers; others treat in this way only materials that are visibly contaminated; and others dispose of only grossly bloody articles in hazardous-waste containers. As definitions of hazardous waste and research relating to infection from hazardous waste are further delineated, the issue will be clarified.

How much draping is required to provide a safe, economic area of sterility? If an eye is the area of surgery, does the entire patient need to be covered with drapes? Use of standard surgical drape routines for procedures that are classified as clean-contaminated, such as oral, vaginal, or anal procedures may or may not require full draping for infection control (Patterson, 1991). Overdraping is common. As the issue is evaluated more critically, guidelines should provide direction for what is optimum draping.

Reusable and disposable products raise questions about which is the most cost-effective and ecologically sound for daily practice. Are reusable drapes more cost-effective than disposable drapes, which require hazardous-waste disposal through incineration or landfill? Further definition is needed as to which disposables may be reused safely and what type of processing is required (O'Neale, 1992).

REFERENCES

Anonymous. (1993). Tests evaluate barrier effectiveness of gowns. *OR Manager, 9*(5), 1, 7.

Association of Operating Room Nurses. (1993a). Regulated medical waste definition and treatment: a collaborative document. *AORN Journal, 58*(1), 110–114.

Association of Operating Room Nurses. (1993b). *Standards and Recommended Practices.* Denver: AORN.

Atkinson, L. (1992). *Berry and Kohn's Operating Room Technique.* 7th ed. St. Louis: C. V. Mosby.

Bartley, J. (1993). Operating room air quality. *Today's OR Nurse, 15*(5), 11–18.

Baumgardner, C., Maragos, C., Walz, M., Larson, E. (1993). Effects of nail polish on microbial growth of fingernails. *AORN Journal, 58*(1), 84–88.

Belkin, N. (1992). Personal protective equipment in aseptic technique and universal precautions. *Today's OR Nurse, 14*(6), 15–20.

Bruning, L. (1993). The bloodborne pathogens final rule: understanding the regulation. *AORN Journal, 57*(2), 439–464.

Crow, S. (1990). It's second nature to me now. *Today's OR Nurse, 12*(10), 6–8.

Fay, M., Dooher, D. (1992). Surgical gloves: measuring cost and barrier effectiveness. *AORN Journal, 55*(6), 1500–1519.

Fox, V. (1992). Clinical issues: passing surgical instruments, sharps without injury. *AORN Journal, 55*(1), 264–266.

Fox, V. (1993). Clinical issues: preventing glove tears, sharp injuries. *AORN Journal, 57*(3), 703–706.

Garber, N. (1993). OSHA regulations for the OR nurse. *Today's OR Nurse, 15*(1), 27–30.

Giordano, B. (1993). Let's put our fear of HIV in proper perspective. *AORN Journal, 57*(4), 822–824.

Gruendemann, B. (1990). Surgical asepsis revisited. *Today's OR Nurse, 12*(10), 10–14.

Hubbard, S., Wadsworth, K., Telford, G., Quebbeman, E. (1992). Reducing blood contamination and injury in the OR. *AORN Journal, 55*(1), 194–201.

Jackson, M., McPherson, D. (1992). Blood exposure and puncture risks for OR personnel. *Today's OR Nurse, 14*(7), 5–10.

Johnson and Johnson Medical Inc. (1992a). *Programmed Instruction in Asepsis I: Basic Microbiology.* Arlington, Texas.

Johnson and Johnson Medical Inc. (1992b). *Programmed Instruction in Asepsis II: Microbiology and Health Care.* Arlington, Texas.

Larson, E. (1988). APIC guidelines for infection control practice: guidelines for use of topical antimicrobial agents. *American Journal of Infection Control, 16*, 253–266.

Laufman, H. (1990). Environmental concerns in surgery in the 1990's. *Today's OR Nurse, 12*(10), 41–48.

Leclair, J. (1990). A review of antiseptics. *Today's OR Nurse, 12*(10), 25–28.

Lisanti, P., Talotta, D. (1992). Hepatitis update: the delta virus. *AORN Journal, 55*(3), 790–800.

Mathias, J. (1993). Experts discuss merits of surgical masks. *OR Manager, 9*(11), 1–10.

McPherson, D., Parris, N. (1992). Reducing occupational exposure to blood in the OR. *Today's OR Nurse, 14*(10), 23–27.

McVeigh, P. (1993). Medical waste reduction, reuse and recycling. *Today's OR Nurse, 15*(1), 13–18.

O'Neale, M. (1992). Clinical issues: environmental issues concerning sterile reprocessing, disposal practices, recycling. *AORN Journal, 55*(2), 606–608.

O'Neale, M. (1993). Clinical issues: double gloving. *AORN Journal, 57*(5), 1159.

Patterson, P. (1991). *Sacred Cows in the OR. OR Manager.* Boulder, Colorado.

Radke, S., Ford, D. (1993). Aseptic technique monitoring. *AORN Journal, 58*(2), 312–323.

Ritter, M., Marmion, P. (1988). The exogenous sources and controls of microorganisms in the operating room. *Orthopaedic Nursing, 7*(4), 23–28.

Rothrock, J., Meeker, M. (1991). *Alexander's Care of the Patient in Surgery.* 9th ed. St. Louis: C. V. Mosby.

Rutala, W. (1990). Disinfection in the OR. *Today's OR Nurse, 12*(10), 30–37.

Smith, C. (1992). Clinical issues: open sterile fields; implant logs; needle counts; photography and aseptic technique. *AORN Journal, 55*(5), 1254–1257.

Smith, C. (1993). Clinical issues: latex allergies. *AORN Journal, 57*(6), 1445–1447.

Tait, A. (1993). Perioperative control of infection. *Current Reviews for Post Anesthesia Care Nurses, 15*(1), 1–7.

U.S. Dept. of Health, Education and Welfare. (1978). *Minimum requirements of construction and equipment for hospitals and medical facilities.* DHEW publication (HRA) 79-14500. Washington, D.C.

Wenzel, R. (1993). *Prevention and Control of Nosocomial Infections.* 2nd ed. Baltimore: Williams and Wilkins.

Wicher, C. (1993). AIDS and HIV: the dilemma of the health care worker. *Today's OR Nurse, 15*(2), 14–22.

Young, E. (1990). A disinfectant guide. *Urologic Nursing, 10*(3), 7–9.

Practice Scenario 1
Asepsis: Protecting the Patient, Personnel and Environment

by Nancy Girard, PhD, RN, CS

SCENARIO

Jeanette Lewton is an 82-year-old female who is scheduled for a total hip replacement to improve her quality of life by increasing mobility and decreasing pain. Mrs. Lewton is 5 feet 2 inches tall, weighs 98 pounds, and has osteoarthritis. She is also an insulin-dependent diabetic with accompanying vascular complications. However, her health has been relatively good and at present she is in control of her disease processes. She is alert and cognitively intact. She performs blood glucose monitoring and administers her own insulin. Mrs. Lewton states she has had her flu and pneumonia shots because she has a tendency to catch upper respiratory infections rather easily.

PERIOPERATIVE INTERPRETATION

Using what you have just learned in this chapter, as an experienced perioperative nurse, you would consider the following in the care of this patient.

1. Assessment:
   Based upon the nursing preoperative assessment, you recognize that:
   • The patient's weight indicates possible malnutrition, which would decrease her healing ability and predispose her for positioning injuries.
   • The history of insulin-dependent diabetes places the patient at risk for postoperative wound infection owing to impaired cell-mediated and humoral immunity.
   • The patient's age can compromise her healing ability owing to decreased macrophages and neutrophils for fighting an exogenous infection.
   • Age-related bladder and urethra changes such as stenosis, fragile mucosal tissue, and degenerative bladder wall changes decrease the patient's ability to resist opportunistic bacterial infections if an indwelling catheter is inserted.
   • The blood glucose levels have been stable and must remain so during the perioperative period

in order to maintain energy at the cellular level to fight infection and promote healing.
   • Mrs. Lewton's impaired microcirculation and decreased peripheral vascular sensation secondary to her peripheral vascular condition must be considered when positioning.

NURSING DIAGNOSES

   • High risk for postoperative wound infection related to age, diabetes, and nutritional status.
   • High risk for respiratory infection related to fragile respiratory system, risk of aspiration secondary to age-diminished gag reflex, and anesthesia drugs.
   • High risk for urinary tract infection due to catheterization, related to age-related urinary tract changes.
   • High risk for skin breakdown related to compromised microcirculation, weight, and age.

2. Planning:
   • Use the concept of surgical conscience to dictate scrupulous adherence in establishing and maintaining a safe surgical environment.
   • Discuss with the surgeon the plans to use antimicrobial incise drapes to decrease microbial migration toward the wound.
   • Determine methods to minimize traffic and personnel in the room.
   • Plan to monitor for any breaks in aseptic technique and rectify them immediately.
   • Consult with the anesthesiologist about the method and frequency of monitoring the patient's blood glucose levels throughout surgery.
   • Procure the required supplies for positioning to allow the circulating nurse to remain with the patient during induction.

3. Implementation:
   • Wash hands with an antimicrobial solution prior

to touching the patient for any invasive procedure, such as urinary catheterization.

- Position patient and pad all bony prominences.
- Assess peripheral circulation by taking radial, popliteal, posterior tibial, and dorsalis pedis pulses. Assess capillary refill, color, and skin temperature.
- Place a sign outside the operative suite door limiting personnel access to the room during the procedure. Keep movement and conversation in the room to a minimum.
- Procure blood glucose monitoring equipment and test strips and have insulin available. Test blood intraoperatively for blood glucose levels.
- Document in the intraoperative record any breaks in sterile technique and the corrective action taken, the type of prep solution, the use of incise drape if any, the limitation of traffic through and in the room, skin integrity, positioning aids, and blood glucose testing and results.

4. Evaluation:
- Convey to the post-anesthesia care unit nurse the patient's diabetic condition and blood glucose levels, age, presence of osteoarthritis, decreased immune status, and preoperative cognitive level.
- Inspect extremities and bony prominences for any untoward effects of or reactions to positioning.
- Assess vascular circulation, by taking peripheral pulses, capillary filling, color, and skin temperature.

Practice Scenario 2
Asepsis: Protecting the Patient, Personnel, and Environment

by Cyndi Abbott, RN, PhD, CNOR

SCENARIO

Peggy Allen is a 63-year-old retired elementary school teacher with a history of lymphoma. The patient has been in remission for 7 years, but a recent physical examination revealed two lumps in the left armpit. The patient is scheduled for a biopsy of the lumps in the same day surgery unit. Dr. Furgate has asked that the pathologist scrub in to view the mass in anatomic site. The patient is 6 feet 1 inch and weighs 175 pounds. Her husband accompanies her to all office visits and plans to drive her home after the surgery. Mrs. Allen states he offers her comfort when she feels down. Blood and urine values are normal. Mrs. Allen has full range of motion in all extremities.

PERIOPERATIVE INTERPRETATION

Using what you have just learned in this chapter, as an experienced perioperative nurse you would consider the following in the care of this patient.

1. Assessment:
   - Given your preoperative assessment and knowledge of the surgical procedure, you know that two doctors and a scrub person will be scrubbed on the procedure. The scrub person is a fairly new surgical technician who has just finished orientation.
   - Knowing the location of the procedure and the surgeon's preference, the sterile team will be sitting down during the biopsy. Potential breaks in sterile technique could occur if the surgical team changes positions between standing and sitting.
   - The pathologist's familiarity with gowning and gloving must be considered because he does not scrub often and may be unfamiliar with the principles of aseptic technique.
   - The patient's height poses a problem with positioning on the surgical bed.
   - The patient's spouse appears to provide adequate emotional support for the patient. The patient appears to be relaxed and not experiencing any undue anxiety.

NURSING DIAGNOSES

High risk for injury related to hyperextension of the left arm
High risk for infection related to breaks in aseptic technique

2. Planning:
   - Provide additional staff member to assist the pathologist with surgical scrubbing and donning of sterile gown and gloves.
   - Procure extra gowns and gloves, draping materials, and extra personnel to allow the left arm to be prepped and drape-free for manipulation during the surgical procedure.
   - Procure a hand table and sitting stools and review with the sterile surgical team the need to avoid changing position during the surgical procedure.
   - Obtain a footboard to provide an extension to the surgical bed to facilitate the patient's positioning on the surgical bed.
3. Implementation:
   - Prior to placement of the patient on the surgical bed, place the footboard at the end of the bed to extend the surface of the surgical bed. Pad the footboard so the surface is the same height as the bed's mattress.
   - Instruct the assistant holding the patient's arms during the prepping to avoid placing undue stress on the brachial plexus.
   - Assess the team members' sterile technique in donning sterile gown and gloves. Immediately verbalize breaks in technique and provide gowns/gloves to correct the problem.
   - Monitor that the surgical team remains seated throughout the entire procedure. If team members change position during the procedure, offer a change in sterile attire.

- Verbalize breaks or punctures in surgical gloves. Take action to cover or replace the torn gloves. To cover the gloves, don a sterile glove the same size or use a glove a half-size larger than the glove worn. To replace a glove, the circulating nurse removes the original glove while wearing a glove. The sterile person uses the open-gloving technique to replace the glove, or another sterile person gloves the team member.
- Monitor the position of the patient's left arm during the procedure to prevent hyperextension on the hand table.
- Document on the intraoperative record the position of the patient and positioning aids used. Record the surgical personnel involved in the procedure. Reclassify the patient's surgical wound classification to the next level in the event of a major break in sterile technique.

4. Evaluation:
- Report to the post-anesthesia care unit nurse the outcome of the surgical procedure and nursing interventions used during the intraoperative phase.
- Assess the patient's ability to extend her left arm postoperatively as compared to the preoperative base line. Assess the patient's comfort.
- During the postoperative telephone call the next day, evaluate the condition of the surgical site and the presence of any fever.

Chapter Four

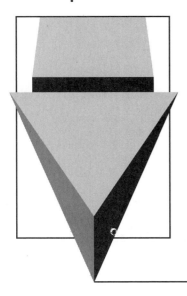

Sterilization/ Disinfection: Equipment and Instruments

Connie Diane Brown, RN, BSN, CNOR

Prerequisite Knowledge   Prior to beginning this chapter, the learner should review concepts of microbiology.

Chapter content is correlated with several AORN recommended practices. These recommended practices may be considered a prerequisite prior to beginning the chapter or a refresher upon completion of the chapter.

Recommended practices for aseptic technique

Recommended practices for surgical attire

Recommended practices for disinfection

Recommended practices for protective barrier materials for gowns and drapes

Recommended practices for safe care through identification of potential hazards in the surgical environment

Recommended practices for the care of instruments, scopes, and powered surgical instruments

Recommended practices for the selection and use of packaging systems

Recommended practice for sanitation in the surgical practice setting

Recommended practice for sterilization, steam, and ethylene oxide (EO)

Recommended practices for traffic patterns in the surgical suite

Recommended practices for universal precautions in the perioperative practice setting

Chapter Outline

Learning Objectives

1. List various methods of sterilization and disinfection used in health care facilities.

2. Discuss the preparation of instruments for decontamination.

3. Discuss methods used in the decontamination process of soiled instruments and medical devices.

4. State the criteria used in instrument preparation for sterilization.

5. Describe the criteria to determine the material to be used when packaging instruments for in-hospital sterilization.

6. List sterilization process monitors.

7. Discuss the relevance of shelf life of sterile items.

8. Discuss the fundamentals of various sterilization methods.

9. Describe various methods of disinfection.

Scope of Sterilization and Disinfection

Methods of sterilization and disinfection are the foundation upon which infection control is based. Their efficacy is reliant on several factors, primarily encompassing the level of decontamination. Measures implemented for the prevention of surgical wound infection involve providing instruments, supplies, and equipment free of contamination at the time of use. Since medical devices used in patient care are potentially contaminated with infectious pathogenic microorganisms (Table 4–1), an understanding is needed to identify the most appropriate type and level of decontamination.

Decontamination is a process that removes as many microorganisms as possible from an item by physical, mechanical, or chemical means. The desired outcome is a medical device free of pathogenic microorganisms and safe to handle without wearing protective attire. A health care facility usually provides several methods of decontamination, each offering a different level of microbial reduc-

TABLE 4-1. **PATHOGENIC MICROORGANISMS**

CLASSIFICATION	PATHOGENIC MICROORGANISMS
Spore-forming bacteria	*Bacillus anthracis*
	Clostridium botulinum
	Clostridium tetanus
Vegetative bacteria	*Salmonella choleraesuis*
	Pseudomonas aeruginosa
	Staphylococcus aureus
	Mycobacterium tuberculosis
Viruses	Herpes simplex
	Poliovirus
	Hepatitis B
Fungi	*Candida albicans*
	Coccidioides
	Aspergillus
	Alternaria

Good Hospital Practice: Handling and Biological Decontamination of Reusable Medical Devices, AAMI, 1992d, ST 35, Vol. 1: Sterilization, Arlington, Virginia.

tion. When determining the type and level of decontamination needed, three basic factors should be considered:

- type of patient contact
- manner in which the device is used
- probability of biologic hazard to health care personnel (AAMI, ST 35, 1992d).

Cleaning, the physical removal of organic material, is considered the initial step of a decontamination process. Cleaning is usually done with water and detergent; however, many health care facilities use a presoak enzymatic solution that separates blood, bone, and tissue from surgical instruments. The purpose of cleaning is to remove or reduce bioburden rather than to destroy microorganisms (CDC, 1981). Effective cleaning and decontamination practices are critical for the provision of quality disinfection and sterilization processes as explained later in this chapter.

DISINFECTION

Disinfection, recognized as the intermediate state between physical cleaning and sterilization, is accomplished by using thermal processes or chemical germicides (Garner, 1985). Chemical disinfection is usually performed by submersing an item in a covered basin of germicidal solution for a designated length of time to achieve the desired level of microbial kill. However, disinfection may also be achieved through automated equipment such as washer-decontaminators or washer-disinfectors. Common methods of disinfection are listed in Table 4-2.

Disinfection ordinarily eliminates many or all pathogenic microorganisms on inanimate objects, with the exception of bacterial spores. To understand the rationale for cleaning, disinfecting, or sterilizing, levels of disinfection (known as Spaulding's process classification) should be identified. The Centers for Disease Control and Prevention (CDC) publication *Guideline for Handwashing and Hospital Environmental Control* (Garner, 1985) defines them as:

- high-level disinfection
- intermediate-level disinfection
- low-level disinfection.

The levels represent various degrees of antimicrobial activity (see Table 4-2). Chemical disinfectants should be registered with the U.S. Environmental Protection Agency (EPA) and approved for marketing by the Food and Drug Administration (FDA). The label of every disinfectant product should contain the

TABLE 4-2. **STERILIZATION AND DISINFECTION: HOW ARE THEY DIFFERENT?**

CATEGORY	STERILIZATION	DISINFECTION
Purpose	To destroy all forms of microbial life	To destroy many or all pathogenic microorganisms on inanimate objects, usually not bacterial spores.
Antimicrobial Activity	Destruction of all vegetative bacteria, fungi, viruses, and spores	**High-level disinfection:** purposed to destroy all microorganisms, with exception of large populations of bacterial spores (some chemicals may be used as sterilants depending upon the length of contact time).
		Intermediate-level disinfection: purposed to inactivate *Mycobacterium tuberculosis*, many viruses (hepatitis B), vegetative bacteria, and most fungi. It does not necessarily kill bacterial spores.
		Low-level disinfection: has the ability of killing most bacteria (vegetative), some viruses, and some fungi. It is not reliant to destroy resistant microorganisms, i.e., tubercle bacilli or bacterial spores. This level of disinfection is commonly referred to as sanitization.
Application	**Critical item classification:** items used in contact with sterile tissue or the vascular system: *Examples:* surgical instruments/medical devices, catheters, implants, and needles	**Semicritical items:** used in contact with mucous membrane or nonintact skin (generally require high-level disinfection). *Examples:* Respiratory therapy and anesthesia equipment, and endoscopes **Noncritical items:** used in contact with intact skin but not mucous membranes (requires low-level disinfection). *Examples:* Reusable item or equipment for external contact, i.e., external positioning aids, bedpans, blood pressure cuffs, bed rails, patient furniture, etc.
Methods	**Thermal:** Steam or dry heat (washer-sterilizers included) **Liquid chemical sterilants:** peracetic acid 6% hydrogen peroxide 2% glutaraldehyde solutions chlorine dioxide (efficacy reliant upon prolonged contact time, refer to MR*) Ethylene oxide	**Thermal:** Washer-disinfector/sanitizer **Chemical agents** High-level disinfectants: glutaraldehyde solutions hydrogen peroxide chlorine dioxide peracetic acid Intermediate-level disinfectants: phenolics iodophor compounds chlorine Low-level disinfectants: quaternary ammonium compounds mercurial compounds

*Manufacturer recommendations.
Rutala, 1990; Garner, 1985; Perkins, 1983; AAMI, 1994d; Reichert, 1993.

spectrum of antimicrobial activity. The EPA requires a hospital disinfectant to have the ability to kill *Mycobacterium tuberculosis*. This should be stated on the product label along with the recommended contact time and temperature requirements (AAMI, ST 35, 1992). Does this disinfectant inactivate hepatitis B virus (HBV) and human immunodeficiency virus (HIV) as well as *Mycobacterium tuberculosis*? What is the required contact time to achieve the desired level of disinfection? It is critical that all users of chemical disinfectants carefully read the label to identify antimicrobial activity and projected end results. The label should also inform them of how to safely use and dispose of the product.

Patient-care items are categorized on the basis of risk of infection involved and the level of decontamination needed. The CDC describes them as

- critical
- semicritical
- noncritical.

Each category recommends the level of disinfection needed to prevent the risk of infection. *Critical items* are those in contact with sterile tissue or the vascular system. These items present a high risk of infection if contaminated with any microorganisms, especially bacterial spores; therefore, all items of this category must be sterile.

Semicritical items come into contact with mucous membranes and do not ordinarily penetrate body surfaces. Mucous membranes are usually resistant to infection caused by bacterial spores but are susceptible to infection caused by other organisms. A high-level disinfection process is recommended. It destroys vegetative microorganisms, most fungal spores, tubercle bacilli, and small nonlipid viruses (Garner, 1985).

Noncritical items touch only intact skin. The risk of these articles in transmitting disease or infection is very rare; consequently, low-level disinfection is sufficient. Refer to Table 4–2 for examples of items in each category. It is important that each item, whatever the category, be meticulously cleaned before the disinfection is implemented. Improper cleaning and organic debris are among many factors that have been known to nullify or limit the efficacy of this process (Rutala, 1990).

With information about the risk of infection, the perioperative nurse can assess the appropriate process of sterilization or disinfection to provide the optimal care for his/her patient.

STERILIZATION

Sterilization is the process of killing all forms of microbial life. Common hospital processes that destroy all vegetative bacteria, fungi, viruses, and spores are found in Table 4–2. *Steam sterilization* or moist heat in the form of saturated steam is considered the most economical and efficient form of sterilization. The rapid processing time is a major advantage because it allows the frequent availability of a medical device. This method of sterilization is purposed for items that can tolerate high temperatures and moisture. Three components that are critical to insure the effectiveness of steam sterilization are time, temperature, and moisture. The two common types of steam sterilizers that are discussed in this chapter are the prevacuum or pulsating vacuum sterilizers and the gravity displacement sterilizers.

Chemical sterilization is commonly used on items that are heat sensitive. Sterilizers utilizing peracetic acid and hydrogen peroxide plasma are designed to safely sterilize delicate instruments and a wide variety of cameras and endoscopes. These sterilizers operate at low temperatures in relatively short cycles.

Ethylene oxide (EO) sterilization is most acknowledged for its ability to sterilize heat-labile and/or moisture-sensitive medical supplies without causing damage or deterioration. There are various factors to consider when using ethylene oxide:

- toxic and flammable nature of EO
- lengthy processing/aeration time
- safe work environment for personnel
- environmental concerns
- high cost.

Different ethylene oxide sterilizers use different EO concentrations—some use 100% concentrations of EO, while others use mixtures of EO with hydrochloro-fluorocarbons (HCFC) and other inert gases. These factors, along with other issues surrounding the use of ethylene oxide, are explained later in the chapter.

By following these processes of cleaning, decontamination, disinfection, and sterilization, the perioperative nurse can effectively implement safe work practices that reflect the efficacy of sterile processing. The following sections take the reader through the routine phases of sterile processing from decontamination to sterile storage.

Preparation of Instruments for Decontamination— Perioperative Role

The initial reduction of gross soil on surgical instruments and medical devices is performed by the scrub person intraoperatively or at the point of use. The jaw, blade, serrations, and box locks are anatomic features of instruments that commonly retain a high level of bioburden (Fig. 4–1). While coordinating the needs of the surgical team, the perioperative nurse removes blood and tissue with a moistened sponge and sterile water. This simple task decreases the number of microorganisms and reduces nutrient material that may promote microbial growth. It also minimizes the potential for environmental contamination and removes substances, including blood, saline, iodine, and so forth, that cause damage by initiating corrosion (AAMI, ST 35, 1992). Responsibilities for providing proper care and handling of instruments do not cease at the end of a surgical procedure. Preparations for transport should be handled in a manner that minimizes any chance of contamination of the worker and the environment.

Note: Creutzfeldt-Jakob disease (CJD) is a rare, usually fatal degenerative neurologic disease that requires important precautions in preventing nosocomial transmission and bloodborne exposures. The CJD pathogen is difficult to destroy; therefore, health care workers associated with supposed CJD patients need to carefully follow the recommended practices stated subsequently or follow recommendations of the health care facility's infection control representative.

- Sterilize potentially contaminated materials prior to discarding, cleaning, or resterilizing them.
- Contaminated instruments should not be handled or washed until they have been sterilized for 1 hour in a steam sterilizer at 132°C, followed by routine decontamination processes. For instruments that cannot endure steam sterilization, a 1-hour submersion in 1N sodium hydroxide is suggested. Manufacturers recommendations should be followed (Rutala, 1990).
- Disinfect contaminated inanimate surfaces with 0.5% sodium hypochlorite (1 : 10 dilution of household bleach) prior to routine cleaning.

POSTOPERATIVE INTERVENTION: ORGANIZATION OF INSTRUMENTS

The scrub person should prepare the instrumentation and all other items for the necessary phases of decontamination. The goal is to maximize the surface areas of all medical devices. This promotes the effectiveness of the cleaning mechanism and agent. The recommended practices that should be followed are

- Place instruments in a mesh bottom tray to allow full exposure of the cleaning mechanism.
- Open jointed instruments at box locks to maximize surface area.
- Disassemble instruments composed of more than one part.

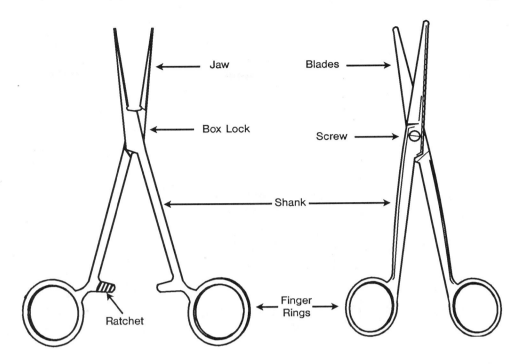

Serrations

TYPES

Horizontal   Longitudinal   Diamond

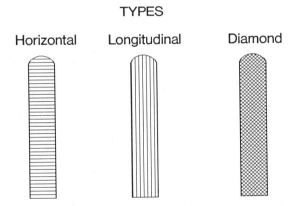

FIGURE 4–1. "Anatomical Features" of Hinged Instruments (Courtesy of Baxter V-Mueller and Mary A. Seithers, Baylor Media Services)

- Separate delicate scissors and microsurgical instruments from heavier instruments to avoid damage.
- Remove and appropriately discard disposable sharps (Fig. 4–2).
- Place reusable sharps in a puncture-resistant, leakproof container appropriately labeled for sharps; they should be stored or processed in a manner that prevents the worker from blindly reaching into containers where sharps are placed (OSHA, 1992).
- Suction canisters should be sealed and secured for transport (Fig. 4–3).

The type of container needed for transport depends on the items being transported. Containers must prevent spillage or leakage of liquids. Impermeable bags, bins with lids, and closed-case cart systems are methods used alone or in

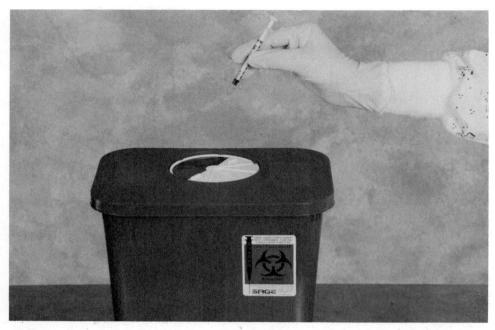

FIGURE 4–2. Sharps should be disposed in appropriate sharps container. (Courtesy of SAGE Products Inc.) Crystal Lake, Illinois.

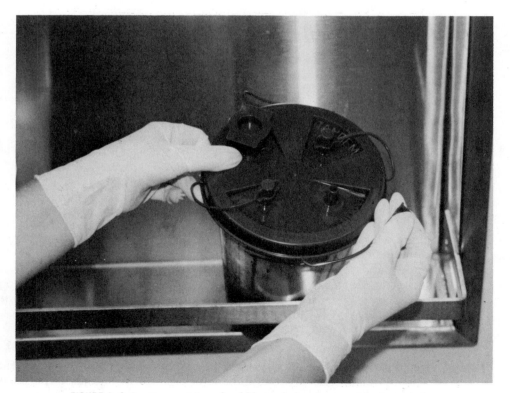

FIGURE 4–3. Suction canisters should be sealed and secured for transport.

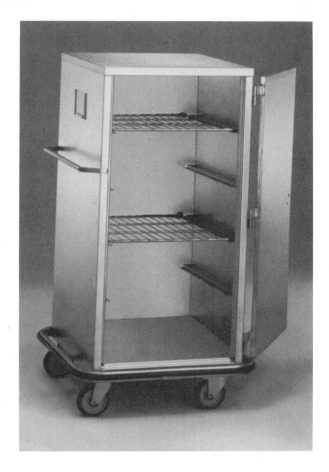

FIGURE 4-4. Confine and contain contaminated items during transport.

combination to prevent inadvertent personnel contact or exposure to these contaminated items (Fig. 4-4).

Decontamination Process

DECONTAMINATION AREA

The Association for the Advancement of Medical Instrumentation (AAMI) defines the decontamination area as a location designated for the collection, retention, and cleaning of soiled instruments. It should be physically separate from all other processing areas. This separation decreases the risk of cross-infection by reducing the incidence of exposure to personnel and supplies to soiled items. The air from the decontamination area should be exhausted to the outside atmosphere and not recirculated because contaminated aerosols and dust particles can be carried from "dirty" areas to "clean" areas by air currents.

ATTIRE

Personnel working in the decontamination area as well as all other processing areas should wear clean surgical attire. This should be changed whenever wet or soiled. All head and facial hair should be covered with surgical hair caps. If shoe covers are worn, they should be removed and discarded when leaving the area and replaced when returning from other areas of the facility. These guidelines should also apply to hair coverings.

Specific personal protective equipment is crucial for those working directly in the decontamination area. The Occupational Safety and Health Administration (OSHA) has established the following guidelines concerning the implementation of personal protective equipment.

Gloves—rubber heavy-duty or household-type; if torn, should be immediately replaced after thorough handwashing; if reusable, should be daily cleaned and inspected for tears and holes; should be discarded if any evidence of barrier breach is found

Mask—high filtration (96% or greater); should be worn properly or discarded; could be considered mode of transferring microorganisms

Protective eyewear—face shield, goggles, or safety glasses with solid side shields; should be worn when exposed to potential splashing or aerosolization

Fluid-resistant covering—impermeable apron, jumpsuit, or gown

Shoe covers—fluid-resistant shoe covers or rubber boots

The operating room personnel and the processing staff need to comply to these safety requirements.

Controlling access to the decontamination and processing areas will assist in minimizing the transfer of microorganisms. The infection control committee of each facility should clearly define in their protocol and enforce the appropriate attire to wear when leaving and returning to these areas.

As stated earlier, the initial performance of gross decontamination is when the scrub person removes organic debris from instruments intraoperatively. Immediately following the surgical procedure, a presoak enzymatic solution or spray is frequently used to loosen soil, tissue, and other bioburden from instruments. This activity usually occurs in a matter of minutes and is often substituted for manual cleaning. If a presoak is initiated within the operating room, care must be taken to safely contain and transport solutions to the decontamination area. An initial cold water rinse also facilitates the removal of blood and debris. Otherwise, manual or mechanical methods of cleaning and decontamination are implemented.

Note: Consult the manufacturer's instructions to determine whether their devices can tolerate high temperatures or liquid immersion.

MANUAL CLEANING

Manual cleaning is recommended for delicate items that are heat sensitive. Personnel engaged in manual cleaning should wear complete personal protective equipment as previously described.

- Instruments are cleaned under water in a nonabrasive neutral pH detergent.
- While cleaning, keep instruments submerged, especially if using a brush. This minimizes the risk of aerosolization and splashing (Fig. 4–5).
- Special attention should be given to difficult-to-clean areas of instruments such as serrations (especially vascular serrations, i.e., DeBakey or Cooley) and box locks.
- Items containing lumens should be cleaned with brushes of appropriate size and flushed under water.
- Detergents need to be low-sudsing and should not leave a residue when rinsed.

Note: Recommendations concerning pH levels are less than 7 for inorganic debris and greater than 7 for organic debris (Reichert, 1993).

Manual cleaning can be followed by high-level chemical disinfection, depending on the integrity of the medical device. If the item is heat tolerant, a mechanical decontamination or sterilization process should be followed. The purpose of decontamination is to remove as many microorganisms as possible, rendering the item safe to handle.

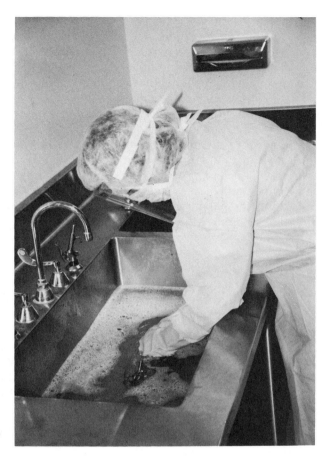

FIGURE 4–5. Instruments should be cleaned under water.

ULTRASONIC CLEANERS

The ultrasonic cleaner is one of several methods of mechanical cleaning (Fig. 4–6). Energy from high-frequency sound waves causes vibration with the implosion of bubbles, loosening organic material from the instrument. This process, known as cavitation, enables the removal of soil from serrations and box locks

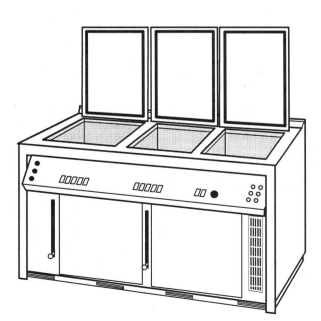

FIGURE 4–6. Ultrasonic Cleaner (Courtesy of Mary A. Seithers, Baylor Media Services)

and other hard-to-clean areas. This system *must follow* a mechanical washer or decontaminator process to adequately remove gross soil and debris. The worker should understand that the ultrasonic washer is a cleaning process — not a disinfection process. Soil should be removed prior to use because it interferes with the sonic energy that enables the removal of fine debris.

Ultrasonic units may have one or several chambers. The first is usually a wash chamber followed by a rinse chamber. The basket of instruments is immersed in a solution of warm water and low-sudsing detergent. It is rinsed with deionized or distilled water. Each time the chamber is filled with water, it should be degassed to remove dissolved air, which reduces the effectiveness of the process (Reichert, 1993). The wash water should be changed at least once every 8 hours and when it becomes cloudy (ASHCSP, 1986). This minimizes the chance for microbial growth and limits particle contamination from the wash water to the instruments. The second chamber is used for rinsing, and if there is a third chamber, it is designated for drying.

The ultrasonic cleaning process should be initiated prior to exposure to the high temperatures of a washer-sterilizer. This will provide adequate cleaning and debris removal that would otherwise be "baked" on. CDC states in its *Guidelines for the Prevention and Control of Nosocomial Infections* (CDC, 1981) that reusable objects must be thoroughly cleaned before any process designed to establish sterility because organic materials, such as blood, mucus, bone, and urine, as well as proteins, will coagulate on items and will protect microorganisms from the sterilant and sterilization. Even though the washer-sterilizer is not the final sterilization process prior to patient use, a system that provides optimal cleaning and decontamination is one of the most effective tools in infection control.

An antimicrobial, water-soluble lubricant should be provided for instruments cleaned in this machine because the cavitation process removes the preexisting lubrication. Lubrication should be implemented prior to packaging and sterilization.

THERMAL MECHANICAL DECONTAMINATION

Thermal disinfection involves hot water to decontaminate reusable medical devices and instrumentation. Moist heat and time have been proved to effectively destroy microorganisms. Vegetative bacteria are known to be the least resistant to heat, whereas bacterial spores and some viruses are generally most resistant (followed by most fungi and some viruses) (AAMI, ST 35, 1992). There are several types of mechanical decontaminators or washers that effectively reduce bioburden or the number of microorganisms on an object (Fig. 4–7). These units closely resemble a dishwasher in performance. They wash, rinse, and disinfect a high volume of instrument trays with minimal personnel contact. The temperature ranges are significantly lower (60–95°C) than those in a washer-sterilizer (132°C). As the temperature increases, so does the level of microbial destruction. Forceful agitation of hot water in combination with an adequate detergent is effective in destroying microorganisms. Ordinarily, these machines provide an intermediate-level of disinfection.

Automatic indexed washer-decontaminators are units consisting of several chambers, each providing a separate function in the decontamination process (Figs. 4–8, 4–9). The initial chamber may provide a cold water prerinse and wash, followed by an ultrasonic cleaner. This automated system offers a wash, rinse, and lubrication process to which instruments are mechanically advanced by means of a conveyor. The advantage of an indexed unit is its ability to process a large number of instruments with a streamlined work flow. This system functions with minimal contact from personnel, which reduces the potential for exposure to infectious microorganisms.

The *washer-sterilizers* wash, rinse, and use gravity steam sterilization (Fig.

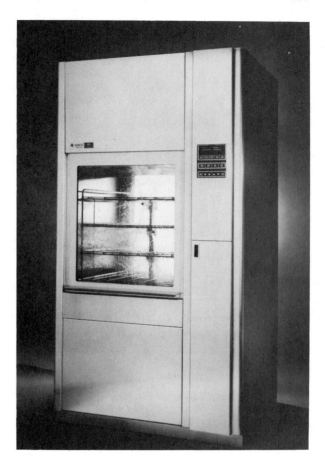

FIGURE 4–7. Mechanical Washer (Courtesy of AMSCO, Erie, Pennsylvania)

4–10). The high temperature (132°C) and steam leads to the total destruction of microorganisms. Staff should refer to the instrument manufacturer's instructions before placing items in a washer-sterilizer. Many items may be sufficiently heat tolerant to withstand various types of mechanical washers but not washer-sterilizers.

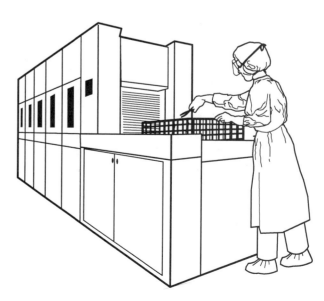

FIGURE 4–8. Automatic Indexed Washer-Decontaminator (Courtesy of Mary A. Seithers, Baylor Media Services)

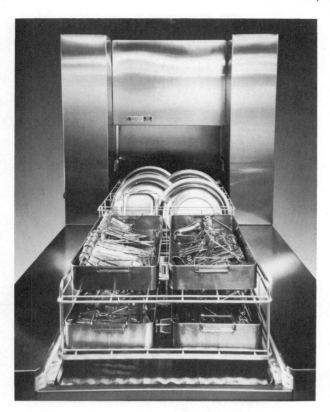

FIGURE 4-9. AMSCO Automatic Indexed Washer (Courtesy of AMSCO, Erie, Pennsylvania)

Note: Instruments should not be considered ready or safe for patient use, because this process utilizes steam sterilization. They must be inspected for cleanliness and workmanship and properly assembled and prepared for terminal sterilization.

The assurance of effective cleaning and removal of bioburden prior to the exposure in a washer-sterilizer is of vital importance. Any tissue or debris not re-

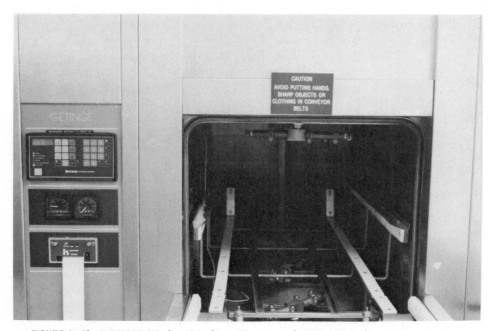

FIGURE 4-10. GETINGE Washer-Sterilizer (Courtesy of GETINGE, Lakewood, New Jersey)

moved during the wash cycle may be baked on during the sterilization cycle. As previously stated, not only will the device be difficult to clean, but it will also harbor microorganisms. The advantages to a washer-sterilizer are

- increased penetration capability due to utilization of saturated steam
- exposure of higher temperatures to all surface areas
- greater incidence of microbial lethality (Reichert, 1993)
- automatic time-released lubrication cycle in many units, which helps maintain the instruments.

Once instruments have been exposed to effective decontamination processes, they are considered safe to handle without risk of exposing patients and health care personnel to bloodborne pathogens.

Preparation for Sterilization

INSPECTION

The individual inspection of instruments provides the assurance of effective cleaning and proper workmanship. This process involves the examination of several critical items:

- cleanliness; absence of soil (especially pertaining to items with lumens); absence of corrosive substances
- free motion of hinged instruments; absence of stiffness or stress corrosion
- proper alignment of jaws and teeth
- proper tension with closed ratchet
- sharpness of blades, trocars; absence of burrs and gouges
- clean screws and pins secured in appropriate tray or holder
- general integrity of instrument; absence of cracks, dents, chipping, and worn areas
- intact insulation sheathing on specialized instrument; absence of tears, insecure or loose sheath
- items composed of more than one part are complete and parts fit together securely
- powered surgical instruments appropriately lubricated and tested for proper functioning; cords checked for absence of cracks or cuts; all components complete and fit together securely.

Many processing areas employ lighted magnifying lamps to enhance the inspection process. Personnel implementing this task should be trained to identify and demonstrate the proper function of the instruments they are inspecting. This step reduces the risk of a medical device malfunctioning at the point of use.

ASSEMBLY OF ITEMS TO BE STERILIZED

The preparation of items for sterilization should be done in a manner that protects the instruments and allows the sterilant to contact all surface areas. When preparing an instrument set, all hinged instruments must be opened and secured with stringers or pins in a wire mesh basket (Fig. 4–11). The weight of an instrument set should be evenly distributed to avoid a collection of moisture during the sterilization process. A towel or other absorbent material may be positioned in the tray to facilitate revaporization of condensate. It might be helpful to have pictures of the correct assembly and placement of instruments for standardization. Delicate instruments may require tip guards or foam sleeves to prevent damage (Fig. 4–12). The worker should always consult the manufacturer's recommendations to insure that these protective items are permeable to the sterilant.

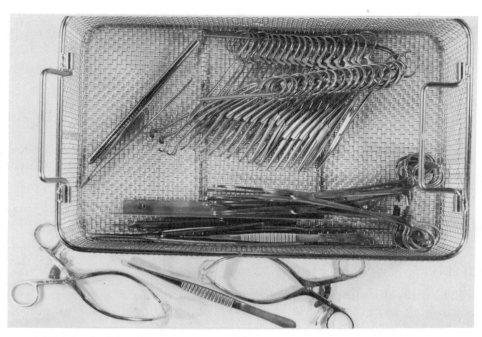

FIGURE 4-11. All hinged instruments must be open and secured prior to sterilization.

Note: Items that are intended for single use should not be resterilized or reused, unless the manufacturer has provided written instructions or scientific data to show that they will be as safe and effective as in their original state (AAMI, SSSA, 1992). Most manufacturers will not assume liability for proper workmanship and sterilization of a device that a health care facility has resterilized for reuse. In addition, the Joint Commission for the Accreditation of Healthcare Organizations (JCAHO) recommends that disposable items not be reused.

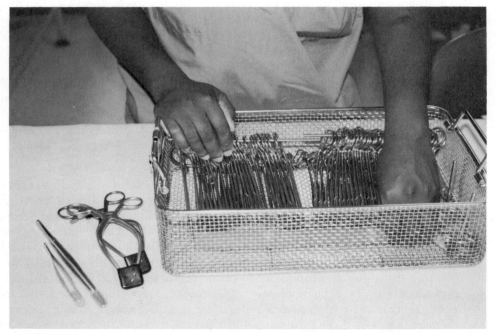

FIGURE 4-12. Instruments using Protect-a-Caps With Air Slits (Courtesy of Key Surgical, Inc. Minneapolis, Minnesota)

DATE:_____ O.R._____ SCRUB NURSE:_____

PROCEDURE:_____ CIRCULATOR: _____

INSTRUMENT COUNT SHEET
Major Set A

Rev 02-18-94

Std	Instruments	Initial Cnt #	+	Comments	Closing Cnt #	Std	Instruments	Initial Cnt #	+	Comments	Closing Cnt #
	Stringer #1						**Tray**				
2	Rt Angles					2	#3 Knife Handles				
3	Munyons					1	Oral Suction				
2	7" Needle Holders					1	ABD Suction				
2	6" Needle Holders					4	Sponge Sticks				
10	Allis					2	White Drape Clips				
6	Oschners					2	Bovie Holsters				
2	Babcocks										
1	Straight Mayo Scissor						**Forceps**				
1	Curved Mayo Scissor					1	Lg Debakey				
1	Regular Metzenbaum					1	Lg Thumb				
1	Small Metzenbaum					2	Medium Debakeys				
1	Wire Scissors					2	Adsons with teeth				
						2	Tissues with teeth				
	Stringer #2					2	Ferris-Smith				
12	Large Towel Clips										
14	Halsteads						**Extra**				
10	Kellys						LC 200 Applier				
							LC 400 Applier				
							Harrington Retractor				
							Army-Navy				

CS Count	
Initial Count	
Closing Count	

FIGURE 4-13. Standard Instrument Count Sheet (Courtesy of Baylor University Medical Center, Dallas, Texas)

Many processing areas have an inventory list or count sheet to enforce standardization of instruments (Fig. 4-13). It contains the type and number of every item in a set, which should be kept to a minimum to eliminate difficulties in counting. This practice greatly enhances the flow of the surgical procedure by minimizing unanticipated problems.

Packaging Materials

Reusable medical devices, supplies, and most other items prepared for in-hospital sterilization must be packaged in a manner that maintains their sterility until the time needed. The implementation of appropriate packaging material is reliant on many variables. The size, shape, number, and density of items to be packaged are among many factors to consider. Three basic principles of packaging must be recognized by the worker.

- It must allow effective sterilant penetration to insure sterilization of the packaging material and its contents.
- It must contain the sterility of the processed items.
- It must allow aseptic presentation of contents.

Refer to Table 4–3 for specific requirements of effective packaging materials.

Health care facilities employ several types of packaging. They consist of textiles, nonwoven materials, peel-pack pouches, and rigid sterilization container systems. Packaging materials should be stored at room temperature (18°C to 22°C) and at a relative humidity ranging from 35% to 70%. Exposure to these conditions will permit penetration of the sterilant and prevent superheating (AAMI, SSSA, 1992). If packaging materials are stored in an area of high humidity, the packaging may become overhydrated, which can affect the integrity of adhesives and seals of peel packages. An extremely dry environment with high temperatures may result in dehydration of packaging materials. They can become brittle and easily tear, removing their ability to provide and maintain asepsis.

Textiles

Textile or woven material commonly known as muslin was the standard reusable wrapping material for many years. Even though it allows for sterilant penetration and air removal, it is not recommended as a barrier material. Moisture can be absorbed, providing a pathway for microorganisms. This four-layered 100% cotton with 140 thread count has been replaced by an improved 100% polyester wrapper (Reichert, 1993). The significance of the textile polyester wrapper is in its fluid repellency properties. Woven materials should be freshly laundered. This prevents the fabric from superheating and facilitates effective sterilization. A quality improvement program should be established to detect holes and tears. Heat-sealed patches, which allow for penetration of ethylene oxide and steam, are applied for repair.

Nonwoven Materials

Nonwoven wrappers are made of spun-bonded polyolefin fibers (Fig. 4–14). This fiber product is more durable and resistant to moisture, punctures, and tears. It is a single-use, low-linting, disposable wrapper that conforms well to items needing

TABLE 4–3. REQUIREMENTS OF EFFECTIVE PACKAGING

FACTORS TO CONSIDER	REQUIRED PACKAGING CRITERIA EFFECTIVE PACKAGING MUST:
Sterilization	Withstand physical conditions of selected sterilization process Enable penetration of the sterilant Allow adequate air removal Allow for removal of sterilant
Integrity	Be visually tamperproof by containing a secure closure or seal Completely enclose an item (adaptable to its size and shape) Be durable to resist tears and punctures from normal handling Maintain reliable barrier qualities throughout selected sterilization process Demonstrate fluid repellency properties
Asepsis	Allow for aseptic presentation of contents at point of use
Safety	Be free of nonfast dyes and toxic substances (Reichert, 1993) Allow for appropriate labeling Protect the contents from physical damage

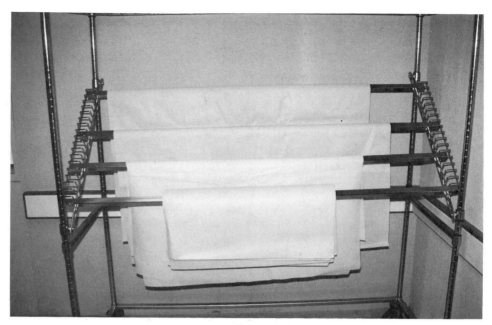

FIGURE 4–14. Nonwoven Wrappers (Courtesy of Kimberly Clark, Roswell, Georgia)

packaging. "Memory" can be a concern with certain nonwoven wrappers. When opened, the edges will try to return to the original fold, risking contamination of the contents. Items prepared with woven as well as nonwoven material should be sequentially double wrapped. This provides a tortuous path for microorganisms and allows for aseptic presentation of contents. The envelope wrap and the square wrap are common techniques (Figs. 4–15, 4–16).

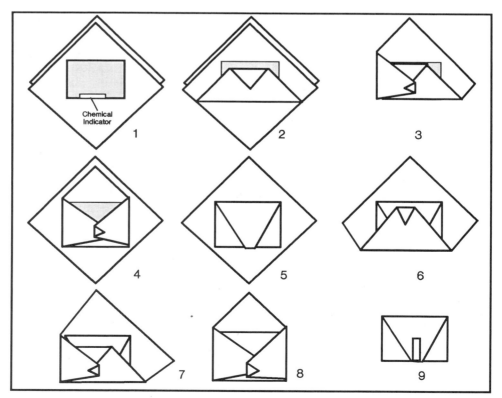

FIGURE 4–15. Envelope Wrap (Courtesy of Good Hospital Practice: Steam Sterilization and Sterility Assurance, AAMI, Arlington, Virginia and Mary A. Seithers, Baylor Media Services)

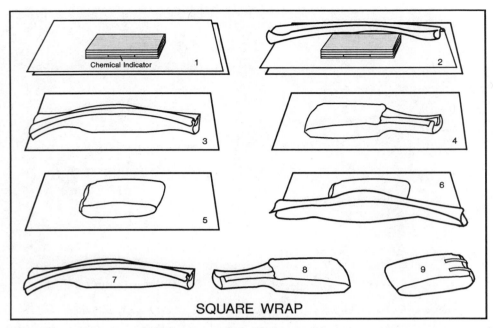

FIGURE 4–16. Square Wrap (Courtesy of Good Hospital Practice: Steam Sterilization and Sterility Assurance, AAMI, Arlington, Virginia and Mary A. Seithers, Baylor Media Services)

Paper-plastic Package Systems

Peel packages consist of a paper-plastic combination pouch that allows for proper sealing to secure the contents within the package. Before sealing, this system should have as much air removed as possible to facilitate effective sterilization and to prevent damage to the package. Double-peel packages should be sequentially sized and sealed to allow for proper fit of the inner pouch (Fig. 4–17). The paper sides of both packages are positioned together to allow adequate penetration of the sterilant, air, and moisture. Double-peel packaging is used when multiple items need to be packaged together. The inner package limits excessive movement and enhances aseptic delivery to the sterile field. Baskets with support racks should be available to hold these packages on edge and allow for adequate spacing during sterilization.

Rigid Sterilization Container Systems

Rigid container systems have replaced nonwoven disposable wrappers in many large hospital facilities. Reduction in cost (over time) and management of waste

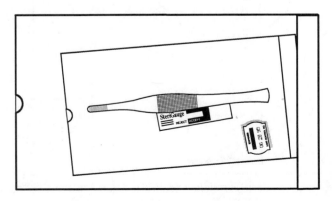

FIGURE 4–17. Double-peel packages should be sequentially sized and sealed. (Courtesy of Mary A. Seithers, Baylor Media Services)

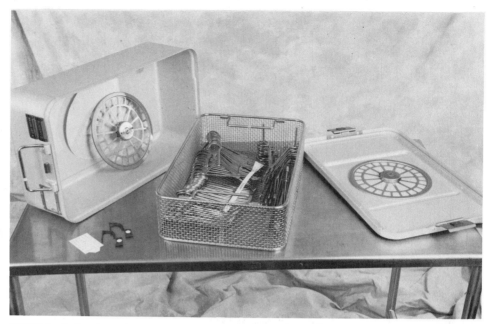

FIGURE 4–18. Rigid Sterilization Container Systems (Courtesy of Aesculap San Francisco, California)

are current issues to consider for justifying this change. These containers are made from aluminum, heat-resistant plastics, stainless steel, or a combination of these materials. Perforations in the lid and bottom are covered with disposable bacterial filters and secured by a filter holder. Filters allow the sterilant to penetrate and contact the items within (Fig. 4–18). Some containers have valve-type closures, which require the manufacturer's instructions to insure proper assembly and function. Tamperproof locks and identification labels assist in assessing the status of the container contents. Manufacturer's recommendations need to be followed concerning weight and density, sterilization cycles and times, and loading practices.

Before use, inspection for proper function of valves or filter holders and locking systems is needed. Seals should be checked on the lids to insure a secure fit to the base of the container. Proper decontamination measures should be implemented after each use.

Rarely utilized wrapped items may be placed in an enclosed sterile storage cabinet or placed in a plastic heat-sealed dust cover. This provides additional barrier protection and extends shelf life. A heat-sealed dust cover should be applied after sterilization and before the item is placed in sterile storage.

All packages prepared for sterilization should be initialed by the preparer. This provides accountability and is an effective quality control measure.

Sterilization Process Monitors

CHEMICAL MONITORS

Chemical monitors or indicators can monitor one or more process parameters of a sterilization cycle to detect failures in packaging, loading, or sterilizer function (AAMI, TIR 3, 1992). The indicator consists of a sensitive chemical or ink dye that develops a visual change or "end-point response" after the exposure to certain physical processing conditions (e.g., temperature and humidity). Chemical monitors should be placed on the outside of every package before processing. An ex-

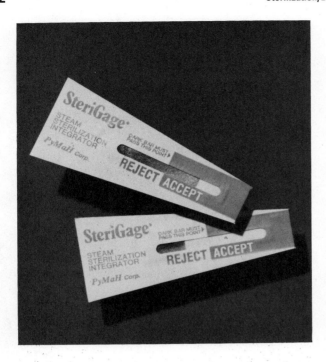

FIGURE 4–19. Chemical Monitors —SteriGage Sterilization Integrator—Steam Sterilization (Courtesy of PyMaH Corporation, Somerville, New Jersey)

ception would be when the packaging allows the user to visualize the internal indicator, as in a peel package. Many brands of peel packages contain a chemical indicator incorporated into the external paper side of the pouch. Chemical indicators are manufactured in several forms, such as tapes, strips, labels, or legends. These need to be examined after sterilization and before use to make certain the item was exposed to the sterilization process (Figs. 4–19, 4–20).

Internal and external indicators need to be on every package for in-hospital sterilization. Internal monitors are placed in the area of greatest challenge within the package. They should be easily visible once the package is opened. Nothing should be presented to the sterile field until all indicators are found to be acceptable. Both external and internal indicators reflect exposure of an item to one or

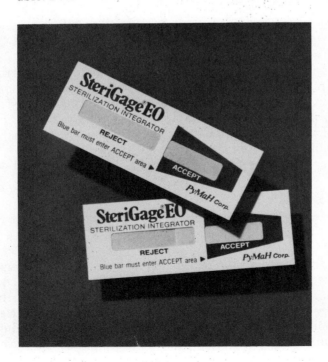

FIGURE 4–20. Chemical Monitors —SteriGage Sterilization Integrators—EO Gas Sterilization (Courtesy of PyMaH Corporation, Somerville, New Jersey)

more sterilization parameters. They do not guarantee sterility. If a discrepancy exists, proper exposure to sterilization is questionable, and the items should not be used. The immediate detection of a potential sterilization failure is a major advantage of chemical indicators.

It is essential that the worker understands what a specific indicator should reveal about the sterilization process. Various brands differ in their performance characteristics. Some of the monitors must be exposed to steam for a minimal amount of time to achieve the end-point response. Others are affected by temperature, moisture, or a combination of these. Understanding the significance of single and multiparameter indicators will help identify problems resulting from indicators with an unsatisfactory reading. The perioperative nurse should be able to quickly read and interpret the indicator's end point. The manufacturers can provide specific performance characteristics of their monitoring systems.

Integrators are chemical monitors, which according to the manufacturer, offer results based on the integration of all parameters of a sterilization cycle. Whatever type of chemical monitor a health care facility uses, they all reflect an exposure to sterilization conditions and should assist in identifying an ineffective sterilization cycle.

BIOLOGIC MONITORS

A biologic monitor is a standardized preparation of known microorganisms highly resistant to a specific mode of sterilization. Its purpose is to reveal evidence of the efficacy of a sterilization cycle by utilizing a high number of resistant spores to challenge the function of the sterilizer (AAMI, SSSA, 1992). Biologic monitors are considered the most reliable monitors, because they respond to conditions of sterilization much like natural organisms.

The spores for steam sterilization are *Bacillus stearothermophilus*; those for gas sterilization are *Bacillus subtilis*. These microorganisms are impregnated on paper strips or capsules and placed within a chamber for exposure to the appropriate sterilization cycle (Fig. 4–21) (AAMI, SSSA, 1992). The biologic monitors may be in special test packs or in wrapped items within the sterilizer. When the sterilization cycle is complete, they are removed and placed in an incubator where microbial growth is observed. Required incubation times may vary, depending on the product and manufacturers' recommendations. A negative biologic monitor contains no growth and indicates that conditions necessary for sterilization and microbial kill were met. If growth is detected by a positive biologic indicator result, the supervisor should be immediately notified. Appropriate documentation should be made, and further testing and investigation are needed to determine the viability of the organisms and the efficacy of the sterilization cycle. A control biologic monitor, which has the same lot number as the test and has not been exposed to a sterilization cycle, is also incubated and examined for growth. A control monitor should reflect growing organisms, indicating a viable lot.

A biologic monitor is available for 270°F (132°C) gravity displacement steam sterilization cycles, which offers results after a 1-hour incubation period. This monitor is purposed for flash sterilization cycles not to exceed 10 minutes (Fig. 4–22). Manufacturers' instructions should be followed with all sterilization monitoring systems.

The Association for the Advancement of Medical Instrumentation (AAMI) recommends the weekly (preferably daily) routine use of biologic monitors for steam sterilization, with every load containing implantable items, during initial installation testing of sterilizers and after major sterilizer repairs (Table 4–4). Biologic indicators for ethylene oxide sterilization should be utilized with every load. When an implantable device is sterilized, it should be quarantined until the test results are available. When emergency situations occur and a quarantine pe-

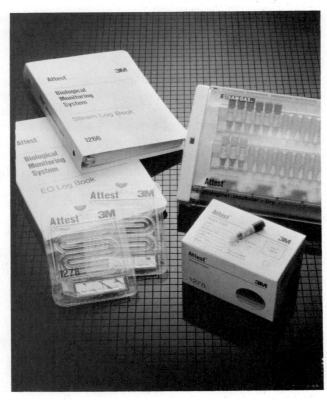

FIGURE 4–21. Biologic Monitoring System (Courtesy of 3M Health Care, St. Paul, Minnesota)

riod is not possible, documentation and close monitoring are necessary to provide the sterility assurance of that implantable device. Although many hospitals employ commercially prepared biologic test packs, AAMI gives several examples of routine test packs (AAMI, SSSA, 1992).

The steps in making a test pack for steam sterilization are (Fig. 4–23)

- Use 16 freshly laundered absorbent towels (16″ × 26″).
- Fold each towel into thirds (lengthwise) and then in half.
- Place towels in a stack, with folds opposite each other.
- Center one or more appropriately labeled biologic indicators between the seventh and eighth towels along with chemical indicators if used.
- Secure the pack with tape. The pack should weigh approximately 3 pounds and have a height of approximately 6 inches.

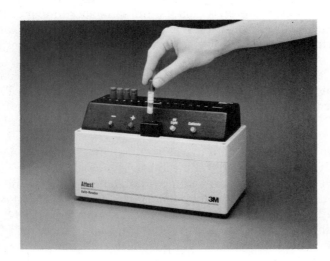

FIGURE 4–22. Rapid Readout Biologic Monitoring System for Gravity Displacement Sterilizers (Courtesy of 3M Health Care, St. Paul, Minnesota)

TABLE 4-4. ROUTINE BIOLOGIC MONITORING

FREQUENCY OF USE
    During installation of sterilizer or after major repairs
    Steam: routinely at least once a week, preferably daily
    Gas: with each load
    With each load containing implants

HOW TO USE
    Appropriately labeled:
        sterilizer identification
        date
        load number
    Placement:
        Steam: in loaded chamber over drain or coolest point of sterilizer
        Gas: in middle of loaded chamber
    Incubation usually 48 hours or according to manufacturer's instructions (monitor available with
        1-hour incubation for gravity displacement steam sterilizer)
    A control with the same lot number also labeled and incubated

HOW TO INTERPRET RESULTS
- Negative: after required incubation, no bacterial growth indicated
- Positive: after required incubation, bacterial growth indicated (further testing and investigation required)

Further steps in making a test pack for ethylene oxide are (Fig. 4–24)

- Use syringe containing appropriately labeled biologic indicator.
- Position plunger in syringe, not touching indicator.
- Remove tip from syringe.
- Wrap syringe in freshly laundered surgical towel.
- Place syringe in peel package or wrapper.

Effective teaching and training are critical to all personnel who operate a sterilizer and work in any area of sterilization processing. Sterility assurance heavily relies upon the operator and his/her understanding of the fundamentals of sterilization and monitoring.

MECHANICAL MONITORS

Mechanical monitors, usually in the form of charts, printouts, or gauges, reflect the current status of cycle parameters during sterilization (time, temperature, and pressure) (Fig. 4–25). The operator should assess these monitors for proper

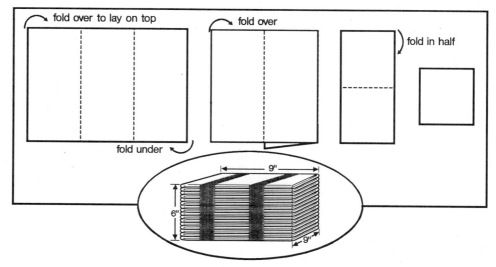

FIGURE 4-23. How to Prepare a Test Pack for Steam Sterilization (Courtesy of Good Hospital Practice: Steam Sterilization and Sterility Assurance, AAMI, Arlington, Virginia and Mary A. Seithers, Baylor Media Services)

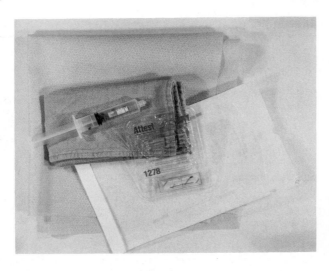

FIGURE 4–24. Items needed for the preparation of a test pack for EO gas sterilization (Courtesy of Propper Manufacturing Co., Long Island, New York)

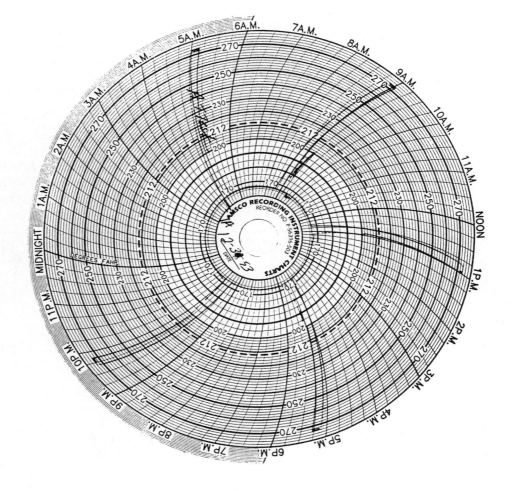

```
==========================
======= D A R T =======
==========================
CYCLE START AT  9:50:26A
            ON  1/26/94

CYCLE COUNT   05177
   OPERATOR   C.Z.
  STERILIZER  VAC05

    STER TEMP = 270.0°F
 CONTROL TEMP = 273.0°F
    STER TIME =  3.5 MIN
    DRY  TIME =  1   MIN

                    P=psig
- TIME        T=°F  V=inHg
--------------------------
C  9:50:26A  131.1    1P
C  9:51:26A  245.0   19P
C  9:54:19A  225.3   10V
C  9:54:59A  264.1   26P
C  9:56:40A  215.4   17V
C  9:57:20A  264.3   26P
C  9:58:48A  203.7   22V
C  9:59:35A  264.2   26P
C 10:01:01A  202.9   23V
S 10:03:02A  270.1   29P
S 10:03:33A  270.4   29P
S 10:04:33A  270.8   29P
S 10:05:33A  270.9   29P
S 10:06:33A  271.0   29P
E 10:06:33A  270.9   30P
E 10:06:59A  218.4    3P
E 10:08:00A  192.6   23V
Z 10:09:25A  186.7    3V


LOAD            12602

  TEMP MAX=271.0°F
  TEMP MIN=270.0°F

CONDITION  =12:57
STERILIZE  = 3:31
EXHAUST    = 2:52
TOTAL CYCLE=19:00
```

FIGURE 4–25. Mechanical Monitors from Steam Sterilizers (Courtesy of Good Hospital Practice: Steam Sterilization and Sterility Assurance, AAMI, Arlington, Virginia and Mary A. Seithers, Baylor Media Services)

setting and function prior to their use. Following a sterilization cycle and before retrieval of sterilized items, the operator must verify that the cycle parameters were met by initialing the charts or printouts. These are kept as permanent records according to the policies of the health care facility. An advantage to mechanical monitoring is the ability to show possible sterilizer malfunction during the actual cycle, which will result in immediate intervention. Sufficient education and training are needed among personnel in central processing and the operating room to insure accurate documentation and monitoring.

Item Identification: Lot Control Number

When the perioperative nurse assesses the integrity of a sterile package prior to opening, an identification or a lot control number should be found. Every item sterilized in the hospital must have a lot control number located on the outside of the package. This control number may be placed on the package before or after the sterilization cycle according to the protocol of the health care facility. It helps locate supplies that have been processed in an inadequate sterilization cycle, usually identified by a process monitor. Whenever there is evidence of sterilization failure, retrieval of items in that specific load must occur. The control number consists of

- identification number of sterilizer
- cycle number
- sterilization date.

The supervisor should contact infection control or risk management personnel to insure appropriate follow-up procedures. Every facility should have a written protocol on product recall to insure patient safety and retrieval of items with questionable sterility.

DOCUMENTATION

Documentation is essential in providing an effective sterility assurance program. Records of sterilization cycles and process monitor results should be kept according to the hospital's protocol. Many facilities have a printed folder to log and contain necessary information concerning a specific sterilizer, its contents, and the results of all process monitors. A separate file should reflect all requested repairs and preventive maintenance. The importance of accurate documentation should be included in the education programs of all personnel who operate sterilizers.

Sterilizer records should contain the following:

- lot control number and corresponding load list
- grafts and charts containing time and temperature recordings (must be initialed by operators for verification of cycle parameters)
- results of chemical and biologic indicator
- implantable biologic test results and documentation of quarantine
- any unsatisfactory or inconclusive response
- air evacuation test results (i.e., Bowie-Dick for prevacuum cycles only).

Shelf Life of Sterile Items

Many hospitals are now adopting the AORN concept of "shelf life of a packaged sterile item is event related." The perioperative nurse is giving more consideration to the integrity of the package, how it is stored, and how many times it is handled, rather than just a quick glance at the expiration date. The expiration date can certainly be noted to insure proper inventory control. However, the expiration date alone is insufficient as an indicator of sterility assurance. Joint Commission's *Accreditation Manual for Hospitals* requires facilities to provide written policies for the shelf life of all stored sterile items. An explanation of how shelf life is determined and how it is indicated on the package (e.g., date, color-coded system) should be included in the policy statement (Mathias, 1992).

AORN RECOMMENDED PRACTICES FOR STEAM AND ETHYLENE OXIDE (EO) STERILIZATION

Before a package is considered sterile, the perioperative nurse must assess the following:

- integrity of packaging material
- how often package is handled
- how package is stored (especially during transport) and conditions of the storage area (e.g., traffic patterns, humidity)
- use of dust covers (Fig. 4–26).

The perioperative nurse should follow facility protocol when receiving sterile items from technical sales representatives. Finding out how the items were stored and transported is valuable information that will assist in determining whether or not the item is sterile and ready for use. Any unsterile reusable device brought in for an evaluation should be decontaminated and sterilized according to the manufacturer's instructions. In-service and education programs on sterility assurance should be required annually to insure safe practices.

Evaluation of the Sterilization Process

Sterilization, or a process that destroys all forms of microbial life, can be accomplished by several methods within a health care facility. It is essential for the perioperative nurse to be able to identify the various sterilization methods avail-

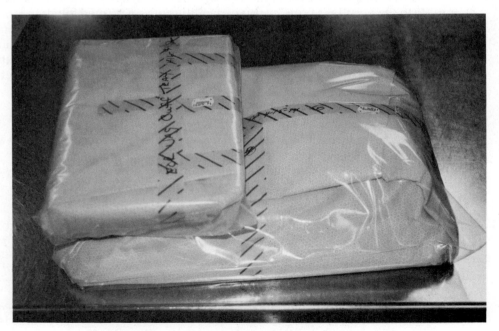

FIGURE 4–26. Sterilized items placed in heat-sealed dust covers

able, as well as to obtain an understanding of the fundamentals of each. Once the full scope of sterile processing is understood, an improvement in work practices will have an impact on the quality of patient care.

STEAM STERILIZATION

Steam sterilization is the most common, cost-effective, and rapid means of sterilization available in hospitals today. A high percentage of instruments, medical devices, and supplies are able to withstand the moisture penetration and high temperature needed for saturated steam.

A steam sterilizer comprises a tightly constructed chamber that is able to withstand high pressures and temperatures. The external chamber walls are usually heated prior to a cycle, preventing condensation within the chamber as the steam is introduced. Heating the external walls of the chamber is accomplished by steam circulating within a jacket space surrounding the chamber (Fig. 4–27). Some small sterilizers do not have a means to preheat the chamber; it is simply heated with each cycle. In general, in a steam sterilization cycle, steam enters the chamber and displaces all air. As the pressure increases, the saturated steam contacts all surfaces, penetrates the packages, and forces the air out through a drain at the bottom of the sterilizer. Sterilization is initiated once all of the air is removed. The high temperature of the saturated steam causes microbial destruction. Proper loading of a sterilizer is crucial because items must be arranged to allow the steam to freely circulate throughout the chamber.

The major components of steam sterilization are *time, temperature, and moisture.* These parameters interrelate to provide the conditions for microbial destruction. For example, the temperature affects the time of exposure in that the higher the temperature, the less exposure time is required. As the pressure increases in a closed chamber, so does the temperature. If these parameters are not optimally represented in a cycle, sterilization will not occur.

Two types of saturated steam sterilizers are gravity displacement steam sterilizers and prevacuum steam sterilizers. There are sterilizers that offer both cycles — gravity displacement and prevacuum (Fig. 4–28). It is important to accurately monitor, utilizing chemical, biologic, and mechanical methods, the sterilizer according to the cycle it presents.

Cycle phases are the same; however, there is a difference in how the air is removed. As the name implies, a gravity displacement cycle allows the steam to enter, and the air removal occurs by the force of gravity. With a prevacuum cycle, a vacuum system pulls the air from the chamber and load contents.

Note: A daily air removal test, commonly referred to as a "Bowie-Dick," is routine in prevacuum sterilizers to insure proper function of the vacuum and detect any air leaks. This chemical monitor is placed on the bottom rack in the sterilizer over the drain before the first processed load of the day. A regular cycle, without drying, is run. A satisfactory test should result in a

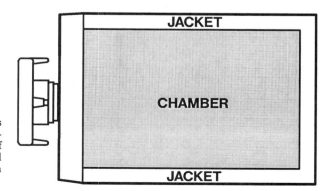

FIGURE 4–27. Steam circulates within a jacket space surrounding the chamber. (Courtesy of AMSCO, Erie, Pennsylvania and Mary A. Seithers, Baylor Media Services)

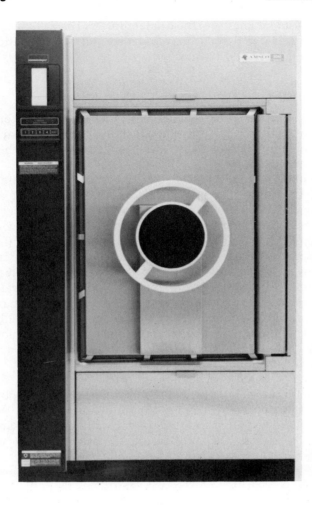

FIGURE 4–28. Steam Sterilizer (Courtesy of AMSCO, Erie, Pennsylvania)

uniform color change of the monitor (Figs. 4–29, 4–30). Results should be documented and filed with other sterilization records. The following section describes each phase of a steam sterilization cycle.

Cycle Phases

Educated personnel who operate sterilizers need to understand what transpires within a sterilizer once the chamber door is locked and a cycle has been initiated. Most sterilizers have a control panel and various types of mechanical monitors to assist the operator with the function of the unit and to reflect the current status of the cycle.

CONDITIONING In a *gravity displacement* cycle, steam enters the chamber and gradually displaces the air, penetrating all packages, forcing the air out (Fig. 4–31A). As more steam is admitted into the chamber, it pushes the air out the bottom drain of the sterilizer. Air is heavier than steam. Steam contacts items in the chamber, and heat is transferred to the contents. During the conditioning phase, both condensate and air escape from the chamber (Reichert, 1993). In a *prevacuum* cycle, pulses of steam are injected into the chamber. As the amount of steam increases and mixes with air, the pressure builds and reaches a level that automatically opens the drain. Air is then forced out by a vacuum pump. Steam is repeatedly introduced as air and condensate are being removed, usually by four or more of these pulses. Complete air removal results and steam penetrates the contents of the load. *Pulsating gravity sterilizers* utilize pulses of steam

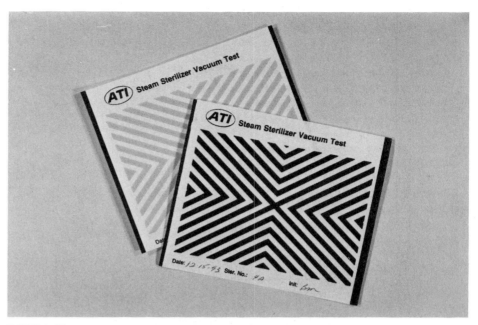

FIGURE 4-29. Air Evacuation Monitor (Courtesy of PyMaH Corporation, Somerville, New Jersey)

to remove the air but do not contain a vacuum pump to aid with air removal following each pulse. Because of these differences, the prevacuum sterilizers are more efficient with air removal and less dependent on position and configuration of load contents. The chamber eventually closes the drain lines after achievement of preset temperature and pressure parameters.

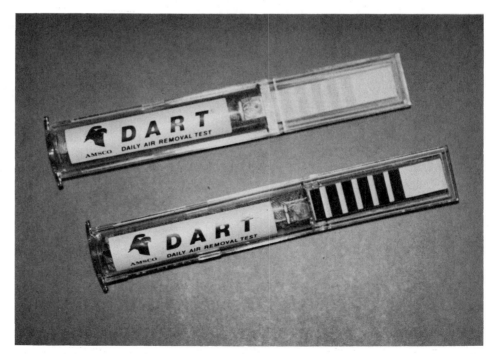

FIGURE 4-30. Air Evacuation Monitor (Courtesy of AMSCO, Erie, Pennsylvania)

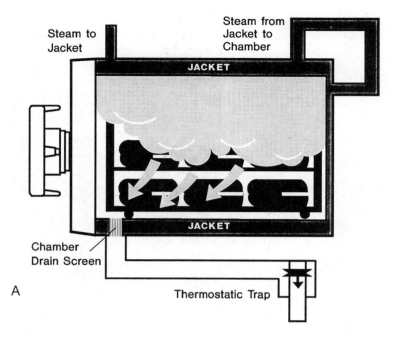

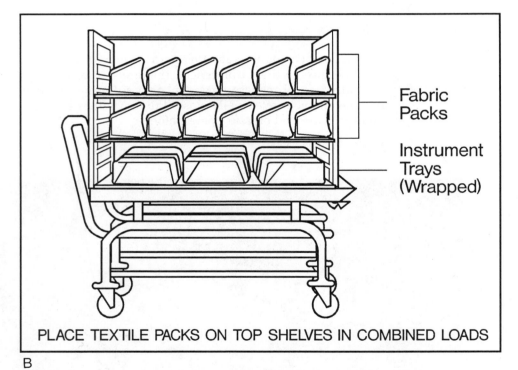

PLACE TEXTILE PACKS ON TOP SHELVES IN COMBINED LOADS

B

FIGURE 4-31. *A*, Steam gradually displacing air from chamber (Courtesy of AMSCO, Erie, Pennsylvania) *B*, Metal supplies should be placed *below* fabric. (Courtesy of AMSCO, Erie, Pennsylvania and Mary A. Seithers, Baylor Media Services)

EXPOSURE   Steam continues to enter the chamber increasing the internal pressure. This pressure causes the temperature to increase attaining the preset sterilization temperature. This load must now be heated to the preset sterilization temperature for the minimum time required to destroy the highly resistant spores of *Bacillus stearothermophilus*. The temperature must be consistent throughout the cycle in order to be effective. The gravity displacement sterilizer

TABLE 4-5. **TIME AND TEMPERATURE EXPOSURES FOR WRAPPED ITEMS**

STERILIZER TYPE (OR CYCLE)	TEMPERATURE	TIME (MINUTES)
Gravity-displacement	270°F–275°F (132°C–135°C)	10–25 15—typical for wrapped instrument/container sets and wrapped basins*
	250°F (121°C)	15–30 30—typical for all wrapped items, linen, and so forth
Prevacuum	270°F–275°F (132°C–135°C)	4

*Reichert, 1993.
Note: Sterilization container systems or powered surgical instruments may require an extended exposure period. The manufacturer's instructions and established hospital policies for exposure guidelines should be followed.

has a longer conditioning and exposure phase because of the slower heating and air evacuation process. AORN suggests common temperature and time guidelines for gravity and prevacuum cycles (Table 4-5).

EXHAUST PHASE   When the exposure time has elapsed, the bottom drain in the sterilizer opens and steam is exhausted. The chamber then returns to atmospheric pressure as filtered air re-enters. If no drying time is needed, the cycle is complete as later explained with the sterilization of unwrapped items.

DRYING PHASE   As the pressure regulates within the chamber, the filtered dry heat along with the existing heat of the chamber will revaporize existing moisture and remove it from the contents of the load. If an abundance of moisture is formed during conditioning, the heated air presented in this phase may not be sufficient and wet packs will result. Proper loading techniques will result in dry articles at the end of a cycle.

Flash sterilization is used in special clinical situations: when there is no alternative and time does not allow an item to be processed by the conventional wrapped method. The items are usually not wrapped, but placed in an opened mesh bottom tray for adequate contact of steam. (Some facilities may have a container system specifically designed for flashing instruments and transport.) Items are usually wet at the completion of a flash cycle, due to little or no drying time. A single wrapped method may be employed in situations only if supported by the sterilizer manufacturer's instructions. Items processed in a flash sterilization cycle should be utilized immediately, with no indication of shelf life. They should be transported to the point of use as safely and effectively as possible, eliminating all potential means of contamination. The encompassing practices that surround this process, such as proper cleaning and methods of transport, are often lacking in their efficacy and may require some reassessment. Considerations for evaluating effective flash sterilization practices are as follows:

- Proper cleaning and decontamination practices
- Location of sterilizer—close proximity to point of use, in a restricted, low traffic area away from splashing and aerosolization
- Adequate monitoring of sterilizer and verification of cycle parameters
- Method of transport (influenced by location of sterilizer)—sterilizer container system, open or covered system, single wrapped method (with specific manufacturer's instructions)
- Air exchange and air filtration of transport area
- Immediate use, no shelf life.

Following the recommended guidelines, flash sterilization is a safe and effective sterilization process. The AAMI recommended guidelines for flash sterilization are given in Table 4-6.

TABLE 4–6. **TIME AND TEMPERATURE EXPOSURES FOR FLASH STERILIZATION OF UNWRAPPED ITEMS**

STERILIZER TYPE (OR CYCLE)	TEMPERATURE	TIME (MINUTES)
Gravity-displacement	270°F–275°F (132°C–135°C)	3—metal instruments, no porous items or lumens
		10—metal instruments/with lumens, porous items (i.e. rubber, plastic)
Prevacuum	270°F–275°F (132°C–135°C)	3—metal instruments, no porous items or lumens
		4—metal instruments/with lumens, porous items (i.e. rubber, plastic)

Note: The Centers for Disease Control and Prevention (CDC) recommend that implantable items should not be flash sterilized (Garner, 1985).

Proper Loading Techniques

Understanding the fundamentals of steam sterilization, the perioperative nurse can more effectively plan and implement correct loading techniques. Preventing the formation of air pockets and obstructions to the circulation of steam will facilitate conditions for an optimal steam sterilization cycle.

Considerations for correct loading techniques include

- Linen packs—positioned laterally on loading rack with ample space between each pack
- Basins and solid-bottom trays—positioned on edge, to allow drainage of moisture
- Load containing fabric and metal items—metal supplies placed *below* fabric, to prevent condensate from contacting other items in the load (Fig. 4–31B).
- Peel packages—placed in wire mesh basket designed to allow adequate spacing and maintain position of edge—all packages positioned in the same direction to allow circulation of the sterilant.

Proper Unloading Techniques

After the cooled loading rack is removed from the sterilizer, it should be placed in a well-monitored sterile storage area. The hot packages are allowed to cool before being handled; otherwise, moisture will form upon contact and cause contamination (strikethrough) of the contents. In addition, the perioperative nurse should not place hot items on metal or cool surfaces, because the formation of condensation will contaminate the sterile package.

ETHYLENE OXIDE STERILIZATION

Ethylene oxide is a colorless, noncorrosive, and highly penetrative gas common in health care facilities. The significance of ethylene oxide is its ability to sterilize materials that are sensitive to high concentrations of moisture and/or heat without causing damage or deterioration. It can be used in 100% concentrations or in mixtures with inert diluent gases such as EO/hydrochlorofluorocarbon (HCFC).

Note: Ethylene oxide causes microbial destruction by a process known as alkylation. With the appropriate conditions of time, temperature, EO concentration, and relative humidity, a chemical exchange develops. This alteration (exchange of hydrogen atoms) results in the inability of a cell to normally metabolize and/or reproduce (Perkins, 1983).

Owing to its toxic nature, appropriate aeration is required to remove residual EO from the contents at the completion of a cycle. Improper usage or handling can present a hazard to patients and health care workers who are involved in EO processing or handling EO sterilized materials (Code of Federal Regulations, 1992). Because EO exhibits toxic and flammable properties, it must be handled by highly trained personnel.

The efficacy of EO sterilization is based on four major components: *time, temperature, EO concentration, and relative humidity.* Exposure times usually range from 105 to 300 minutes. They are greatly influenced by the remaining three components (AAMI, ST 41, 1992). Variations in the density, permeability, and configuration of items to be processed are all important factors related to penetration of the sterilant. The temperature determines the amount of time necessary for EO exposure. A lower temperature requires a longer exposure period. By increasing the concentration of gas, the rate of cellular inactivation also increases. Humidity (45% to 74%) is needed to condition or moisten the cell. This factor enables EO to penetrate the cellular walls, resulting in microbial destruction.

Note: The sterilizer operator should always refer to the manufacturer's instructions for specific cycle parameters.

Loading Procedures

Items are placed on metal racks or in wire baskets in a manner that facilitates air removal, maintenance of humidity, EO penetration, and removal of the sterilant during aeration. Peel packages are vertically positioned with the plastic sides facing the same direction. Instrument sets are placed flat on the loading basket. The operator should refer to the manufacturer's instructions for loading recommendations for rigid container systems. Care must be taken to avoid overloading the chamber, which can compromise the efficacy of the cycle.

100% EO

As previously stated, EO is supplied in 100% concentration or in mixtures with inert gases. The 100% EO is provided in small unit dose cartridges containing less than 5 fluid ounces. This may vary with size of chamber (Figs. 4–32, 4–33). It is used in small nonpressurized automatic sterilizers. The cartridge is positioned in its holder within the chamber. Once the door is locked and vacuum is sufficient, the cartridge is punctured and vaporized EO is released.

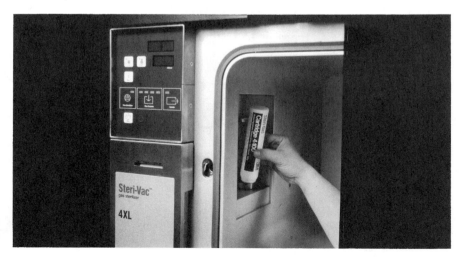

FIGURE 4–32. 100% EO Sterilizer/Aerator (Courtesy of 3M Health Care, St. Paul, Minnesota)

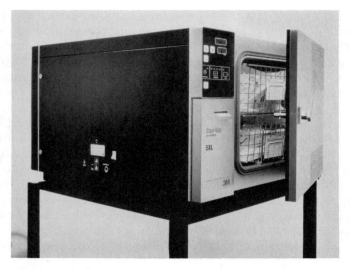

FIGURE 4-33. 100% EO Sterilizer/Aerator (Courtesy of 3M Health Care, St. Paul, Minnesota)

Note: If the cartridge is mishandled and accidentally punctured into open air space (other than a confined small area), the amount of EO in the cartridge would not produce the flammability range of 3.6% in air (Danielson, 1986). The National Fire Protection Agency places 100% EO in the class I flammable liquid category. Their guidelines and the instructions of the supplier of EO should be followed for safe storage practices.

Cycle Phases/100% EO Sterilizers

The unit dose cartridge is correctly positioned in the carrier of a loaded chamber. The door is locked, initiating the preconditioning phase. Automatic air evacuation occurs within the chamber and its contents. Preheating and moisture intro-

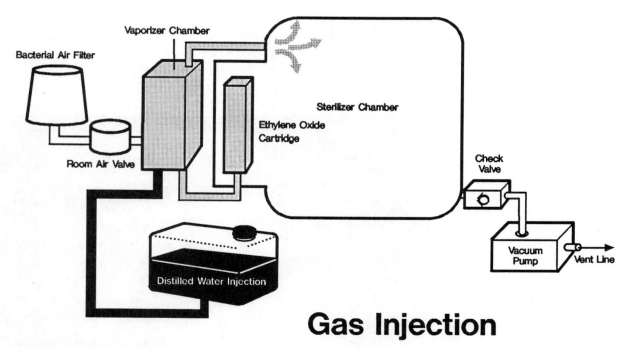

FIGURE 4-34. Gas Injection in 100% EO Sterilizer (Courtesy of 3M Health Care, St. Paul, Minnesota)

TABLE 4-7. **APPROXIMATE TIME AND TEMPERATURES FOR 100% EO STERILIZERS**

Warm cycle	55°C	2 hr 45 min
Cool cycle	37°C	4 hr 45 min

Note: Times and temperatures may vary with each sterilizer.

duction (45%–55% humidity) prepare the items for exposure to the sterilant. Following preconditioning, the cartridge is automatically punctured, and EO permeates items within the chamber (Fig. 4–34). The time and temperature are preset and automatically controlled by the sterilizer (Table 4–7). These units operate under negative pressure throughout the cycle. If a leak develops, air is drawn into the sterilizer instead of the EO escaping out into the work area. At the end of the exposure phase, purge cycles begin to remove the gas. The sterilization cycle is complete. Aeration is needed to further reduce EO residuals to a safe level.

HCFC/EO

The flammable and explosive properties of EO are greatly reduced when it is contained in a mixture of hydrochlorofluorocarbons (HCFC). The proposed HCFC/EO is a 91/9 combination, 91% HCFC to 9% EO (3M, 1993). Owing to concerns that HCFCs are ozone-depleting chemicals, the Clean Air Act passed in 1990 proclaimed their phaseout to begin in 2015 with production to end in 2030. As research continues to focus on environmental issues, such as ozone depletion, restrictions presumably will become more severe.

This mixture, HCFC/EO, is contained in large compressed-gas tanks or cylinders and is utilized in sterilizers, usually larger than 5 cubic square feet, requiring a mild amount of pressure (Fig. 4–35). These supply tanks must be

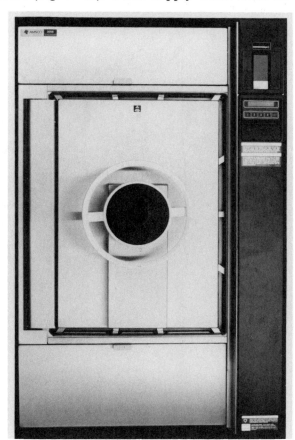

FIGURE 4-35. EO Sterilizer/Aerator uses EO mixture (Courtesy of AMSCO, Erie, Pennsylvania)

changed by educated personnel who follow safety and protective guidelines as established by OSHA and recommended by the sterilizer manufacturer. The Environmental Protection Agency (EPA), under the Federal Insecticide, Fungicide and Rodenticide Act, classifies ethylene oxide as a pesticide. All manufacturers of EO must have their products registered by the EPA. All containers of EO should have an approved EPA label. If there are signs of alterations on the label, the container should not be used and should be immediately returned to the supplier.

Cycle Phases/EO Sterilizers Using HCFC-124

Supply tanks containing EO mixtures are usually located in a recessed area or separate room with adequate ventilation. They must be stored in upright position, secured by safety chains or straps to a solid structure (Fig. 4–36). This protects the valves from damage, reducing potential EO exposure. Preconditioning begins with air evacuation from the chamber. Pulses of steam begin to heat and humidify the contents. A predetermined amount of EO is released and circulates throughout the chamber, permeating porous items within the load. Positive pressure is maintained during this period. Purging cycles remove EO from the contents. Filtered air is admitted into the chamber, returning it to atmospheric pressure. This completes the sterilization cycle. Items must be prepared for aeration, by either remaining in the sterilizer or being transferred to an aerator, depending on the needs of the facility and the capability of the sterilizer.

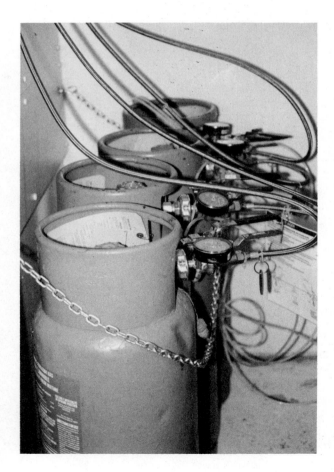

FIGURE 4–36. Supply cylinders properly secured

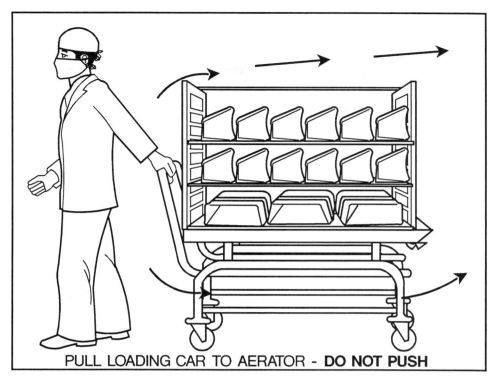

PULL LOADING CAR TO AERATOR - **DO NOT PUSH**

FIGURE 4–37. Proper Transfer of Sterilized Items from Sterilizer to Aerator (Courtesy of AMSCO, Erie, Pennsylvania and Mary A. Seithers, Baylor Media Services)

Unloading EO Sterilized Items and Transfer to Aerator

If items remain in the chamber, levels of EO may increase owing to degassing. This is why it is critical that the contents be unloaded and transferred immediately following a sterilization cycle. OSHA requires the worker to wear appropriate personal protective attire when transferring the basket or contents of the sterilizer. Special EO-resistant rubber or butyl gloves are recommended. When moving a loading rack, it should be *pulled* and not pushed (Fig. 4–37). The air flow and offgassing should move away from the operator, reducing EO exposure.

Aeration

It is critical that every item sterilized with EO, *including implants*, undergo aeration to remove EO and its by-products to a safe level both for the worker and the patient. Continuous currents of warm filtered air act to remove EO, usually over a 12-hour period at a temperature of 50°C (120°F) or an 8-hour period with the aerator at a temperature of 60°C (140°F). Effective aeration times depend on many variables:

- the size and composition of the items and the wrapping material
- the arrangement of items within the aerator as well as the permeability of each.

Specific parameters of the sterilization cycle should be taken into account before setting aeration times and temperatures.

Note: When preparations are made for sterilization, all items should be dry before being placed in the sterilizer. If an item contains an excess amount of moisture because personnel used improper techniques or an inadequate aeration cycle, a toxic by-product, ethyl glycol, is formed. This may not be reduced during aeration and may cause chemical irritation or burn to the worker or patient (Danielson, 1986).

Environmental Monitoring

PERSONNEL MONITORING   When working in an environment with toxic chemicals or gases such as EO, the concentration of airborne contaminants in the breathing zone of individual workers must be identified.

- An EO-exposure monitoring device, which detects exposure levels of EO, is worn for an 8-hour shift. The monitor is interpreted and the results are expressed as a time-weighted average (TWA) concentration.
- Permissible exposure limits (PEL) as described by OSHA, state that "no employee is exposed to an airborne concentration of EO in excess of *one (1) part EO per million parts of air as an 8 hour time-weighted average*" (Code of Federal Regulations, 1992).
- The term "action level" refers to airborne EO concentrations of 0.5 parts per million (ppm) as an 8-hour TWA. If personnel exposure is revealed to be at or above the action level, but equal to or below the TWA, monitoring must be repeated at least every 6 months. If concentrations are greater than the 8-hour TWA, monitoring should be repeated at least every 3 months.
- No employee should be exposed to EO concentrations in excess of 5 parts of EO per million parts of air (5 ppm) as averaged over 15-minute short-term exposures. If these results were above the 15-minute exposure level, they should be repeated at least every 3 months. Refer to the Code of Federal Regulations, 29 CFR 1910.1047, *Ethylene Oxide*, for further information.
- The employee shall be notified in writing of monitoring results.

ENVIRONMENTAL MONITORING   General concentrations of EO also need to be identified in the work area where EO processing is performed. Monitoring devices containing single and multipoint sampling detectors are placed throughout the work area, especially in the immediate area of the sterilizers. By continuously monitoring the airborne EO concentrations, these sensitive detectors will produce an alarm in the event of EO exposures. Health care facilities should have written policies for implementing safety and emergency measures when there is evidence of EO exposure.

Ventilation

Compliance with federal standards regarding effective ventilation of EO from the workplace is the responsibility of the health care facility. Even though EO sterilizers should be located in a well-ventilated area (10 or more air exchanges per hour), all airflow patterns must be directed to minimize possible exposure to the employees. A venting system includes exhaust to the outside air and an emission control system that is monitored by the Clean Air Emission Division of the EPA.

A potential source of EO exposure occurs during the process of changing the compressed gas cylinders. Only educated employees who have a working knowledge of the safety practices and hazardous properties of EO should be allowed to perform this task. Protective clothing and respirator requirements as stated by OSHA should be worn before disconnecting the supply cylinder or any part of the supply line in sterilizers using EO mixtures.

Health Hazards of EO

Studies have shown exposures of ethylene oxide to be associated with multiple diseases such as cancer, reproductive disorders, chromosome damage, and neurotoxicity. Overexposure to EO in the liquid form may cause eye irritations or corneal injury. Contact with the skin could develop into irritation, blistering, or frostbite. Respiratory irritation, lung injury, headache, and nausea are health hazards from overexposure to ethylene oxide vapors. All employees working with ethylene oxide must be made aware of the potential health hazards. OSHA requires that notice of EO hazards be posted in regulated areas or entrances to regulated areas. Signs must contain the following information:

> Danger: ethylene oxide
>
> Cancer hazard and reproductive hazard
>
> Authorized personnel only
>
> Respirators and protective clothing may be required to be worn in this area

OSHA's Hazard and Communication Standard

All containers of EO that have a potential for causing employee exposure must be appropriately labeled with a warning against inhaling airborne concentrations and the following:

> Danger: contains ethylene oxide
>
> Cancer hazard and reproductive hazard

- The employer should have appropriate documentation of individual and environmental monitoring results.
- Material safety data sheets from the manufacturers of EO should be on file and made available to all employees.
- Employees are to attend training programs before they are assigned to work areas with the potential for exposure to ethylene oxide.

Emergency First Aid Procedures

Eye Exposure: Eyes are washed with copious amounts of water flushing both upper and lower eyelids, followed by immediate medical attention. Contact lenses should not be worn in areas where EO is used.

Skin Exposure: Exposed area should be washed immediately in a deluge shower if necessary. If clothing has been penetrated, it can easily ignite, so immediately remove it while in a deluge shower. Contaminated shoes are also removed. Leather shoes can absorb and retain EO and need to be discarded if contaminated.

Inhalation: Move to fresh air immediately; if breathing has stopped, initiate cardiopulmonary resuscitation. Immediate medical assistance is needed.

Swallowing: The person should be given large amounts of water, and vomiting should be induced. Immediate medical attention is needed.

Rescue: The affected person should be moved away from the hazardous exposure area. If he/she has been overcome, another person should be notified before initiating emergency rescue procedures.

OSHA has developed specific regulations purposed to establish a safe working environment and work practices for all who work with EO.

PERACETIC ACID STERILIZATION

Peracetic acid (PA) is a chemical compound composed of acetic acid, hydrogen peroxide, and water (Crow, 1992). This oxidizing agent adversely reacts with the protein and enzymes of a microorganism, penetrating the cell wall and causing destruction (Janssen, 1992).

The sterilant is provided in a tamperproof, unit dose concentration of 35% PA and anticorrosive agents. It is utilized in a tabletop sterile processor, designed to sterilize a variety of endoscopic devices, cameras, and accessories (Fig. 4–38). Processing trays designed for flexible endoscopes and transport trays designed for rigid scopes and their accessories are unique to this sterilizer. As with any other sterilization process, the instruments need to be cleaned and prepared according to the manufacturer's instructions before being placed into the unit. The unit dose container of PA is secured in a designated location within the sterilizer. Pulsating streams of hot water and PA flow within the contents of the tray, contacting all surfaces. This phase is followed by a sterile water rinse. During a cycle, the sterilant mixes with water, which reduces the concentration to 0.2%. The entire process takes less than 30 minutes, depending on the water pressure and the time needed to achieve an adequate temperature level. This sterilizer is equipped with a computerized printout, documenting the process parameters. An area is provided for the operator to initial for verification that the parameters were met. Biologic and chemical monitors are available to test the efficacy of the

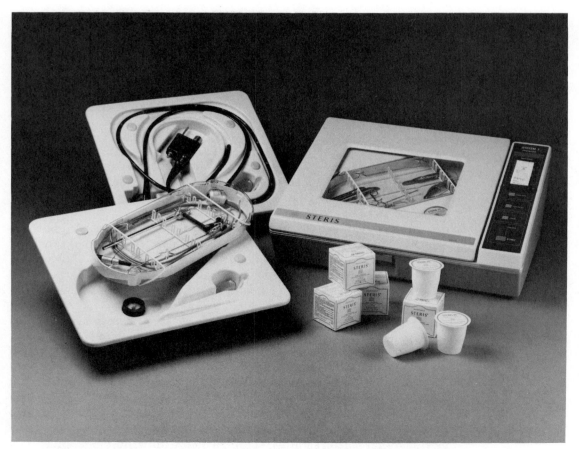

FIGURE 4–38. Steris System Processor and Accessories (Courtesy of STERIS Corporation, Mentor, Ohio)

cycle and sporicidal properties of the sterilant. Peracetic acid is recognized by the Federal Food and Drug Administration as an effective means of sterilization. Endoscopic instruments can be safely sterilized in an automatic, cost-effective, tabletop sterilizer.

HYDROGEN PEROXIDE GAS PLASMA STERILIZATION

Hydrogen peroxide gas plasma is a new sterilization technology that rapidly destroys microorganisms utilizing low temperatures without leaving toxic residues on sterilized items. It is purposed for heat- and moisture-sensitive items. The ambient temperature in the chamber is less than 50°C in a low-moisture cycle.

Plasma is a fourth state of matter, distinguished from solid, liquid, and gas (Jacobs, 1993). Naturally occurring plasma is found throughout the universe. An example of plasma that occurs on earth is the aurora borealis or the northern lights.

In this technology (Fig. 4–39), plasma is generated by the introduction of radio frequency energy to vaporize hydrogen peroxide. Through this reaction and secondary reactions, a variety of reactive species are formed that collide and/or react with and kill microorganisms. This high energy state produces a visible glow. The activated particles recombine to form oxygen, water, and other nontoxic by-products. The plasma state exists for the amount of time required to achieve sterilization and remove residuals.

Cycle Phases

- A cassette containing 58% aqueous hydrogen peroxide is properly positioned in the sterilizer. Safeguards built into the system prevent direct contact with or exposure to hydrogen peroxide. Decontaminated items, wrapped or assembled in special tray systems, are placed in the plasma sterilizer chamber. The chamber door is secured, and a vacuum is initiated.

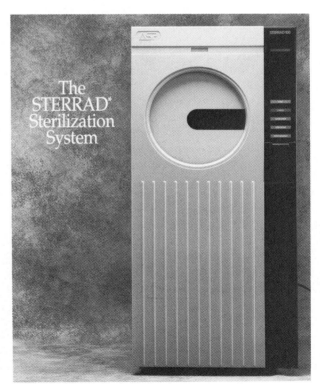

FIGURE 4–39. Low Temperature Plasma Sterilization (Courtesy of Advanced Sterilization Products, Irvine, California)

- Hydrogen peroxide is automatically injected and vaporized within the chamber, surrounding all items to be sterilized.
- Radio frequency energy is applied, creating low-temperature gas plasma.
- During this plasma phase, sterilization occurs. Reactive species are formed that interact with cellular membranes and disrupt the life functions of microorganisms (Jacobs, 1993). These reactive particles recombine to form predominately oxygen and water as by-products.
- Following the sterilization phase, the radio frequency energy is turned off. The vacuum is released, and the chamber returns to atmospheric pressure.

This method of sterilization occurs over approximately 1 hour. It is indicated for metal and nonmetal instruments and supplies, with the exception of linens, other cellulosic materials, powders, and liquids. This system necessitates the use of nonwoven polypropylene wrapping material or specific instrument tray systems (refer to manufacturer's recommendations). For narrow lumens that are longer than 12 inches (31 cm) or narrower than ¼ inch (6 mm), a special adaptor is needed to ensure sterilization of the lumens.

Chemical and biologic (*Bacillus subtilis*) indicators specifically designed for this sterilizer must be employed. As with other sterilizers, it is important for the health care worker to monitor and document results of chemical, biologic, and mechanical monitors.

Hydrogen peroxide gas plasma as a sterilant received FDA clearance in 1993. It is considered to be environmentally safe and effective as a noncorrosive agent for heat- and moisture-sensitive devices.

Factors of Disinfection

Disinfection is defined as the destruction of microorganisms by thermal and chemical means. It is not as lethal a process as sterilization because of its inability to kill large populations of microbial spores. Cellular destruction occurs with the coagulation of protein within the cells (Perkins, 1983). The major differences between sterilization and disinfection are found in Figure 4–1 of this chapter.

Every disinfectant should have an EPA registration number. The label must list the active chemicals and their range of biocidal activity (fungicidal, bactericidal, virucidal, or sporicidal). Some high-level disinfectants have the ability to kill all classes of microorganisms *only upon extended exposure*, as in 2% glutaraldehyde. The perioperative nurse must check the manufacturer's instructions for specific concentrations and exposure times.

Safety precautions should be established in the policies and procedures of every department utilizing chemical disinfectants. The health care worker should wear personal protective equipment (gloves, eye protection, masks) when performing a procedure. This should be done in a well-ventilated area with at least ten air exchanges per hour, or under a vent hood to remove possible hazardous vapors from the chemical. There are several issues affecting the efficacy of the disinfectant that the user must know. The perioperative nurse should know the answers to the following questions about using a disinfectant:

- What are the label claims for microbicidal activity?
- Is this a single-use disinfectant or can it be reused? What is the activated life expectancy?
- Is the user wearing the appropriate personal protective equipment?
- Has the item to be disinfected been thoroughly cleaned and dried?
- What are the manufacturer's recommendations concerning temperature and exposure times?
- Does exposure to light decrease the effectiveness of the disinfectant? Does the soak container have a lid with a secure fit?

- Is the procedure for rinsing effective for the removal of residual disinfectant solution?
- Does the health care facility have specific policies regarding work practices when implementing the disinfection process?

Semicritical medical devices contaminated with blood or body fluids from patients infected with HIV or HBV or with pulmonary tuberculosis are also effectively inactivated by chemical germicides with the capability of high-level disinfection (Rutala, 1990). Glutaraldehyde (2%) is a widely used high-level disinfectant for endoscopic instruments that do not enter a sterile cavity (i. e., semicritical). Care should be taken to effectively clean and dry these delicate instruments without causing damage to the workmanship. The manufacturer's recommendations should be consulted for the appropriate immersion time to insure high-level disinfection.

Many chemical disinfectants are used in health care facilities. The Association for Practitioners in Infection Control, Inc. (APIC) guidelines for selection and use of disinfectants provide information on chemical disinfectants and their usage. Establishing safe and effective practices of infection control will continue to be one of the major goals of perioperative nursing.

Note: The organism that causes Creutzfeldt-Jakob disease may not be inactivated by a high-level disinfection procedure. Items possibly contaminated with this disease must be sterilized according to recommendations mentioned earlier in this chapter.

Postoperative Disinfection of Operating Room Equipment

The operating room environment should be kept as free from exogenous microorganisms as possible. One of the first postoperative activities the perioperative nurse should perform is to clean and disinfect furniture, equipment, surgical lights, positioning aids, and other items needed during the procedure (Fig. 4–40).

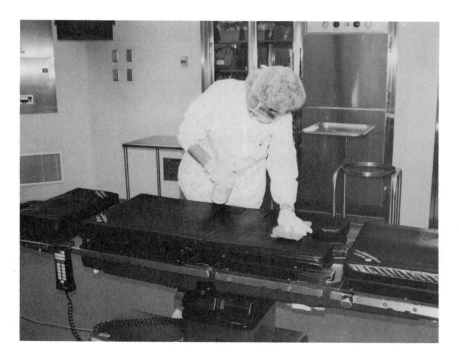

FIGURE 4–40. Disinfecting Operating Room Equipment

METHODS OF STERILIZATION AND DISINFECTION

Object	STERILIZATION		DISINFECTION		
	Critical items (will enter tissue or vascular system or blood will flow through them)		High level (semicritical items; will come in contact with mucous membrane or nonintact skin)	Intermediate level (some semicritical items, and noncritical items)	Low level (noncritical items, will come in contact with intact skin)
	Procedure	Exposure time (hr)	Procedure (exposure time ≥ 20 min)[b,c]	Procedure (exposure time ≤ 10 min)	Procedure (exposure time ≤ 10 min)
Smooth, hard surface[a]	A	MR	C	H	H
	B	MR	D	K	I
	C	MR	E	K	J
	D	6	F[d]		K
	E	6	G		L
Rubber tubing and catheters[c]	A	MR	C		
	B	MR	D		
	C	MR	E		
	D	6	F[d]		
	E	6			
Polyethylene tubing and catheters[c,e]	A	MR	C		
	B	MR	D		
	C	MR	E		
	D	6	F[d]		
	E	6			
Lensed instruments	B	MR	C		
	C	MR	D		
	D	6	E		
	E	6			
Thermometers (oral and rectal)[f]				H[f]	
Hinged instruments	A	MR	C		
	B	MR	D		
	C	MR	E		
	D	6			
	E	6			

Modified from Rutala, W. A. In Wenzel, R. P., ed. (1987). *Prevention and Control of Nosocomial Infections.* Baltimore: Williams & Wilkins. (pp. 257–282) and from Simmons, B. P. (1983). *Am J Infect Control* 11:96–115.

A, Heat sterilization, including steam or hot air (see manufacturer's recommendations)
B, Ethylene oxide gas (see manufacturer's recommendations)
C, Glutaraldehyde-based formulations (2%) (A glutaraldehyde-phenate formulation at full strength also has been shown to sterilize items that are soaked for 6 ¾ hours. Caution should be exercised with all glutaraldehyde formulations when further in-use dilution is anticipated.)
D, Demand-release chlorine dioxide (will corrode aluminum, copper, brass, series 400 stainless steel, and chrome, with prolonged exposure)
E, Stabilized hydrogen peroxide 6% (will corrode copper, zinc, and brass)
F, Wet pasteurization at 75°C for 30 minutes after detergent cleaning
G, Sodium hypochlorite (1000 ppm available chlorine; will corrode metal instruments)
H, Ethyl or isopropyl alcohol (70% to 90%)
I, Sodium hypochlorite (100 ppm available chlorine)
J, Phenolic germicidal detergent solution (follow product label for use-dilution)
K, Iodophor germicidal detergent solution (follow product label for use-dilution)
L, Quaternary ammonium germicidal detergent solution (follow product label for use-dilution)
MR, Manufacturer's recommendations.

[a]See referenced text for discussion of hydrotherapy.
[b]The longer the exposure to a disinfectant, the more likely it is that all microorganisms will be eliminated. Ten minutes' exposure is not adequate to disinfect many objects, especially those which are difficult to clean, because they have narrow channels or other areas that can harbor organic material and bacteria. Twenty minutes' exposure may be the minimum time needed to reliably kill *M. tuberculosis* with glutaraldehyde.
[c]Tubing must be completely filled for disinfection; care must be taken to avoid entrapment of air bubbles during immersion.
[d]Pasteurization (washer disinfector) of respiratory therapy and anesthesia equipment is a recognized alternative to high-level disinfection. Some data challenge the efficacy of some pasteurization units.
[e]Thermostability should be investigated when indicated.
[f]Limited data suggest that at least 20 minutes' exposure time is necessary. Do not mix rectal and oral thermometers at any stage of handling or processing. From Rutala, W. A. (1990). APIC guidelines for selection and use of disinfectants, *American Journal of Infection Control, 18*(2), 99–117.

A tuberculocidal chemical disinfectant will greatly reduce the risk of contamination between patient and health care worker.

Personal protective equipment should be worn to prevent direct exposure to blood or body fluids while cleaning. This includes

- gloves
- gown

- protective eyewear
- face shield or mask.

A lint-free cloth moistened with a disinfectant solution should be used to clean items and remove bacteria. Mechanical friction and scrubbing enhances the effectiveness of cleaning. The table and footstools are commonly contaminated with blood and body fluids during a surgical procedure and may require initial cleaning before disinfection (Fig. 4–40). The surgical team must employ safe practices while preparing the operating room.

- All contaminated disposable items are placed in leakproof, tear-resistant, labeled containers to prevent personnel and environmental contamination.
- Contaminated linen is handled as little as possible and discarded in labeled or color-coded leakproof bags or containers. This safely confines and contains potentially infectious microorganisms.
- Disposable sharps should be placed in puncture-resistant, labeled hazardous-waste containers.
- Specimens should be placed in clean, leakproof, labeled hazardous-waste containers for transport. It is important to keep the outside of the container as well as the lab forms or requisitions free from contaminants.
- Suction canisters should be secured and sealed for transport.
- All exposed instrumentation should be contained in a way that prevents inadvertent personnel contact or exposure.
- The floor should be cleaned with hospital-grade disinfectant/detergent to remove soil and debris. A wet-vacuum system is recommended as the most effective means of sanitization (AORN, 1994).

Cleaning and disinfection of operating room equipment, furniture, and other items should occur immediately following the transfer of each patient. This provides a safe environment for the patient and health care worker.

Note: Packaged sterilized items that have been issued to an operating room and not used, as long as the integrity of the package has not been altered, may be returned to sterile storage. However, the package must be intact with no evidence of contamination (AAMI, SSSA, 1992).

Achieving Competency in Sterilization and Disinfection Practices

In-service and education training programs should be an annual requirement of all staff involved with decontamination, sterile processing, and disinfection. Quality improvement programs and documentation of competency in these practices are critical for the safety of the worker as well as the patient. Some areas to consider are

- education and in-service training on all processing equipment with follow-up on the implementation of correct practices
- problem solving techniques and/or correct reporting policies
- availability of manufacturer's instructions and recommendations for equipment, sterilant, and sterilization supplies for all staff
- annual review of written policies and protocol on methods of sterilization and disinfection
- thorough orientation program for new employees
- annual review of safety practices
- Compliance with OSHA regulations and standards on bloodborne pathogens (29 CFR part 1910) concerning chemicals in hospital sterilization and disinfection processing.

ISSUES FOR FUTURE DEVELOPMENT

Sterilization technology continues to develop as medical devices and instruments become so highly specialized. Practicality, cost-effectiveness, and environmental safety are among the greatest concerns health care facilities voice reguarding sterilization.

Ethylene oxide sterilization has undergone many changes and will continue to replace the HCFC/EO mixture, which has a phase-out date of year 2030 or sooner. EO/CO_2 (10% EO/90% CO_2) mixtures are being re-introduced to replace HCFCs. This is not a new technology. It may prove to be more environmentally safe but would result in increasing sterilization times by 50% (3M, 1993).

As perioperative nurses, it is crucial to remain current on issues affecting sterilization and disinfection. This enables the quality of patient care to continue to reach its highest level.

REFERENCES

3M Health Care Div. St. Paul, MN. (1993). Low temperature sterilization technologies in the 1990's. *Infection Control Rounds, 16*(3), 9–11.

3M Medical-Surgical Division. (1992). Steri-Vac 5XL Gas Sterilizer/Aerator Operator's Manual. St. Paul, MN. (pp. 7–27).

American Society for Healthcare Central Service Personnel. (1986). *Training Manual for Central Service Technicians.* Chicago: American Hospital Association.

American Society for Hospital Central Service Personnel (ASHCSP). (1986). *Ethylene Oxide Use in Hospitals.* (2nd ed). Chicago: American Hospital Association.

Association for the Advancement of Medical Instrumentation. (1992). *Good Hospital Practice: Ethylene Oxide Gas—Ventilation Recommendations and Use.* GVR. Vol. 1: Sterilization. Arlington, Va.: AAMI. (pp. 409–423).

Association for the Advancement of Medical Instrumentation. (1992). *Good Hospital Practice: Ethylene Oxide Sterilization and Sterility Assurance.* ST 41. Vol. 1: Sterilization. Arlington, Va.: AAMI. (pp. 371–395).

Association for the Advancement of Medical Instrumentation. (1992). *Good Hospital Practice: Flash Sterilization—Steam Sterilization of Patient Care Items for Immediate Use.* ST 37. Vol. 1: Sterilization. Arlington, Va.: AAMI. (pp. 203–215).

Association for the Advancement Medical Instrumentation. (1992). *Good Hospital Practice: Handling and Biologic Decontamination of Reusable Devices.* ST 35. Vol. 1: Sterilization. Arlington, Va.: AAMI. (pp. 677–689).

Association for the Advancement of Medical Instrumentation. (1992). *Selection and Use of Chemical Indicators for Steam Sterilization Monitoring in Health Care Facilities.* TIR 3. Vol. 1: Sterilization. Arlington, Va.: AAMI. (pp. 225–265).

Association for the Advancement of Medical Instrumentation (AAMI). (1992). *Good Hospital Practice: Steam Sterilization and Sterility Assurance.* SSSA. Vol. 1: Sterilization. Arlington, Va: AAMI. (pp. 159–191).

Association of Operating Room Nurses. (1994a). *Standards and Recommended Practices. Recommended Practices for Care of Instruments, Scopes, and Powered Surgical Instruments.* Denver: AORN. (pp. 177–184).

Association of Operating Room Nurses. (1994b). *Standards and Recommended Practices. Recommended Practices for Sanitation in the Surgical Practice Setting.* Denver: AORN. (pp. 227–232).

Association of Operating Room Nurses. (1994c). *Standards and Recommended Practices. Recommended Practices for Selection and Use of Packaging Systems.* Denver: AORN. (pp. 201–205).

Association of Operating Room Nurses. (1994d). *Standards and Recommended Practices. Recommended Practices for Sterilization, Steam and Ethylene Oxide (EO).* Denver: AORN. (pp. 245–252).

Centers for Disease Control. (1981). *Guidelines for the Prevention and Control of Nosocomial Infections.* Atlanta: U.S. Department of Health and Human Services, Public Health Services, Centers for Disease Control and Prevention.

Code of Federal Regulations. Occupational Safety and Health Administration. (1992). Title 29, Chapter XVII, 1910.1030 *Bloodborne Pathogens* (pp. 306–322) and 1910.1047 *Ethylene Oxide* (pp. 231–243). Washington, DC: Office of the Federal Register.

Crow, S. (1992). Peracetic acid sterilization: a timely development for a busy healthcare industry. *Infection Control and Hospital Epidemiology, 13*(2), 111–113.

Danielson, N. E. (1986). *Ethylene Oxide Use in Hospitals.* 2nd Edition, American Society for Hospital Central Service Personnel of the American Hospital Association. American Hospital Publishing, Inc. (pp. 5–137).

Garner, J. S., Favero, M. S. (1985). *Guideline for Handwashing and Hospital Environmental Control.* Atlanta: U.S. Department of Health and Human Services, Public Health Services, Centers for Disease Control and Prevention. (pp. 1–20).

Jacobs, Paul T. (1993). A New Technology for Instrument Sterilization, STERRAD Sterilization System. Johnson & Johnson. Advanced Sterilization Products. Mission Viejo, Ca: (pp. 1–12).

Jacobs, Paul T. (1993). Plasma sterilization. EtO Alternatives. Johnson & Johnson. Advanced Sterilization Products. Mission Viejo, Ca.

Janssen, D. W., Schneider, P. M. (1992). Cold sterilization beyond 1995: a look at the alternatives to 12/88 EtO. *Journal of Healthcare Materiel Management, 10*(8), 31–59.

Johnson, M. E. et al. (1992). Sterilization methods keeping up with health trends. *Review & Outlook, 3*(1), 1–2.

Mathias, J. M. (1992). Sterility assurance replaces expiration dating. O.R. Manager, *8*(3), 1–3.

Perkins, J. L. (1983). Principles and Methods of Sterilization in Health Sciences. (2nd ed). Springfield, Il.: Charles C. Thomas. (pp. 312–326).

Reichert, R., Young, J. H. (1993). *Sterilization Technology for the Health Care Facility.* Gaithersburg, Md.: Aspen Publishers, Inc.

Rutala, W. A. (1990). APIC guidelines for selection and use of disinfectants. *American Journal of Infection Control, 18*(2), 99–117.

Rutala, W. A. et al. (1991). Disinfection practices for endoscopes and other semicritical items. *Infection Control and Hospital Epidemiology, 12*(5), 282–287.

Practice Scenario 1
Sterilization/Disinfection: Equipment and Instruments

by Barbara Crim, RN, MBA

PATIENT SCENARIO

Jack Thornhill is a 28-year-old white male motorcycle enthusiast. He received a compound fracture of his right tibia and fibula and compound fracture of his left ankle 2 years ago in a motor vehicle accident. At that time, his tibia and fibula were treated with a closed reduction and cast application. The left ankle was fused and is still painful. The treatment resulted in a nonunion of his right tibia. Dr. Davis has scheduled Jack for a right tibia intramedullary nailing with bone graft.

PERIOPERATIVE INTERPRETATION

Using what you have just learned in this chapter, as an experienced perioperative nurse, you would consider the following in the care of this patient.

1. Assessment
   - Based on your knowledge of the surgical procedure, you know that the intramedullary nail that Dr. Davis is planning on using is not stocked by the hospital and does not come sterile.
   - Image intensification and fluoroscopy will be used during the procedure. Radiation safety devices should be used to protect the operating room personnel and patient during the procedure.
   - Since the patient's left ankle is still painful, positioning on the orthopedic operating room bed should be considered to reduce any additional discomfort.

NURSING DIAGNOSES

High risk for infection related to inappropriate preparation of the surgical implant
   Alteration in comfort related to painful left ankle

2. Planning
   - Procure radiation safety devices, such as lead aprons with thyroid shields and gonad shields.

- Assemble the necessary surgical instrumentation.
- Contact the orthopedic sales representative to assure that the surgical implant is available for adequate preparation and sterilization.

3. Implementation
   - Position the patient on the orthopedic operating room bed after anesthesia induction to reduce the patient's discomfort.
   - Place a gonad shield on the patient's scrotum after induction of anesthesia. Check its placement after any repositioning of the patient.
   - If the surgical implant has been sterilized by the manufacturer,
      Check that the implant label states that the item is sterile unless the outside packaging has been entered.
   - If the surgical implant has *not* been sterilized by the manufacturer and arrived in the operating room more than 48 hours prior to the planned surgical procedure,
   *Check the cleanliness of the surgical implant.
   *Select the packaging material appropriate for the implant and the sterilization method.
   *Wrap the surgical implant, using the facility approved chemical indicator, and label the package identifying the contents and sterilization date.
   *Ensure that a biologic indicator was processed with the surgical implant package and confirm that the indicator was negative by verifying the facility policy on sterilization.
   *Open the sterile package in a way that preserves the sterility of the contents.
   - If the surgical implant has *not* been sterilized by the manufacturer and arrives in the operating room just before the planned surgical procedure,
   *Check the cleanliness of the surgical implant.
   *Select the appropriate sterilization tray that will allow presentation of the surgical implant to

the sterile field without contamination and place a facility-approved chemical indicator in the tray with the implant.

*Place a biologic indicator that provides results in 1 hour in the autoclave with the sterilization tray containing the implant.

*Process the surgical implant according to the facility's sterilization procedure.

*When the sterilization process is complete, check the external sterilization readout/graph to ensure that the appropriate sterilization parameters were obtained. Process the sterilized biologic indicator according to the facility's procedure.

*Present the surgical implant to the sterile field after the biologic indicator has been obtained and indicates that the sterilization process was achieved.

• Document in the intraoperative record the radiologic protective devices used for the patient and special positioning interventions to reduce the patient's discomfort.

• Include in the medical record the implant label provided by the manufacturer, and document in the intraoperative record the surgical implant used, catalog number, and manufacturer lot number.

4. Evaluation

• If the implant was sterilized in the operating room prior to the surgical procedure,

Validate the achievement of the sterilization parameters on the outside of the sterilizer.

Record the implant sterilized, sterilizer used, and results of the biologic/chemical indicator in the sterilization log per facility policy.

• Convey to the post-anesthesia care unit nurse the patient's discomfort in the left ankle and need to assess the patient's perception of pain in this ankle after surgery when awake.

Practice Scenario 2
Sterilization/Disinfection: Equipment and Instruments

by Debbie Woodard, RN, BSN, CNOR

PATIENT SCENARIO

James Hyde is a 72-year-old male admitted to Southern Medical Center for right lower extremity claudication and pain. The patient is 5 feet 10 inches tall and weighs 265 pounds. He smokes one pack of cigarettes daily. Your assignment is to circulate for Mr. Hyde, who is scheduled for a femoral-posterior tibial bypass graft. Although the scrub person has only been in surgery for 3 months and is unfamiliar with this procedure, he/she did participate in a femoral-popliteal bypass graft the day before. As you are bringing the patient into the operating room, Dr. Johnson tells you his partner, Dr. Stone, will be coming to help. Twenty minutes into the procedure, Dr. Stone comes in with a new pair of vascular forceps and scissors. He says he want to use them on this case, but they need to be sterilized.

PERIOPERATIVE INTERPRETATION

Using what you have just learned in this chapter, as an experienced perioperative nurse, you would consider the following in the care of this patient.

1. Assessment
   - Based upon the nursing preoperative assessment of this patient, you know that smoking and obesity can contribute to a prolonged or abnormal healing process.
   - All items used on the sterile field must be sterile.
   - Since you are already 20 minutes into this procedure, these instruments need to be sterilized as soon as possible.
   - Items to be sterilized should have as low a bioburden as possible.
   - Check the flash sterilizer to ensure proper functioning.

NURSING DIAGNOSIS

High risk for infection related to the inappropriate preparation of instruments.

2. Planning
   - Need to assess the instruments for cleanliness and possibly arrange to have them handwashed.
   - Need to determine when you would be able to start the sterilization process.
   - Knowing the scrub person may not have adequate time to remove the instruments from the sterilizer, you plan on using a flash sterilization container with a lid.

3. Implementation
   - Handwash and dry instruments, since they appear to be clean.
   - Place the opened scissors and forceps in the flash sterilization container.
   - Put a chemical indicator in with the instruments.
   - Place the flash sterilization container in the gravity displacement steam sterilizer. Close and secure the sterilizer door.
   - Set the sterilizer at 270°F for 10 minutes, since the forceps and scissors are made of metal and were handwashed.
   - Using protective gloves, an unsterile person would carry the flash sterilization container into the room and present the contents to the scrub person in a sterile manner.

4. Evaluation
   - When the sterilization cycle is complete, examine the time-temperature recording chart to see if the sterilizer maintained the correct temperature and exposure time.
   - Sign the recording chart prior to removing the flash container from the sterilizer.
   - Upon removal of the flash container, check the chemical indicator to verify exposure to the sterilization cycle's parameters prior to delivering the instruments to the sterile field.
   - The patient will need to be assessed 24 to 48 hours postoperatively for the presence or absence of infection.

Chapter Five

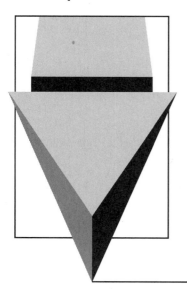

Environmental Safety in the Surgical Suite

Lois M. Bruning, RN, BSPA, CNOR

Prerequisite Knowledge   Prior to beginning this chapter, the learner should review concepts of universal precautions.

Chapter content correlates with several AORN recommended practices. These recommended practices may be considered a prerequisite prior to beginning the chapter or a refresher upon completion of the chapter.

Recommended practices for disinfection

Recommended practices for electrosurgery

Recommended practices for protective barriers for surgical gowns and drapes

Recommended practices for safe care through identification of potential hazards in the surgical environment

Recommended practices for care of instruments, scopes, and powered surgical instruments

Recommended practices for laser safety in the practice setting

Recommended practices for reducing radiologic exposure in the practice setting

Recommended practices for sponge, sharp, and instrument counts

Recommended practices for steam and ethylene oxide (EO) sterilization

Recommended practices for universal precautions in the perioperative practice setting

Chapter Outline

Risk Management
Regulation of hazards
The JCAHO
OSHA's hazards communication standard
OSHA's bloodborne pathogen standard
Organization safety program
Benefits
Surgical counts

Electrical Safety
Types of electricity
Safety measures
Electrosurgery

Laser Safety
Background
Potential hazard sources
Interventions for patient protection
Staff protection

Fire Safety
Essential elements of fire
Oxygen enriched atmospheres
Ignition sources
Fuel sources
Fire prevention/intervention
Flammability ratings

Radiologic Safety
Ionizing radiation
Radium implants
Nonionizing radiation

Chemical Safety
OSHA hazards communication standard
Anesthetic gases
Other agents

Occupational Safety
Common physical injuries
Preventing injuries
Motion economy principles

Biologic and Hazardous Materials Safety
Definitions
Biologic risks
Handling sharps
Regulated waste
Interventions

Learning Objectives

1. Describe the benefits to be derived from a safety program.
   - Identify requirements of a safe work environment.
   - List regulatory agencies impacting safety in health care.

2. Identify equipment that could be a source of electrical hazard.

3. Describe ten safety precautions in the use of electrosurgical units.

4. Specify the source of greatest danger related to laser surgery.

5. List five laser safety precautions.

6. List the three essential elements of a sustained fire.

7. Identify the major causes of fires in operating rooms.

8. Describe three potential side effects of excessive radiation. List five protective devices to minimize patient and personnel exposure to radiation.

9. Define personal protective equipment personnel should wear to provide protection from chemicals.

10. List the ten principles of motion economy.

11. Discuss OSHA's *Occupational Exposure to Bloodborne Pathogens: Final Rule* impact on health care providers.
    - Relate four examples of engineering and work practice controls.
    - Specify four components of regulated medical waste.

Risk Management

Risk management is a program that seeks to improve the working conditions and the health and safety of employees by enforcing safety procedures, monitoring activities, correcting faults, and documenting incidents for follow-up. The goal is to reduce or prevent accidents. Risk management requires investigation into mishaps to determine appropriate actions to prevent future occurrences. Actions may include repair of faulty or malfunctioning equipment or training and education of employees. Risk management activities prevent accidents through in-service programs related to hazards and safeguards; maintenance of equipment; and enforcement of regulations, standards, guidelines, and laws.

Many professional organizations and governmental agencies participate in the formation of guidelines, standards, and recommended practices addressing safety (Table 5–1). In addition to reaching compliance with the general safety requirements of federal, state, and local regulations, hospitals are subject to scrutiny unique to the health care industry. Hospitals receive direction from the American Medical Association (AMA) and the American Hospital Association Joint Committee on Health Programs for Hospital Personnel (AHAJCHP). And that is only the beginning. All health care institutions are subject to examination.

REGULATORY AGENCIES

The Occupational Safety and Health Administration (OSHA) is a federal regulatory body that addresses all aspects of employee safety for all employers, not only health care employers. The Safe Medical Devices Act (SMDA) mandates the reporting of adverse experiences with medical devices to the U.S. Food and Drug Administration (FDA). The FDA classifies medical devices into three groupings, relative to the potential risk of the device, and regulates the commercial use of items that are life sustaining or life supporting. The Joint Commission on Accreditation of Healthcare Organizations (JCAHO), an organization in which participation is voluntary, focuses on the safety of patients and, to a small degree, of staff in health care facilities. In many instances, hospital accreditation from the JCAHO is required for an institution to receive reimbursement from the federal government. The American National Standards Institute (ANSI) develops voluntary guidelines for evaluating occupational health and safety in health care institutions. The Association of Operating Room Nurses (AORN) establishes standards and recommended practices for perioperative nursing and is considered an expert resource for the OR. Other organizations addressing safety issues are the National Institute for Occupational Safety and Health (NIOSH), Centers for Disease Control and Prevention (CDC), Association for Advancement of Medical Instrumentation (AAMI), National Fire Protection Agency (NFPA), and National Safety Council (NSC).

TABLE 5–1. **AGENCIES CONCERNED WITH HOSPITAL SAFETY**

REGULATORY AGENCIES

EPA	Environmental Protection Agency
FDA	Federal Drug Administration
OSHA	Occupational Safety and Health Administration

VOLUNTARY AGENCIES

AAMI	Association for Advancement of Medical Instrumentation
AHAJCHP	American Hospital Association Joint Committee on Health Programs for Hospital Personnel
AMA	American Medical Association
ANA	American Nurses Association
ANSI	American National Standards Institute
AORN	Association of Operating Room Nurses
CDC	Centers for Disease Control and Prevention
JCAHO	Joint Commission on Accreditation of Healthcare Organizations
NFPA	National Fire Protection Agency
NIOSH	National Institute for Occupational Safety and Health
NSC	National Safety Council

These organizations have a focused goal of helping and/or mandating employers to protect patients and staff. They encourage the practice of risk management, which includes hazard abatement strategies to avoid the risk of harm. Many of the regulatory agencies monitor health care facilities for compliance to certain rules and regulations.

The Joint Commission on Accreditation of Healthcare Organizations

The JCAHO exercises a great deal of influence because many hospitals have a high percentage of Medicare and Medicaid patients whose medical expenses are subsidized by the federal government; it is essential for these institutions to maintain their accreditation status. In keeping with its stated mission to improve the quality of patient care, the JCAHO includes in its accreditation manual a segment addressing safe environments (JCAHO, 1995). Health care facilities are required to measure the four criteria listed as follows.

1. *There is a safety management program that is designed to provide a physical environment free of hazards and to manage staff activities to reduce the risk of human injury.* This means the governing body must monitor policies and procedures for safety in all departments and services. A facility-appointed safety officer directs a safety committee in the development, implementation, and monitoring of the safety program. Among other duties, the program pays special attention to hazards related to the ages of patients; includes a system for reporting and investigating safety incidents; designs practices for the identification and control of hazardous materials and waste; and establishes a program to manage the consequences of natural disasters that disrupt hospital care and treatment.

2. *There is a life safety management program designed to protect patients, personnel, visitors, and property from fire and the products of combustion and to provide for the safe use of buildings and grounds.* Beginning in January 1993, every building that provides overnight care to patients is required to comply with the NFPA's 1991 edition of the *Life Safety Code* or to provide equivalent protection. Organizations must develop a correction plan if not meeting these requirements. An ongoing program for fire safety that includes maintaining fire detection equipment and fire fighting equipment is also required.

3. *There is an equipment management program designed to assess and control the clinical and physical risks of fixed and portable equipment used for the diagnosis, treatment, monitoring, and care of patients and of other fixed and portable electrically powered equipment.* The safety program must include written criteria related to equipment function, maintenance, clinical application, incident history, inventory, testing procedures, user-training programs, problems or failures, and user errors. If information is received that indicates the equipment may have contributed to a patient injury, death, or illness, the organization must report the information as required by the Safe Medical Devices Act.

4. *There is a utilities management program designed to assure the operational reliability, assess the special risks, and respond to failures of utility systems that support the patient environment.* This requires written criteria that will identify utilities used including life support, infection control, environmental support, and equipment support; will assure a reliable, adequate emergency power system to provide electricity in the event of a power outage; and will require an accurate inventory, operational plans, and documentation and recordkeeping.

Each of these four criteria requires institutions to identify problems, specify actions to correct problems, document the actions, and evaluate the actions for effectiveness (JCAHO, 1995). Violation or noncompliance with the standards could mean loss of accreditation for hospitals (Newman, 1991).

Food and Drug Administration

In November 1991, health care institutions for the first time were required by the SMDA to maintain implant tracking and to report device-related incidents to the FDA. Anything used in the treatment or diagnosis of a patient that is not a drug is considered a device (Koch, 1992). Any device that causes a serious accident or illness to a patient must be reported within 10 days to the manufacturer or to the FDA if the manufacturer is unknown. Any device that contributes to the death of a patient must be reported to the FDA and to the manufacturer within 10 working days. Each facility is required to keep records of these reports and file a summary each January and July. The reports must include

- The name of the institution or facility
- Identification of the product, including its serial and model numbers, if applicable
- The name and address of the manufacturer, if known
- A description of the event

Manufacturers are required to track all devices when the failure of a permanently implanted device would have serious consequences. To complete the tracking and ensure proper notification of problems, health care facilities are required to document and record patient information. Operating room managers and nurses must be cognizant of the regulation. Fines of up to $15,000 may be imposed for noncompliance with the reporting requirements. More than half of all device-related incidents are caused by human error emphasizing the need for a thorough investigation of all accidents.

HEALTH CARE FACILITY SAFETY PROGRAM

As a general rule, communities believe that their health care facilities are safe, antiseptic facilities, staffed by skilled, nurturing physicians and nurses. However, only 8% of health care facilities are able to comply *fully* with the guidelines published by NIOSH (Newman, 1991). Potential health hazards are numerous in health care and include falls; burns; electrocutions; repetitive motion injuries; and exposure to steam, radiation, gases and other chemicals, and biologic pathogens. The AORN's *Recommended Practices for Safe Care Through Identification of Potential Hazards in the Surgical Environment* (1994a) provides optimum guidelines for providing safe care to patients.

While establishing a risk management program may be perceived as costly, health care administrators must remember the expense of treating an employee who is injured at work. The National Safety Council estimates the average cost of a disabling injury to be $18,000 (National Safety Council, 1991). The follow-up care to someone who experiences a needle stick with no resulting infection ranges from $200 to $900 and from 5 to 7 hours lost work time. Follow-up care to an employee who becomes infected as a result of an exposure may exceed $500,000 and workmen's compensation, plus the possibility of litigation. Health care institutions must train and educate their employees and enforce compliance with safety precautions. Employers cannot afford the financial repercussions of accidents or illnesses (Weisman, 1993).

Experts estimate that as many as 85% of the health problems encountered by health care providers may be attributed to environmental factors, many of them affecting the reproductive systems of both men and women. Numerous studies over the years have tried to document exactly how great the risk is. These studies have helped to formulate some of the guidelines and standards that exist today.

Most of the research has looked at issues of pregnancy and spontaneous abortions; over 60% of women aged 18 to 64 are in the workforce. Health care facilities employ a high percentage of women and therefore have an increased responsibility to be aware of health hazards to women of childbearing age. It is important for health care administrators to be aware of the particular hazards that might be encountered by pregnant females. Interventions that should be employed include

- Providing factual information related to the environmental hazard and the possible effects of exposure
- Instructing and enforcing the use of appropriate safety precautions
- Requiring personnel to report possible pregnancies to their manager as early as possible to prevent or minimize exposures
- Requiring personnel to utilize biologic monitoring devices while at the work site.

Occupational Safety and Health Administration

Employer responsibility for providing a safe workplace for all employees is mandated by federal law. The Occupational Safety and Health Act of 1970 was enacted for the specific purpose of reducing work-related injuries and illnesses. The OSHA formulates the law and has the authority to make and enforce safety and health regulations in all workplaces. Noncompliance by a health care institution can result in large monetary penalties.

A first step in reaching compliance is to establish policies and procedures for safe work practices. This information must be monitored and enforced consistently throughout the institution. Although the risk manager is usually the best person to formulate health care safety policies, the individual unit managers are usually the best persons to monitor and enforce safety procedures in a particular area. They are familiar with the employee and the employee's duties and have the authority to invoke behavior changes. Managers are responsible for preparing action plans addressing building evacuation routes, first aid, and potential hazards. They should use incident records and safety reports to identify trends to prevent future incidents. An alert and knowledgeable manager can anticipate and prevent accidents. Shrewd health care administrators provide managers the opportunity to learn safety performance measurement and other safety techniques through a college or university course as a first step in developing a safety-conscious team. Once the management team is educated, they can set the example and train their own staff. The education on safety techniques must be provided to employees during orientation and be repeated at regular intervals. Constant reinforcement maintains a high level of employee awareness—awareness that can prevent tragedies from happening.

Successfully run safety programs utilize employees' input to develop rules that are practical and enforceable based upon their own work situation. Empowering employees to set safety goals helps them feel responsible and builds good will. Safety-conscious teams identify potential hazards and plan strategies to control or eliminate them. Team members make sure first aid equipment is readily available. If an accident does occur, it is fully investigated and recorded, and the information is used as a tool to prevent future incidents (National Safety Council, 1991). Recognition given to departments who hold the best accident-free record will be motivating to other departments.

Prevention of illnesses from bloodborne pathogens encountered in the workplace is a responsibility specific to health care institutions. The OSHA bloodborne pathogens standard, which went into effect July 6, 1991 addresses health care workers' need for protection against occupationally acquired diseases (OSHA, 1991). Education and training related to bloodborne diseases must be provided to all employees who have occupational exposure. It must be presented during normal work hours in a method employees can understand regardless of their educational level. Managers must ensure that the employees are trained before they assume their job responsibilities to prevent accidents due to ignorance.

The OSHA standard also requires employers to provide employees with immunization against hepatitis B. The vaccination series must be offered free of charge to every employee who is identified as having occupational exposure and must be administered according to the guidelines of the U.S. Public Health Service. Employees who decline the vaccine or fail to finish the inoculation series must sign a declination statement, which becomes part of their medical record. Employers are responsible to provide free follow-up medical care to employees who become ill as a result of their occupational exposure. Employers have both a moral and legal responsibility to protect the health of their patients and employees (Newman, 1991).

BENEFITS OF RISK MANAGEMENT

While it is not uncommon to hear administrators complain about the costs of health care programs, the benefits of a successful risk management strategy are numerous. Demonstrating concern about employee safety can improve morale and generate feelings of security. Behaviors that result in fewer accidents mean less absenteeism and better productivity. When an employee is ill or injured, a heavier burden is placed on coworkers. An accident-free work site creates less stress on employees, and fewer accidents mean fewer disruptions to surgical procedures. Many accidents are caused by equipment failure and human error. Less equipment downtime due to operator error results in improved service to patients and their families. Insurance companies frequently offer discounts to establishments that can prove safe practices — for example, a nonsmoking facility. Some insurance companies go so far as to refuse coverage unless they can conduct a training program within the facility. Fewer accidents or illnesses mean less money will be spent on employee emergency care and follow-up treatment. Fewer accidents also mean less time will be spent investigating and reporting accidents. Violations of safety rules and regulations established by governing bodies can be costly. Noncompliance with federal, state, and local regulations can result in fines for deficiencies. Serious accidents in an institution inevitably receive attention from the media. A successful safety program is the proven answer for preventing accidents and the undesirable negative publicity (National Safety Council, 1991).

SURGICAL COUNTS

The AORN publication *Recommended Practices for Sponge, Sharp, and Instrument Counts* (1994) advises that sponges, sharps, and instruments be counted for all surgical procedures; that the counts be documented on the intraoperative record; and that counting be enforced through written policies and procedures. The entire surgical and nursing team, including the relief crew, is responsible for correct counts. Because a retained foreign substance in a patient presents an almost indefensible legal case, such cases are rarely brought before a jury (Murphy, 1991). Litigations of this type are generally settled out of court. Accurate counts and accountability of the team involved are critical to the welfare of the patient. Everyone involved in the surgical procedure could be held liable by a court of law if the patient initiates legal action.

To achieve an accurate count, the scrub person and the circulating nurse should conduct audible counts together. Visualization of each item by both parties is a requirement. Sponge counts typically include 4 × 4-inch and 4 × 8-inch folded gauze and larger absorbent fabrics called tapes, laps, or packs. X-ray–

detectable sponges should be used in all open wounds and for packing. Dissecting sponges such as peanuts, Kitners, and tonsil sponges should be included in the count as well as cottonoid patties and pledgets. As each pack of sponges is opened, it should be counted by the scrub person and the circulating nurse and recorded. Some hospitals have a wall board to keep track of counts during the procedure and record only the results of the counts on the operative record. Other institutions record everything on the patient's record. Either approach is correct.

As sponges are used, they must be carefully confined and contained — either by the scrub person on the back table or by the circulating nurse in impervious containers. This practice prevents indirect contamination of other areas in the room. Care must be exercised not to discard counted sponges in the trash while the procedure is in progress. At the end of the case the sponges can be disposed of with the other regulated waste. The room should be thoroughly inspected at the end of each procedure to ensure that all sponges are removed before beginning the next case. Sponges remaining in the room could cause the next procedure to have an incorrect count.

Sharps also must be counted. Sharps, which include scalpel blades, surgical needles, injection needles, safety pins, trochars, and electrosurgical needles and blades, are difficult to monitor. Each item or package should be counted as it is added to the surgical field. Suture packets can remain closed until they are needed. Sharps should be given only on an exchange basis to the surgeon. Whenever possible the used sharps should be confined in a sharps-counting device; many efficient devices are available on the market. Loose sharps should never be permitted on the surgical field. A sharp that punctures a glove must be passed off the surgical field to the circulating nurse. Counted sharps should not be allowed to leave the room during the surgical procedure. Broken sharps must be carefully examined to prevent any missing pieces from being left in the wound. OSHA requires disposable and reusable sharps to be placed in containers that are leakproof, puncture resistant, and colored red or labeled with the biohazard symbol. Containers for disposable sharps must have tight-fitting lids to allow safe handling during transportation. Containers for reusable sharps are not required to have lids but must separate the sharps from the other surgical instruments prior to decontamination. OSHA considers reusable sharps to include any instrument that can easily cut or puncture. This definition may include items such as skin hooks, rakes, Gelpi retractors, pointed scissors, or perforating towel clips.

Instrument counts should be performed for all procedures. However, in some facilities policies may designate specific procedures for which counts may be eliminated. Instrument counts should be mandated for procedures where a body cavity is entered or where the incision is large enough to allow an instrument to be accidentally left in the patient. Reducing the number and types of instruments and establishing the standard sets will facilitate the counting procedure (Fig. 5–1). Instruments should not be separated until they are counted. Those with detachable parts should have all the pieces counted, and counts should be recorded on standardized records. The initial documentation can be started by the person who assembles the set; the scrub person verifies the count when the set is opened; the scrub person and the circulating nurse together count the instruments; and the circulating nurse records these and any instruments added during the procedure.

Sponge, sharps, and instrument counts are recognized as safety practices by health care professionals. Policies and procedures must be established addressing action to be taken if a count must be omitted. A hospital that fails to do so exposes itself to potential legal action if a count is not taken. The potential need for bypassing surgical counts exists in extreme emergency situations and should be documented in the operating room's policy and procedures manual. The specific situations and how they are to be handled should be approved by the surgical

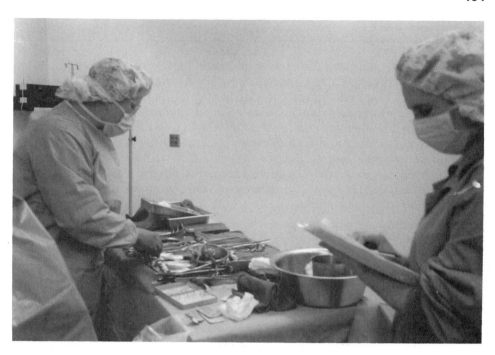

FIGURE 5-1. Counting Instruments

committee with administrative and legal input. The omission and rationale should be documented on the patient's intraoperative record.

Counts are conducted in the OR and documented at the following times:

- Prior to the beginning of the surgical procedure
- During the procedure as additional items are added to the field
- Before the closure of a body cavity or deep incision
- Before the closure of a cavity within a cavity, e.g., a cesarean section
- A final count during the subcuticular closure or during the skin closure.

Incorrect counts must be followed by specific procedures:

- Immediately inform the surgeon and begin a search for the missing item
- The scrub person searches the sterile field, Mayo stand, and back table; the circulator searches the unsterile areas; the surgeon searches the operative site and surgical wound
- Based upon the patient's condition and the opinion of the surgeon, an x-ray film may be made either before or after the wound is closed, but before the patient leaves the room
- The OR manager should be notified.

Liability for incorrect counts can be placed on any member of the surgical team. The circulating nurse must document the outcome and any unusual circumstances of all counts.

The operating room is one of the most technical areas in a health care facility and contains sophisticated and potentially hazardous equipment, medical devices, and chemicals. This advanced technology is vital to modern surgery and treatment, but careless practices or improper handling of supplies or equipment has the potential to result in injuries or infections. OR environmental factors may contribute risks to patients, staff, and physicians, but recognition of the risk factors and a properly administered risk management program will ensure safety for everyone. Health care administrators must be proactive in supporting risk management programs that will ensure that all departments are in compliance with health and safety regulations.

Electrical Safety

As medical technology advances, more and more electronic equipment is found in the operating room. To function safely within this environment, operating room personnel must have knowledge of safe work practices as related to electricity. Information is readily available. The federal government regulates the performance of electronic medical devices; AAMI recommends standards and practices for users and manufacturers alike; and the JCAHO publishes requirements that must be met for the health care facility to achieve accreditation. While published guidelines and recommendations are helpful, the best defense against an accident is well-informed and conscientious personnel. Understanding a few simple principles of electricity is beneficial.

TYPES OF ELECTRICITY

There are three types of electricity: static, direct, and alternating. Risks from static electricity have diminished significantly in this country because explosive anesthetic agents are rarely provided any longer. Since a static charge can supply the necessary energy to generate a spark, it could energize the fuel for a fire. Static electricity develops from friction and accumulates on objects. When two objects bearing static electricity come into contact, the higher accumulated charge discharges to the lower. Sparks can be created when the accumulated energy is high enough. These sparks have the potential of igniting material or gases. To prevent a dangerous buildup of static electricity:

1. Maintain room humidity at a range of 50% to 60%.
2. Dissipate charges frequently by touching metal surfaces and avoiding friction-causing activities.
3. Avoid wool and synthetic materials that have not received antistatic treatments — use cotton sheets and blankets.
4. Use special antistatic liners in trash receptacles and kickbuckets, if they are available.

Direct and alternating currents (DC and AC) are named from the pattern of movement of charged particles. Current is the rate of flow of electrons through a conductor. Voltage is the force that moves electrons through material and induces current to flow in one direction. The movement is measured in volts — the higher the number of volts, the more direct the path of the current. The ability of material to resist the flow of electrons is measured in ohms. Electricity flows easily through substances like metal, water, and the human body; flow is difficult through rubber, plastic, and glass. Without proper precautions, the patient can become part of an unplanned pathway for electrical current.

Both AC and DC current can leak; expect it and plan for it. Areas such as the OR that treat high-risk patients are required to be constructed with an isolated electrical source. The isolation transformer is usually located in the walls and makes the total circuits smaller, thus minimizing unplanned circuits. Because electricity always follows the path of least resistance, it is important for all equipment to be properly grounded. Grounding systems discharge current directly to ground, bypassing the patient in the circuit and preventing a potential shock or burn.

In patient care areas, copper bars or pipes are used as a ground. Copper is an excellent conductor and absorbs a great deal of current. The third long prong in electrical cords is connected to this copper, providing a means for current to flow to the ground or to the conductive surfaces. Again, remember that electricity always follows the path of least resistance, so if the insulation on electrical cords is broken or frayed, some current will leak. If the equipment is grounded, leakage returns through the ground wire causing no damage.

Isolated power systems isolate the OR electrical circuits from grounded circuits in the power mains; the electrical circuit does not include the ground in its pathway. The current flows from one isolated line to another. The line-isolation monitor checks the degree of isolation by continually measuring resistance and capacity between two isolated lines and ground. If current leakage exceeds safe levels, the alarm sounds alerting personnel of the hazard. If this happens, personnel should at once unplug the last piece of electrical equipment that was plugged in; if the alarm does not silence, continue to unplug electrical equipment in the room until the leaking appliance is found; and if the alarm still does not silence, close the OR suite until biomedical engineers can check for current leakage.

SAFETY MEASURES

Safe practices in the use of electronic equipment will prevent needless electric shock or electrocution of either staff or patients. Recommended practices include the following:

1. Proper monitoring and care of high voltage equipment such as x-ray machines, electrosurgical units (ESUs), lasers, and monitoring devices. Equipment should be checked at least quarterly (monthly is preferred) by a biomedical engineer, and each piece must meet the Underwriters Laboratories safety requirements (Atkinson, 1992).
2. Regularly checking the integrity of the cords and removing any machines with defective cords. Cords should not be stretched taut or be suspended above the floor when in use. If possible, place them so that they are out of traffic lanes.
3. Locating ESUs and lasers as far as possible from monitoring devices. Plugging each unit into a separate outlet.
4. Prohibiting extension cords, because most will leak even if insulated. If their use is unavoidable, only heavy-duty cords with a grounding prong should be permitted.
5. Educating personnel to never set any kind of liquid on electrical equipment. Spills can cause internal short circuits.
6. Instructing personnel to always disconnect a unit by pulling on the plug, never on the cord. Machines should be turned off whenever they are being connected or disconnected.
7. Ensuring that all machines are properly grounded; prohibiting use of unauthorized appliances in the OR, i.e., personal radios should be safety checked before being allowed in the suite.
8. Instructing personnel to avoid the use of needle electrodes for electrocardiogram monitoring.

Electrosurgery Units (ESUs)

Electrocautery as a means of controlling bleeding is practiced in about 95% of surgical procedures today. The benefit of using this tool to cut tissue and coagulate bleeders is recognized by most health care professionals. However, the acceptance of the practice does not mean health care providers should allow themselves to become complacent about necessary safety measures (Table 5–2). Patients and users have been burned at times when equipment failed, but more commonly because of operator error. A correctly functioning generator provides for the current produced by the unit to return to the generator through the electrosurgery grounding pad. If the current returns through an unintended path, an alternate-path burn is likely to result. Ground reference generators may be more susceptible to alternate-path burns than isolated generators. An example of a ground reference generator is a spark-gap generator. Current from this type of

TABLE 5-2. **ELECTROSURGERY SAFETY**

- Schedule frequent preventive maintenance routines
- Check for proper grounding of ESU
- Have adequate cord length for the unit
- Do not use extension cords
- Inspect machines before each use
    Check for functioning safety lights and alarms
    Check cords for exposed wires or frayed insulation
- Document ESU identification number on patient record
- Remove any flammable agents, i.e., prepping solutions
- Confirm power settings verbally
    Use the lowest effective power
- Follow cleaning instructions; protect from spills
- Locate as far as possible from other monitors
- Turn ESU off when not in use
- Avoid using EKG needle electrodes
- Ensure proper placement of manufacturer's dispersive grounding pad
- Place ESU pencil in holder when not in use
- Remove contaminated ESU cords from the field
- Avoid overlapping electric cords or wires
- Avoid using internal temperature probes

unit seeks a return to ground by following the path of least resistance, which could be the surgeon, the patient, the OR bed, or the dispersive grounding pad. Safer are the isolated electrosurgery generators where the current generally flows to the patient's dispersive grounding pad and back to the generator.

Another type of an ESU is the bipolar electrosurgery unit. This unit does not require a dispersive grounding pad because current flows between the tip of the forceps. One side of the forceps is the active electrode and the other side is the ground. The operator uses a foot switch to control bipolar units. A good understanding of safe procedures and good clinical practice can prevent accidents from happening. The AORN's *Standards and Recommended Practices for Electrosurgery* (1994c) includes recommended practices for electrosurgery and provides a resource for safety recommendations.

Each manufacturer of electrosurgical equipment issues operating instructions for their own equipment. Selection of the ESU should include an evaluation of its physical design. The stand should be sturdy and prevent accidental tipping. There should be an audible and visual alarm that alerts staff of any malfunction. Each unit should have adequate cord length to reach electrical outlets without extension cords. The circuitry should be designed to ensure adequate grounding. Each ESU in the suite should be assigned a number for easy identification. This number should be documented on the patient's intraoperative record.

Whenever a new piece of equipment is introduced to the OR suite, all members of the surgical team should receive in-service training. Staff competency can be ensured by requiring return demonstrations from each employee who will utilize the equipment. A copy of the operator's manual should be maintained in the area where the equipment is expected to be used. In addition, attaching detailed written instructions and a problem-solving checklist to the unit provides an immediate refresher in the event of difficulties. In-service training programs should be repeated at least annually for users of the equipment.

Accidents can be decreased by formulating policies and procedures that support the manufacturer's instructions; they should be available to staff and enforced by management. Safe practices include the following:

- The audible and visual safety alarm should never be disconnected or turned so low that the purpose is defeated.

- The manufacturer's recommended active electrodes should be used in preference to all others.
- Proper placement of the patient dispersive grounding pad is essential to prevent burns. It should be positioned as near to the operative site as possible; hairy areas or scarred tissue should be avoided; the hair should be shaved if necessary to guarantee good skin contact with the grounding plate; areas where fluids may pool should be avoided; the dispersive grounding pad should be positioned over a muscle mass, such as the buttocks or upper thighs, avoiding bony prominences like shoulder blades (Fig. 5–2).
- Pediatric grounding pads should only be selected for patients weighing less than 25 pounds. The smaller size of the pad ensures good contact with the patient. Placement depends upon the surgical procedure and should follow the same safety precautions as those for adults.
- The insulation on reusable cords should be carefully inspected for any degradation before use. Cracks in the cord will expose wires and allow current to arc from the wires to patients or staff.
- Limited-life cords must be marked each time they are reprocessed.
- If alcohol-based preparation solutions are used, they must be allowed to thoroughly dry. Flammable agents of any type should be prohibited when electrosurgery is used.
- An electrosurgical pencil should be placed in a safe, nonflammable holder when it is not being used.
- If an electrosurgical active electrode becomes contaminated during the procedure, it should be disconnected from the unit and removed from the sterile field if possible. This will prevent accidental activation.
- Avoid overlapping or crossing electrosurgical cords with other cables or monitoring wires. Leakage current from one wire may transfer to another wire causing a burn. Patients have been burned under the ECG electrode when current has traveled from the electrosurgical cord to the ECG wires.
- Biomedical engineers recommend avoiding the use of internal temperature probes simultaneously with the ESU. Leakage of current can result in a burn at the tip of the temperature probe.

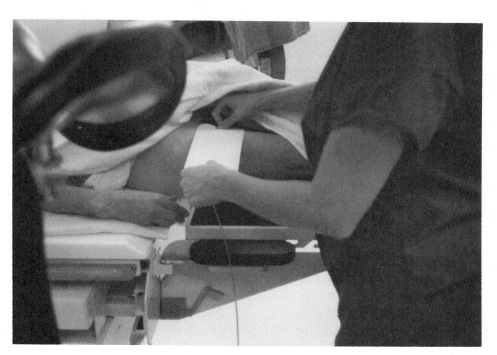

FIGURE 5–2. Grounding Pad Application

- The patient's skin integrity should be evaluated and documented at the end of the procedure.

Open heart surgery and other surgeries requiring two electrosurgical generators at the same time need special consideration. It is critical that each of the patient electrodes be placed as close as possible to its own active electrode without touching the other. The heart may not be positioned between the active electrode and the patient's electrode. A grounding pad is utilized for each generator, applying the same safety precautions as for an individual unit.

Laser Safety

BACKGROUND

The use of lasers in surgical procedures has accelerated dramatically in the last 20 years, and it is predicted that by 1995 roughly 40% of surgical procedures will have a laser in some capacity (Rupke, 1992). In fact, authorities estimate that the U.S. will nearly double its use of lasers between 1989 and 1994. In 1989 an estimated 21,000 units were in use, indicating a projected estimate of 42,000 laser units by 1994. This tremendous growth in use of laser technology requires a rigorously enforced safety program. In spite of documented laser-related operating room accidents and deaths, few states have regulations or guidelines concerning medical lasers. The 12 states that have established formal recommendations for lasers fail to adequately address clinical issues (Rupke, 1992).

Specific guidelines are needed by health care facilities, which have been experiencing the escalating demands to provide laser services. Because national standards do not exist and guidelines are voluntary, safety is often inadequately and inconsistently addressed. The American National Standards Institute has published standards (Z136.3 ANSI Standard) for the safe utilization of lasers in health care facilities, but they are not mandatory standards (ANSI, 1993). The AORN has also published recommended practices for laser safety. Both are widely recognized authorities, but many of their recommendations are ambiguous or discretionary (Smalley, 1991). By balancing their recommendations and other expert opinions, health care professionals can develop a comprehensive safety program.

As in any situation, when there is an increase in the factors capable of causing accidents, the risk of accidents is simultaneously greater. The most effective way to prevent an increase in the number of laser accidents is to have a rigorously enforced laser safety program.

POTENTIAL HAZARD SOURCES

People are the primary cause of laser-related accidents, yet in spite of the potential danger and repeated warnings, complacency exists. To discourage the natural inclination to regard laser surgery as routine, facilities must accept responsibility for maintaining 3 to 4 laser in-service programs per year, hold mandatory annual laser safety updates, and provide ongoing, one-on-one instruction for new users. Programs of this type are not without cost, but facilities cannot lose sight of the fact that costs cannot be cut when it comes to human safety (Rupke, 1992).

One study suggests that laser accidents from equipment malfunction or equipment failure are rare. The study, conducted by six physicians, grouped the accidents occurring during laser surgery into three major categories.

Category 1 included burns caused by the operator when the laser was intentionally being used. Within the operative field, burns were sustained by the patient, surgeon, or surgical assistant.

CONTROVERSY BOX

One of the theorized dangers of laser surgery is laser plume. Laser plume is smoke that is generated as tissue is vaporized; it has been described as a thick malodorous smoke. Numerous publications support the belief that personnel should avoid breathing laser smoke/plume because of the possibility of lung damage; particles in the laser plume are small enough to penetrate to the deepest regions of the lung. Another suspected risk is the possibility of disease transmission. Viral DNA has been recovered in laser debris from the surgical suite; however, no evidence exists to prove a related in vivo viral infection (Wisniewski, 1990).

Recommendations advising personnel to wear a face mask capable of filtering viruses have been published but have been difficult to follow. The filtration efficiency of standard surgical face masks is measured by the amount of bacteria that is filtered as a person exhales. Most of the air that is inhaled comes from the mask edges. Standard surgical face masks are worn to protect patients from health care workers' bacteria as they exhale. These masks are able to filter particles as small as 5 microns, the size of common bacteria. They are not designed to stop particles of laser-plume size (0.5–5.0 microns), and viruses are even smaller (Nezhat, 1987). Viruses range in size from 0.3 to 0.1 microns. A mask capable of filtering particles as small as 0.3 microns may prove to be difficult to find and if found impossible to wear. If a face mask were designed to prevent the inhalation of room air and to filter particles the size of viral DNA, it would not allow enough oxygen through to sustain human life (Wisniewski, 1990). But NIOSH has concluded that laser smoke/plume and ESU smoke are potential health hazards. At this time, there is no mask that is effective against laser plume. The most effective method to minimize laser smoke/plume inhalation is to wear the best filtration mask available and use smoke evacuators to eliminate as much plume as possible (Patterson, 1993).

Both NIOSH and ANSI recommend smoke evacuators during laser surgery. NIOSH additionally suggests venting exhaust outlets for smoke evacuation to the outside and providing personal protective equipment for personnel who service the smoke evacuators. Centralized vacuum systems, available in newer institutions, provide an efficient method for smoke evacuation. Disposable tubing is used in the OR, and the filter is changed in the control room. AORN's *Recommended Practices for Laser Safety in the Practice Setting* (AORN, 1994d) advises that plume and noxious fumes be evacuated through a filter device and that personnel wear high filtration surgical masks. OSHA is concerned about smoke as it relates to worker safety. Although no specific standard exists, the agency has the authority to regulate the hazard under its respiratory protection standard.

How well a smoke evacuator performs depends upon the type of filtration system in place. Triple filters are preferred. They are composed of a prefilter to trap large particles, an ultralow penetrating air (ULPA) filter for particles in the 0.1-micron range, and a charcoal filter to absorb odor and hydrocarbons. The filters are rated by the size of particles they can trap. A UPLA filter is certified at 99.999% for particles of 0.1 microns. A high-efficiency particulate air (HEPA) filter is rated at 99.97% for particles of 0.3 microns (Patterson, 1993). But for any filter to be effective, the evacuation hose must be held very close to the operative site; distance as little as 2 cm away will allow up to 50% of the particles to escape.

Category 2 included burns incurred when the operator was not intentionally using the laser. Burns could be sustained by anyone or anything.

Category 3 included equipment failure. In the study there were no accidents in this category.

The authors reported a total of 13 accidents unrelated to the surgical procedure, out of 141 procedures. Category 2 accidents can be eliminated by having a properly educated individual operate the laser control panel at all times. Category 1 accidents are the most difficult to control because they depend on operator skill and experience, teamwork, and safe instrumentation and drapes. The study criticized the current practice of draping with wet towels for protection from burns. The towels do not ignite but the laser beam can penetrate almost instantly exposing the underlying tissue to the laser beam: "The prevailing belief that a wet drape provides safety is false, as demonstrated by our report." They further stated that except for one disposable drape made from a plastic polymer, polypropylene, "All other currently manufactured drapes of natural or synthetic fibers, wet or dry, will ignite under the intense heat energy of a CO_2 laser beam." Consideration must also be given to the risk of bacterial migration through wet fabric (Brodman, 1993).

INTERVENTIONS

ANSI has published a 55-page standard providing guidelines for the safe utilization of lasers and laser systems in health care institutions (ANSI, 1993). As a first step, an individual must be appointed the laser safety officer (LSO) with the authority to enforce safety standards. This individual should chair the laser committee, which governs laser activity and establishes criteria. The committee should include the OR supervisor, a biomechanical engineer, the chief of surgery or chief of staff, and an administrator. If the endoscopy department is not under the jurisdiction of the operating room supervisor, a representative from the endoscopy department should be included on the committee. The committee is responsible for ensuring the credentialing and certification of medical and nursing staff. The ANSI recommendations include the establishment of a laser safety and training program to be enforced by the LSO.

Generally accepted protective practices enforced by a laser safety committee include

- Wearing wavelength-appropriate eye protection (goggles) at all times
- Installing a flashing light outside of the room to indicate when the laser is in use
- Labeling and signage to identify the type of laser in use
- Assigning in addition to the circulating nurse, a person trained in laser use to the procedure to monitor the laser
- Requiring instruments to be anodized or coated to diffuse reflected light
- Performing routine equipment safety checks before each procedure
- Prohibiting PVC endotracheal tubes; mandating that wrapped silicone or red rubber tubes or laser-safe tubes be used
- Mandating ignition-resistant drapes
- Providing wavelength-appropriate goggles for the awake patient; for the sleeping patient, providing water soluble eye ointments and/or taping the eyes closed
- Ensuring ongoing physician and nurse education programs that provide consistent information to both groups, thus avoiding different interpretations of safe practices
- Installing a safety door switch that deactivates the laser when the door is opened
- Having a fire extinguisher readily available, i.e., on the laser supply cart; fire blankets in each room; wet towels on the back table to smother a small blaze
- Mandating accurate documentation, including the type of laser, power range, tissue type, pulse duration, name of the surgeon, name of the laser operator, safety measures employed, preoperative safety check, instructions given to the patient and the patient's response.

Since surgical lasers are here to stay, it is incumbent upon institutions to provide and enforce safe practices. Consistent training at all levels and cooperation of all members of the surgical team are essential to achieve an accident-free laser program.

Fire Safety

While fires in operating rooms may be rare, they have occurred and there have been patient fatalities. Professionals are of the opinion that reported OR fires do not accurately reflect the actual number or severity of fires in health care institutions. Unless severe, fires are seldom publicized since there are many reasons for involved parties to downplay the actual problem. Experts estimate that there are 15 unreported small fires for every serious fire reported (Paper Drapes and Gowns a Fire Risk, 1992). In addition, Dr. Ralph A. Milliken, professor of anesthesiology, believes there is at least one unreported serious fire for every serious fire that is reported (Price, 1990). Compounding the problem of accumulating data, no central agency gathers data on fire-related injury or death.

Risk managers and health care officials should stress the potential risk of OR fires and enforce safe practices. Invariably litigation follows when a patient is harmed and health care facilities find themselves trying to defend their position. Michael Blau, JD, stated, "To be a defendable occurrence, (hospitals) should take whatever steps are available to reduce the risk of there being a fire. That means if there are known technologies that are available to hospitals and standard equipment used to minimize or eliminate the risk of fire, then those ought to be used in connection with whatever procedure is being performed" (OR Fire Occurrence Low, but Resulting Liability High, 1992).

High-energy devices require health care professionals to use the safest products available, but existing standards and codes are inadequate in addressing fire safety requirements (UCLA Operating Room Fire, 1990). Organizations such as AORN, AAMI, and NFPA are collaborating on recommendations addressing the issue of surgical drapes and flammability. In the interim, health care professionals will have to select safe products employing their own professional judgment. It is unlikely fires will ever be as infrequent as anyone would like; therefore, it is incumbent upon risk managers and health care supervisors to stress fire safety programs.

ESSENTIAL ELEMENTS OF FIRES

A sustained fire requires three components: oxygen, ignition source, and fuel. Eliminate any one of these three and there will be no fire. Unfortunately, the OR environment provides all these necessary components. Flammable anesthetic gases were once a high-risk factor in OR fires, but these gases have generally been replaced with safer agents. In spite of the fact that flammable anesthetic gases are seldom utilized in health care facilities today, the OR suite should still be considered a potentially high fire hazard area.

While the major causes of fires in health care facilities are smoking (28.2%) and arson (12.8%), 57.7% are caused by equipment (12.8%), appliances (11.6%), cooking (11.3%), and electrical distribution (9.2%) (Fig. 5–3). Roughly a hundred fires a year can be attributed to electrical equipment. Fatalities resulting from fires in health care facilities tend to be the patients who are often very close to the point of ignition (Hall, 1991). In the operating room patients are usually helpless as well.

Oxygen-enriched Atmospheres

The assumption that OR fires are more serious because of an oxygen-enriched atmosphere (OEA) is usually not valid. Most operating rooms have an ambient

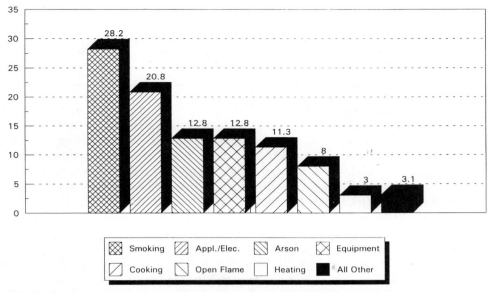

FIGURE 5–3. Major Causes of Fires (Health Care Facilities) (From Hall, J. R. (1991). Causes of fires in facilities that care for the sick. *The U.S. Fire Problem Overview Report Through 1989*, Quincy, MA: National Fire Protection Agency. (pp. 58–60))

oxygen reading of around 21%; the entire operating room is not oxygen enriched. While high concentrations of oxygen can accumulate around the head of a patient if drapes are not adequately ventilated, investigations of serious fires show that OEAs are not usually contributing factors in OR fires. According to Dennis J. Stouffer, when an OEA is a factor, the enriched oxygen levels are generally concentrated around the patient's nose, mouth, and face. Under normal conditions, oxygen will not saturate entire drapes or involve a large area. Following a fatal OR fire in California in 1991, the Los Angeles City Fire Department conducted an extensive investigation over several months. In the final report, the LACFD concluded that an OEA was not a contributing factor in the fire and that exceptionally rapid ignition of paper drapes can occur in a normal oxygen environment (Stouffer, 1991).

Ignition Sources

The frequent use of high-energy devices, such as electrosurgery units (ESUs), disposable hand cauteries, fiber-optic light sources, and lasers, contributes a greater risk of fires in the OR and requires health care professionals to exercise great care and caution with this equipment. Less often implicated in fires, but still carrying a risk, are high-speed drills and saws, which may generate intense heat at the point of use; also defibrillators, heated probes, and warming lights carry a risk. Any equipment capable of creating enough heat to ignite a fuel source should be handled with appropriate safety precautions. Fiber-optic light cords are often inappropriately disconnected from the instruments while the light source is left on. The intense light and resultant heat from the end of the cord is capable of igniting supplies found in the sterile field—items such as gauze, paper drapes, and disposable towels. Bronchoscopy lights, fiber-optic lights, hot cautery tips, ESUs, and lasers have been reported to cause fires.

Reports of fire locations have included some unexpected places. Fires have occurred in patients' intestines owing to the presence of methane gas, usually ignited when the ESU was being used. Much of the intestinal gas can be removed with suction and the bowel packed with wet lap sponges to reduce the risk. Fires

---

ACTION STEPS FOR AIRWAY FIRES

Stop the flow of gas. Disconnect the breathing circuit from the endotracheal tube. Cut the cuff inflation tube and anchor ties.

Remove the endotracheal tube and hand off to another staff member to extinguish. Remove any remaining segments of the tube from the airway.

Care for the patient. Reestablish the airway and resume ventilating with air. If no burning materials are left in the throat, switch to 100% oxygen. Examine the airway for damage and treat accordingly.

Save the tube for later examination. Report the fire to risk management personnel and the fire department (Airway Fires: Reducing the Risk During Laser Surgery, 1990).

---

have erupted in endotracheal tubes (ETTs) during the utilization of a laser with disastrous results. Because of the concentration of oxygen and/or nitrous oxide, the atmosphere inside the tube can produce a rocketlike fire, resulting in severe damage to the patient's trachea, lower airway, and lungs. All OR personnel should be aware of the four steps for extinguishing airway fires. Every second counts so teamwork is essential. Hesitation could mean irreparable damage or even death to the patient.

Fuel Sources

Once the first two essential components of oxygen and an ignition source are present, only fuel is needed to create a sustained fire, and there is a profusion of highly flammable fuels in the average OR. To begin with, most solutions for surgical preps are alcohol based. Alcohol in any form is intensely combustible. Prepping solutions should be given time to evaporate, or if time does not allow this, the site should be towel dried. Ointments, tinctures and aerosols should be judiciously evaluated with regard to potential for ignition and replaced with water soluble products if available.

Nonwoven fabrics made from a combination of cellulose and synthetic fibers are commonly referred to as disposable paper products. They include towels, surgical drapes and gowns, and sterilization wraps. In test situations, ignition times for paper drapes were as short as 0.5 seconds, and once ignited they burned very rapidly (Stouffer, 1991). In the aftermath of the California hospital fire, tests conducted by the city fire department proved that surgical drapes made from paper fabrics will ignite and burn very rapidly (average ignition 3.92 seconds) in a non–oxygen-enriched atmosphere (Stouffer, 1991). According to the NFPA voluntary standard 702-1980, materials having a flame spread of 3 to 7 seconds are rated as class III. An instinctive reaction to the sight of a drape fire is to throw saline or water on the flame. But, because surgical fabrics have been treated with chemicals to be repellant to fluids, trying to extinguish a drape fire with water or saline is ineffective.

Cotton bath blankets, sheets, patient gowns, towels, and other fabrics made from cotton cellulose fibers are also highly flammable. In at least one case, an infant was severely burned when an electrosurgical unit ignited the paper drapes and cotton gauze sponges during an emergency cardiac procedure (OR Fire Occurrence Low, but Resulting Liability High, 1992).

All surgical suites contain innumerable items and products that are flammable. Laparotomy sponges, 4 × 4s, latex tubing, and gauze dressings are commonly found in and around the surgical field. In a few cases, a patient's hair or gastrointestinal tract gases have been implicated as the fuel source. Once a fire starts, even the furniture in the OR has the potential for adding fuel to the blaze.

FIRE PREVENTION: INTERVENTIONS

Since OR suites contain an abundance of the three essential ingredients needed to cause a sustained fire, it becomes apparent that preventing a fire through staff education and safe practices is of utmost importance. The most important factor for fire prevention in the OR is proper handling of the equipment that generates the ignition source and controlling as far as possible the fuels that feed the fires. At the time of this writing, existing standards and codes for high-energy devices are inadequate in establishing safety procedures, workable fire extinguishing devices, and fire resistance of fabrics (UCLA Operating Room Fire, 1990). It therefore becomes doubly important for health care facilities to educate personnel for fire prevention.

Annual education should be carefully planned to avoid interference with the intraoperative care of patients while not placing additional stress on the OR staff. Hospital-wide fire prevention programs fail to address the special conditions of the OR suite. If OR educators edit out the segments that are not applicable to the OR and insert unit-specific needs, they can improve the caliber and effectiveness of the program they facilitate. Planning independent learning activities that require active involvement increases the learners' absorption and retention and also reduces the length of time needed for the formal presentation. An example of an independent activity is one that might require OR members to tour their OR suite themselves and mark the location of all fire extinguishers and alarm boxes on a floor plan (Vidor, 1989).

The following material should be included in a fire safety program for operating room staff:

1. Plan, discuss, and practice action steps needed if a fire does occur. Eliminate any complacency about the possibility of an OR fire. Create awareness of the risks.
2. Explain the physical impact of a smoke-filled room. It may be difficult or impossible to breathe, forcing OR staff to vacate the room — compelling them to leave the patient.
3. Provide practice sessions using the different types of fire extinguisher. The staff must know where extinguishers and gas shut-off valves are located and when to use them.
4. Identify the location of fire hoses, fire alarms, and fire doors. Review evacuation routes and develop a plan for moving unconscious and intraoperative patients. Ask personnel for their response to hypothetical situations.
5. Ensure the availability of adequate portable auxiliary lighting. It may be needed if the fire knocks out the electrical system — smoke can quickly and severely limit visibility.
6. Identify the flammability rating of the surgical drapes and gowns purchased by the institution. Inform personnel of the time elements involved in flame spread.
7. Provide each room in the OR suite with a fire blanket. It should be readily available to extinguish fires of surgical drapes or clothing of personnel.
8. Develop policies and procedures that require wetting patients' hair with water soluble gel or other solutions if the hair will be near the operative site, for example, wetting a beard during facial surgery.

Following its investigation of two serious OR fires, the Los Angeles City Fire Department developed the following recommendations for fire safety in health care institutions:

1. That high-energy heat sources be placed in a holder or other location when not in active use
2. That cords that provide power from ESU generators be disconnected and removed when no longer needed

3. That directly clamping or winding cords to or around any objects be prohibited
4. That patients be continuously monitored for isolation from conductive paths, i.e., metal surfaces; if possible, that OR sheets be secured in a way to prevent contact with metal surfaces
5. That the hospital's operating room staff receive an increased level of fire and life safety training
6. That the hospital's operating room staff be required to periodically review high-energy surgical equipment safety guidelines and usage requirements
7. That hospitals require the use of materials meeting the class I classification according to NFPA standard 702-1980 for
   a. the wearing apparel of all hospital operating and surgical staff when utilizing high-energy surgical heat sources
   b. all draping material utilized to cover or drape equipment within the vicinity of the operating room bed (UCLA Operating Room Fire, 1990).

FLAMMABILITY RATINGS

There are no laws requiring flame-resistant fabrics in operating rooms and no standards for OR attire. NFPA 702-1980 *was* a voluntary standard for wearing apparel, but surgical drapes and gowns are not defined as clothing (Stouffer, 1991). The less stringent Consumer Products Safety Commission (CPSC) standards are intended only for street clothing. Even though the NFPA 702-1980 has been withdrawn as a wearing apparel standard, it still is used in research as a valid method to determine the flammability of fabrics and has been recommended by the Los Angeles City Fire Department. It is up to each institution to decide upon the standard they wish to uphold.

To make a rational decision about fire standards, health care facilities must understand the differences between the retired NFPA standards and the current CPSC ratings (Table 5–3). To earn a Class I rating by NFPA, a fabric was required to have a flame spread time of 20 seconds or more, but a Class I rating by the CPSC allows a fabric to ignite and burn in as little as 3.5 seconds (CPSC, 1990). The daily newspaper will burn at this rate. The CPSC rating should be considered unacceptable for fabrics in high-hazard areas. According to a 1986 report from the Emergency Care Research Institute, most reusables would be rated as Class II and most disposables as Class III. A few synthetic reusables have a Class I rating, but only one disposable, a polypropylene fabric, was rated Class I, outperforming other disposables even under testing conducted in an oxygen-enriched atmosphere.

One method of evaluating flammability of draping material involved response under oxygen conditions ranging from 21% to 100%.

TABLE 5–3. **FLAMMABILITY RATINGS**

NATIONAL FIRE PROTECTION ASSOCIATION 702-1980
CLASS I — RELATIVELY SLOW BURNING — fabric has a flame spread time of 20 seconds or more.
CLASS II — MODERATELY FLAMMABLE — fabric has a flame spread time of 8 to 19 seconds.
CLASS III — RELATIVELY FLAMMABLE — fabric has a flame spread time of 3 to 7 seconds.
CLASS IV — DANGEROUSLY FLAMMABLE — fabric has a flame spread time of less than 3 seconds.
   (From National Fire Protection Association. Test Method 702-1980)

CONSUMER PRODUCTS SAFETY COMMISSION
CLASS 1 — NORMAL FLAMMABILITY — fabric has an ignition time of 3.5 seconds or more.
CLASS 2 — INTERMEDIATE — not applicable for medical textiles.
CLASS 3 — RAPID AND INTENSE BURNING — fabric ignites in less than 3.5 seconds.
   (From Consumer Products Safety Commission. *Standards for Flammability of Clothing Textiles. Federal Register* 16 CFR 1610)

Although choosing safe supplies is important, OR staff cannot rely on product selection alone. Greater importance should be placed on preventing fires through safe practices and education.

Radiologic Safety

IONIZING RADIATION

Background

The benefits of ionizing radiation include cancer therapy, using gamma rays or x-rays to alter tumor cells; and providing diagnostic procedures such as cholangiography, angiography, and fluoroscopy. Excessive exposure can cause cataracts, burns, bone marrow injury, and tissue necrosis. Operating room personnel assisting with invasive x-ray studies or fluoroscopy are exposed to scatter radiation. The effects of radiation may have an extended latency period with symptoms not manifesting for many years. Because the effects are cumulative, it is essential for personnel to both measure their exposure levels and take protective action to avoid unnecessary exposure.

As early as 1898, the dangers of burns due to ionizing radiation were reported by the *International Dental Journal*. The need for a way to detect the amount of exposure health care workers faced was met with devices for utilization in dental radiographs. Concerns about the dangers of ionizing radiation have been growing owing mainly to reports about the Hiroshima and Nagasaki atom bombs and the nuclear plant accidents of Three Mile Island in the U.S. and Chernobyl in the former Soviet Union. Concern about the potential undesirable effects of exposure to radiation has increased dramatically as a result of publicity, and these latter accidents have served to highlight the need for safe work practices in highly hazardous areas.

The National Council on Radiation Protection and Measurement calculated that we receive 82% of our ionizing radiation exposure from natural sources, such as radon gas, naturally occurring radioactive materials on earth, and cosmic (outer space) radiation. Radon gas is responsible for 50% to 75% of this exposure. The remaining 18% of exposure comes from man-made sources, with medical and dental procedures accounting for 75% of these sources, and consumer products accounting for about 20% (Farman, 1991).

Hazards

Following the bombing of Hiroshima and Nagasaki in 1945, studies to evaluate the potential genetic effects of radiation were initiated by the U.S. National Academy of Sciences, the U.S. Department of Energy, and the Japanese Ministry of Health and Welfare. Survivors who received significant amounts of radiation were followed to measure the genetic effects in their children. The study was based on children born between 1946 and 1985. Indicators chosen included stillbirths, major congenital defects, impaired physical development, and development of cancer before age 20. For all the indicators chosen, there was no statistically significant difference between the study groups (Neel, 1991).

Studies to examine possible environmental causes of childhood leukemia and lymphoma reported in the vicinity of the Sellofield nuclear plant in the United Kingdom were reported in 1990. Children of fathers who had occupational exposure to ionizing radiation in a nuclear plant were more likely to develop leukemia than children of fathers in a control group. This did not hold true for the lymphoma cases (Gardner, 1990).

The carcinogenic effects of radiation on physicists and physicians who developed leukemia and skin or bone tumors have been well documented. Patients who receive diagnostic and therapeutic doses of ionizing radiation are more likely to develop breast cancer, thyroid cancer, leukemia, and bone tumors; the greater the exposure, the greater the risk. Women of childbearing age must be especially careful to estimate the possibility of a pregnancy when faced with any type of ionizing radiation exposure. A fetus is at greatest risk of cancer malformation or even death if exposed to radiation during the 2 to 15 weeks' gestation period. Inadvertent fetus exposure can be avoided if procedures are performed during the first 2 weeks of the menstrual cycle, during menses, or if a contraceptive is faithfully used. The latency period between exposure and illness can be as long as 20 years (Farman, 1991).

Fluoroscopy and X-Ray Studies

Because exposure to radiation is cumulative, it is essential for OR personnel to have appropriate protective devices during procedures requiring radiation. Reproductive organs, thyroid glands, and the lenses of the eyes are especially sensitive to radiation exposure. Protective devices, such as lead aprons, are heavy and tiring to wear during long procedures, but they provide essential protection to the body. Sterile team members wear the apron under their sterile gowns. Aprons should always be hung when not being worn — never folded. Folding will crack the lead and ruin the shield. Thyroid collars should be made available to patients for radiation of head, neck, or upper extremities and to anyone within 6 feet of exposure. Lead shields provide the best protection and absorb radiant energy. Team members who cannot leave the room should stand behind a shield. A shield should also be placed behind a cassette holder, to absorb scatter radiation when lateral exposures are required. Holding devices for cassettes should be employed whenever possible. If a single exposure requires the cassette to be held by hand, the person holding the cassette should wear lead impregnated rubber gloves. Lead gloves provide protection and can be sterilized by ethylene oxide. The lens of the eye is particularly susceptible to radiation damage; personnel should wear leaded glasses during fluoroscopy. Long-term exposure of the eyes to radiation can result in cataracts (Smith, 1993).

Exposure to radiation should be measured and limited. When a procedure requires radiation, OR staff should rotate assignments. Pregnant personnel should leave the room during radiation exposure, be adequately shielded, or request reassignment to other cases. If unsterile team members leave the room during exposures, they should first determine that the patient is securely positioned and should maintain visual contact. Exposure can also be limited by standing behind a lead shield, standing 6 feet or more from the patient, or standing out of the direct aim of the beam, whichever is possible. Radiation intensity decreases geometrically in proportion to the square of the distance from the source — double distance equals one quarter intensity (Farman, 1991).

X-ray tubes, fluoroscopes, and image intensifiers should be turned off when not needed. Radiation can be present only when a machine is energized. All personnel who work with or around ionizing radiation on a regular basis or for long procedures, should wear monitoring devices to measure the total accumulated exposure. Film badges are the most common monitoring devices and more than one may be worn to determine the whole body dose — one outside the apron at the neck and the other under the apron. Annual in-service training programs should review the risks and safety measures.

Radium Implants

Radium is radioactive metal employed in the treatment of malignant tumors. Available sources include needles, seeds, or capsules; the type selected depends upon the type of tumor and the anatomic site. In many facilities implantation of these devices takes place in the x-ray department, or an after-loading technique is chosen. With the after-loading technique the patient is prepared for the implant in the OR by the insertion of an unloaded applicator into the tissue. The radiation source is then loaded into the applicator by the radiologist at the patient's bedside. The radioactive elements gradually disintegrate. Many patients have surgery following the implantation. Surgical procedures should be delayed at least 24 hours after a safe radiation level has been reached.

Other safety precautions to observe when working with radium implants are as follows:

1. Radiation elements should remain in or be returned to lead-lined containers and handled as quickly as possible.
2. Radium elements should be handled only with forceps or tools—never with hands.
3. When implanting radium devices, the person should do so from behind a lead screen.
4. Warning signs should be posted on the door during surgery for patients with implants.
5. Body fluids and tissues from these patients should be treated as hazardous waste and quickly confined in appropriate containers.
6. Personnel should limit their time in close proximity to patients with implants.

NONIONIZING RADIATION

Nonionizing radiation is a term given to a group of electromagnetic radiations. This type of radiation is not cumulative in the body; does not require monitoring; and, when properly handled, is not considered hazardous. Nonionizing radiation is usually undetected unless its intensity creates heat. Common sources of nonionizing radiation include radios, television sets, microwave ovens, computers, warmers, and light sources. Common sources of nonionizing radiation in health care facilities include germicidal lamps for disinfection, phototherapy lamps for excessive bilirubin therapy in newborns, diathermy equipment for musculoskeletal disease therapy, hyperthermia equipment for cancer therapy, video display terminals, computer and television monitors, magnetic resonance imaging devices, electrosurgical devices, and lasers (Charron, 1991).

To ensure safety from any nonionizing source, all equipment must be properly maintained and handled; biomedical equipment checks must be maintained on a regular basis; written safety instructions from the manufacturer must be followed; and personnel must use generally accepted safety practices. AORN's *Recommended Practices for Reducing Radiological Exposure in the Practice Setting* (AORN, 1994e) emphasizes the need to provide protection to both staff and patients during x-ray exposures.

Chemical Safety

The health hazard of occupational exposure to waste anesthesia gases, pharmaceuticals, sterilants, and other chemicals is a serious concern. Even though research provides no consistent answers in studies about the risks, OSHA has increased enforcement activity.

HAZARDS COMMUNICATION STANDARD

In 1987, the *Hazards Communication Standard*, 29 CFR 1910.1200, was expanded to include hospitals and health care facilities. The standard mandates

Although the information on the MSDSs was designed for users of large amounts of chemicals, several health care facilities have been cited by OSHA for failure to properly label some chemicals. When chemicals are transferred from their original containers into smaller containers for easier handling, care should be taken to ensure adequate labeling for the secondary container.

ANESTHETIC AGENTS

Waste anesthesia gases are included in the government's hazard communication standard list of products that require MSDSs. The FDA recognizes the recommended exposure levels set by National Institute for Occupational Safety and Health (NIOSH) of 25 ppm for nitrous oxide. Gases and vapors that escape from anesthesia equipment have been the topic of numerous epidemiologic investigations since the 1970s. Although the studies have included cancers, renal hepatic disorders, and the nervous system, far more attention has been directed to the effects on reproduction and spontaneous abortion. Even though anesthesia agents have been targeted as the likely causal agents, these studies have failed to show any cause-and-effect relationship between exposure to gases and adverse effects, mainly because of serious shortcomings in the way the data were compiled. Some studies, however, suggest there may indeed be a deleterious effect from prolonged exposure to nitrous oxide. In 1992, the *Canadian Journal of Anesthesia* (Woods, 1992) reported on a 1984 study (Amos, 1984) which showed that patients and personnel exposed to 50% nitrous oxide for periods as short as 5 hours during cardiac bypass surgery demonstrated dose-dependent megaloblastic changes in bone marrow. Notwithstanding that intravenous techniques for the induction of anesthesia reduce the exposure to personnel, the study concluded that the maximum exposure to nitrous oxide recommended by NIOSH is unattainable in actual practice.

Mounting evidence suggests that exposure to ambient nitrous oxide results in reduced fertility among female dental assistants if exposed for more than 5 hours per week, but the concentration and length of exposure have not been proven. The American Dental Association (ADA, 1992) mandates that scavenging equipment

- reduces ambient N_2O to the lowest possible level
- works effectively regardless of the ventilating system
- achieves the NIOSH and OSHA recommended standards.

Many other factors affect the effectiveness of scavenging devices, including patient behavior (crying or talking), certain dental procedures, improper administration of the gas, and improper fit of the anesthesia mask.

The ADA suggests additional measures to minimize atmospheric contamination by waste gases, including periodic equipment testing, evaluation of building ventilation systems, and adjustment of room air exchanges to ten exchanges per hour with at least partial fresh air mix.

The *American Industrial Hygiene Association Journal* in March of 1992 (Sass-Kortsak, 1992) reported on the exposure of OR personnel to occupational environment factors in seven Toronto hospitals. A total of 291 subjects were included in the study. In measuring exposure to nitrous oxide, anesthetists were found to have significantly higher exposures than the OR nurses. The anesthetists' time-weighted average exposures exceeded the recommended 25-ppm standard in 27% of all measurements, whereas only 14% of the OR nurses' measurements exceeded the recommended standard. The major source of waste gas pollution came from leaking anesthesia equipment, spills, and leaks from the high-pressure delivery system. The age of the equipment was a significant factor in the amount of leakage. Improvement in waste gas pollution can be achieved by updated scavenging systems, increased maintenance and leak detection, and careful anesthetic practices.

The American Association of Nurse Anesthetists (AANA) recommends quarterly checks for implementation of the following:

- Preventive maintenance routines (PMR) by a factory-trained service provider for the anesthesia equipment
- A central vacuum system for scavenging operations (e.g., closed circuit breathing system for anesthesia) and performance
- Testing of ventilation an air conditioning systems to ensure complete room air exchanges of 15 to 20 times per hour
- A system for the measurement of levels of trace/waste gas concentrations.

Studies indicate there is a potential for adverse effects from long-term exposure to nitrous oxide, but much of the methodology of the studies was flawed and failed to demonstrate the nature, degree, and length of exposure that could cause adverse reactions. Even though the studies were inclusive, both NIOSH and OSHA have established standards recommending that exposure levels do not exceed 25 ppm per hour.

OTHER AGENTS

The sterilizing gas ethylene oxide (ETO) is an agent that has been proved to be toxic to all living cells. It is a colorless, noncorrosive, highly penetrative gas, making it an ideal agent to sterilize moisture-sensitive items such as fiber-optic instruments, cameras, rigid and flexible scopes, and plastic or porous items. However, it also has serious disadvantages. Identified as toxic waste by the Environmental Protection Agency (EPA), it is also known to be a carcinogen and mutagen. Chemical burns and cataracts have been caused by contact with skin and eyes. Inhaled, it has caused dizziness, nausea, and vomiting. More serious reactions include neurologic damage, leukemia, chromosomal aberrations, and spontaneous abortions. Additional disadvantages include the flammability and explosive nature of the gas, the increased cost over steam sterilization, and the length of the sterilization cycle, which may be as long as 30 hours (Steelman, 1992).

Sterilization by ETO requires rigid control of the gas concentration and measurement of the exposure time, temperature, and humidity. Items to be sterilized must be dry, since ETO contact with moisture will result in the formation of ethylene glycol. Because of the dangerous nature of ETO, personnel must be extremely cautious and follow the safety instructions of the manufacturer. The only way to remove the gas from the sterilized item is through the process of aeration. This may be accomplished in an ambient air chamber, but it is safer and more efficient to utilize a mechanical aerator, preferably one with a safety lock.

In the 1960s and 1970s, there was insufficient information about these dangers. Sometimes impatience led to premature removal of items from the aerator. It was thought that rinsing in sterile water would complete the detoxification of the item. Patients' reactions to improper or incomplete aeration included chemical burns, tissue inflammation, pulmonary edema, and anaphylaxis, and at least one reported death.

Glutaraldehyde is used to sterilize and disinfect items by soaking them in a solution made by mixing a 2% aqueous solution of activated buffered glutaraldehyde. It is activated by adding powdered buffer to liquid, but mixed solutions gradually lose potency over a period of 14 to 30 days depending on the brand. More commonly selected for disinfection, it allows rapid turnover of specialty instruments such as bronchoscopes and items made from plastic or rubber. Disinfection can be achieved in as little as 10 minutes (depending on manufacturer's recommendations) killing bacteria, fungi, pseudomonas, and viruses including HIV and HBV. A 2% solution at 77°F to 86°F may be 100% tuberculocidal in 45 to 90 minutes, depending on formulation; it is sporicidal in a minimum of 10 hours. Fumes from glutaraldehyde are noxious and irritating to the eyes, nose, and throat. OR personnel have reported contact dermatitis from skin contact (Newman, 1992). Instruments must be carefully and thoroughly rinsed in copious amounts of sterile distilled water, and the water must be discarded after each use. The water should never be used more than once. Inadequately rinsed instruments can cause tissue burns in patients. Glutaraldehyde solutions should be carefully confined in a closed container in a well-ventilated room.

Formaldehyde is usually employed in the OR only as a preservative for surgical specimens. Formalin solution consists of 8% formaldehyde in 70% isopropyl alcohol. It is a proven carcinogen and mutagen. Fumes can be toxic to the eyes, nose, and throat. Prolonged exposure has been shown to cause liver damage. Formalin will kill bacteria, pseudomonas, fungi, Mycobacterium tuberculosis, and viruses within 15 minutes and spores within 12 hours.

Other agents utilized in the OR for disinfecting or cleaning include isopropyl alcohol, phenol, and sodium hypochlorite. Fumes from these solutions may irritate nasal passages, and direct skin contact may cause burns. To protect against accidental exposure, personnel should wear at least goggles and gloves.

Methyl methacrylate is a self-curing thermoplastic acrylic cement commonly called bone cement. By the mixing of liquid and powder polymers, a glue that augments fixation of prosthetic devices is produced. When the mixture hardens, it looks and feels very much like bone and can be used to repair a skull defect. Strong vapors are released during the mixing process. These vapors can be irritating to the eyes and throat and may even cause drowsiness. If splashed in the eye, the liquid solvent can cause a corneal burn; contact with skin may cause an allergic dermatitis. Safety requires gloves that are impermeable to the solvent, goggles, and a scavenging system to exhaust or neutralize the vapors; personnel are advised not to wear contact lenses. A 1992 study (Sass-Kortsak, 1992) indicates that the risk to OR personnel from repeated exposures is small, but pregnant females should follow the advice of their physician.

Antineoplastics, cytotoxic drugs, laser dyes, and pharmaceuticals, as well as chemotherapy drugs can be hazardous to employees. Employers are responsible for identifying all drugs that should be classified as hazardous. Each institution must compile a list of drugs that have any of the following characteristics:

1. Potential for causing genetic abnormalities
2. Potential for causing cancer in animal models, patient population, or both, as reported by the International Agency on Research in Cancer
3. Potential for causing fertility impairment in animal studies or in treated patients
4. Evidence of serious organ or other toxicity at low doses in animal models or treated patients.

The list should provide not only information on the drugs and their toxicity, but recommendations for special handling.

When handling any chemical, safe practices include appropriate PPE such as thick gloves, masks, and goggles; engineering controls, such as laminar flow hoods, during preparation of solutions; enforcement of policies and procedures designed to protect personnel, such as washing hands after handling agents and proper disposal of toxic agents; and routine and thorough education of employees regarding the risks of the substances.

Occupational Safety

Work in the operating room requires a great deal of physical activity. Reaching, stretching, bending, lifting, and moving heavy equipment and patients are a required part of the perioperative role. To circumvent injury and conserve energy, good body mechanics and work efficiency principles should be learned and applied. Avoiding falls, injuries, and strains allows health care workers to feel better and work more productively. Regular reviews of safe work practices will promote employee awareness and improve work performance (National Safety Council, 1991).

COMMON INJURIES

Operating room personnel sometimes sustain injuries as a result of poorly designed work areas. Injuries such as back strain, arm or leg muscle strains, carpal tunnel syndrome, cuts, burns, falls, fractures, abrasions, and contusions are not uncommon. The principles of ergonomics have been employed to reduce the injuries caused by poor design. The principles reduce stress and strain by adapting working conditions and areas to fit the needs of employees. Some ergonomic safety changes are as simple as increasing lighting and raising or lowering work surfaces. These changes can measurably reduce stress and improve function (National Safety Council, 1991). Other changes may be more costly requiring new equipment or even remodeling. These costs, however, are quickly justified when compared with the cost of treating an employee for a work-related injury. OSHA considers ergonomics related injuries as illnesses and has the authority to cite employers for problems under the general duty clause.

Preventing injuries has benefits other than monetary for the employer. Not only will the cost of citations and of treating injuries be prevented, but employees will be more productive. Training to prevent injuries should begin when the employee is hired and should be an ongoing process thereafter. Education should not only teach employees how to reach, lift, and turn; it should teach them how to choose correct materials and arrange work areas for greatest efficiency. Even such simple tasks as mopping floors, moving tables, pushing carts, and adjusting equipment need to be done correctly to avoid accidents. Repetitive motion tasks of the hand and wrist are a common cause of carpal tunnel syndrome, which causes symptoms of burning, numbness, and tingling. If the problem remains uncorrected, eventually the result may be loss of function in the affected hand.

Avoiding Injuries

Some injuries can be circumvented by maintaining good body posture when standing or sitting. Personnel should stand with the back straight and feet slightly apart, weight evenly balanced. Adjusting the work surface to 6 inches below the elbow will eliminate the need to bend over and will prevent back stress. When standing in one place for long periods, shift the weight from one foot to the other. Place one foot at a time on a low riser, such as the base of the OR bed, to reduce lower back fatigue. Reduce the stress of long periods of standing by changing position as frequently as possible. Sitting incorrectly can cause lower back, neck, or shoulder pain. Sit with the back straight, feet flat on the floor, and do not slouch; lean forward from the hips to reduce muscle exertion; maintain good head and shoulder alignment to prevent neck and shoulder fatigue. Lift heavy objects off lower shelves or the floor by using the large muscles of the thighs and hips keeping the back straight. Employ team effort to move patients, using the arm, shoulder, and chest muscles. Push rather than pull heavy items; evaluate the balance of equipment as it is moved to prevent tipping.

Prevent falls by keeping traffic areas clean and free of all unnecessary furniture. Discard outer wrappers and packaging in the proper receptacle; immediately pick up small items such as rubber bands, needle caps, and suture packages. Staff members must frequently move quickly in the OR and with their attention focused on the patient; the smallest objects can be overlooked on the floor and be treacherous underfoot. Wipe up spills immediately; have an antimicrobial agent handy to clean up blood or body fluids. Change shoe covers if they get wet on the bottom. Water may be tracked into the OR from the scrub sink; saline or prep solutions may be spilled—all must receive prompt attention. Coil excess tubing and electrical cords close to the unit. When possible, position tubing in front of the operative team, reducing the potential for a fall when stepping backward. Do not permit lines to be suspended above the floor, and connect them to outlets away from the traffic area if possible. Position unnecessary furniture next to the walls and out of the way. Do not lean unused lifters or step stools against the wall; they should be placed with all four feet flat on the floor.

Steam sterilizers are frequently the cause of contact or steam burns. These safety measures should be followed:

- Make sure the cycle is complete before opening the door.
- Crack the door a few inches and allow excess steam to escape before opening. Open the door as wide as it will allow.
- Use sterile extension handles or an insulated mitt to lift the tray out of the autoclave. Take care to avoid arm contact with the rim of the door (Fig. 5–4).
- Close the door as soon as possible to prevent injury to another person.

MOTION ECONOMY

Economy of motion prevents physical fatigue from body movement and improves work efficiency. There are ten principles of motion economy.

- Motions should be productive.
- Motions should be simple.
- Motions should be curved.
- Motions should be symmetric.
- Work should be within grasp range.
- Hands should be relieved of work.

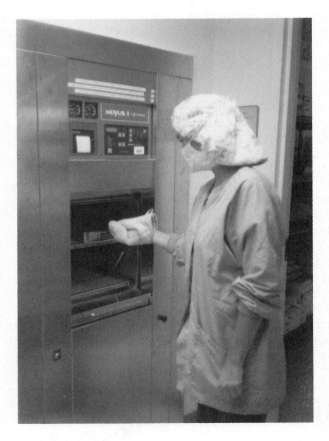

FIGURE 5–4. Autoclave Safety

- The worker should be at ease.
- Work material should be prepositioned.
- Gravity should be used.
- Supplies should be combined.

1. *Motions should be productive.* Work as fast as possible without compromising technique. Neat work areas and standardized instrument sets and table setups eliminate fumbling and rehandling items. Consider work flow to minimize motion.

2. *Motions should be simple.* Reduce body movement to the least possible action to accomplish the task. For example, use only the fingers and knuckles to turn a screw or cut with scissors. Increase the effort and motions only as much as the task requires. Add hand motion to pass instruments, count sponges, or write. The movement of the elbow is required to peel open packages, unfold drapes, or unwrap supplies. Expand the motion to the upper arm and shoulder for opening a door, setting up a Mayo stand, or adjusting an overhead light. Torso muscles are required to move furniture, connect suction tubing, or lift patients.

3. *Motions should be curved.* Circular motion creates less fatigue than push and pull movements; therefore, movements should be circular when possible.

4. *Motions should be symmetric.* Movements should be as smooth and rhythmic as possible. Even when force is required, avoid movements that snap, tug, or wrench. Apply steady, even pressure.

5. *Work should be within grasp range.* The minimum grasp range is the area between the hands in front of the body when the forearms are extended from the elbow and the hands move only on a horizontal plane. The optimum range is the area in front of the body where the arc of the right and left hand overlap when moving on a horizontal plane. The maximum range is the area in front of the body when the arms are extended and shoulder pivotal movement is added.

6. *Hands should be relieved of work.* Hands should be replaced for functions that can be accomplished by other parts of the body. Knees can activate water faucets; feet can activate pedals. Electronic door openers eliminate the need for physical action.

7. *The worker should be at ease.* Good body posture when standing or sitting reduces fatigue. Further elements to consider include ventilation to remove odors, toxic fumes, and waste anesthesia gases. Lighting should be adequate and without glare. Satin finishes on instruments reduce reflection. Softly tinted goggles can decrease eye fatigue. Pastel colors on walls and drapes are less reflective than white. Some operating rooms have wall murals to soften the effect of windowless rooms. Music can be either relaxing or stimulating; it should be carefully selected and played only at low volume. Constant music can be more harmful than beneficial. It should be turned off periodically to prevent mental fatigue. Reduce or eliminate all unnecessary equipment noises. Create as quiet and pleasant a working atmosphere as possible for the benefit of both staff and patient.

8. *Work material should be prepositioned.* Arrange supplies on the tables in the sequence in which they are expected to be needed. Arrange instruments in systematic order, fully assembled. Pass instruments with the handles pointed to the user.

9. *Gravity should be used.* Gravity feed or drop dispensing is a quick efficient method to deliver supplies. Small supplies can be arranged in vertical slots for convenience. Large heavy packs should be on shelves that are slanted slightly to assist with delivery.

10. *Supplies should be combined.* Sterilizer tape holds the package together and indicates exposure to steam at the same time, and only a small amount

of tape is required to do the job. Disposable kits and trays combine all the items needed for a specific procedure. Reusable sets can be prepared on-site to fulfill the same function. Custom procedure trays increase staff efficiency by decreasing the number of individual components that must be opened. They also reduce the number of outer wrappers, cutting down on trash and room cleanup time (Atkinson, 1992).

Biologic Hazardous Materials

DEFINITIONS

To protect health care workers from potential infection, it is necessary to identify causative organisms or toxins capable of causing disease and to employ hazard abatement strategies to avoid, eliminate, or reduce the hazards and exposures. Federal agencies along with state and local agencies all have their own definitions of biologic and hazardous materials. The result is a confusing array of rules and guidelines, some of which are in conflict with each other. As the number of regulating agencies increases, so does the confusion, and no clear-cut definition of medical waste exists (Table 5–4). Health care facilities are faced then with ". . . redundant requirements, inconsistent definitions and increased cost without any apparent risk reduction." For example, OSHA's definition of medical waste states that bandages are not regulated waste unless saturated to the point of releasing blood if compacted, yet feminine hygiene products are generally not considered regulated waste (AHA, 1993). In spite of the cost, most health care facilities rely on overly inclusive interpretations to identify hazardous waste. Until the federal government's definition of what is and what is not infectious waste is put in place, health care facilities will have to comply with their local and/or state regulations.

Instead of overreacting to the remote possibility of an infection from medical waste, regulatory agencies would do well to remember that these four factors are necessary for an infection to occur.

TABLE 5–4. MEDICAL WASTE REGULATIONS AND GUIDELINES

WASTE SOURCE	CDC	EPA	DOT	OSHA	ATSDR
Stocks, cultures, infectious agents	yes	yes	yes	yes	yes
Free-flowing or bulk blood	yes	yes	yes	yes	yes
Items blood soaked or caked			yes	yes	yes
Tissues and organs	yes	yes	yes	yes	yes
Potentially infectious body fluids			yes	yes	yes
All specimens of body fluids			yes		
Used sharps	yes	yes	yes	yes	yes
Unused discarded sharps			yes		yes
Communicable disease isolation		yes	yes		yes*
Contaminated animal waste		**		yes	yes
Surgery and autopsy waste		**			
Dialysis waste		**			
Contaminated equipment		**			

CDC—Centers for Disease Control and Prevention
EPA—Environmental Protection Agency
DOT—Department of Transportation
OSHA—Occupational Safety and Health Administration
ATSDR—Agency for Toxic Substances and Disease Registry
*CDC class 4 only
**Optional
(From AHA, APIC call for end to confusing infectious waste regs. [1993]. *Hospital Infection Control 20*[5], 63.) (Courtesy of American Hospital Association, Chicago, Illinois)

1. Pathogens having sufficient virulence and in sufficient numbers to cause disease must be present.
2. Pathogens must make contact with a person.
3. There must be a portal of entry into the person's body.
4. The person must be susceptible to the pathogen.

The risk is small that all of these factors will come together in the community environment. For example, in the 10 years of known HIV epidemic in the world, there is not a single case of known disease transmission from environmental sources (AHA, 1993).

RISKS

Infection control and health care officials are urging federal agencies to end the aforementioned confusion. The AORN and the AHA, along with other health care organizations, have proposed guidelines for defining regulated waste and for adopting a uniform regulatory approach. The AORN white paper proposes four categories:

- Sharps—used and unused
- Microbiologic waste—including cultures
- Animal waste—such as carcasses and soiled bedding
- Items used by humans infected with class 4 etiologic agents.

Two additional categories of waste that are occupational hazards but do not pose a public health risk and do not need to be regulated are pathologic waste, such as human tissue and organs, and human blood products. If these proposed definitions are accepted there would be no significant change in the way waste in surgery is handled, but it could substantially reduce disposal costs (Regulated Medical Waste, 1993).

Sharps Injuries

OR personnel are at an increased risk of percutaneous injury compared with personnel in other places in the hospital. A study was undertaken (Tokars, 1992) to document the numbers and circumstances of needle sticks and cuts that occur during surgical procedures. The injuries were recorded by direct observation or by voluntary reporting by the participant. The study of 1,382 procedures recorded 99 injuries occurring during 95 (6.9%) of the procedures. A total of 76 injuries were caused by suture needles, and 19 injuries were caused by electric cautery, scalpels, wires, instruments, or bone fragments.

Handling Sharps

OSHA addresses the safe handling of sharps in its standard on bloodborne pathogens. Sharps includes needles, knife blades, razors, broken glass, broken capillary pipettes, and exposed dental wires. Contaminated sharps may not be purposely bent, recapped, or broken by hand, removed from disposable syringes, or otherwise manipulated by hand unless the employer can demonstrate that no alternative is feasible or that such action is required by medical procedure, i.e., blood gas procedures, incremental dose of medication, or blood cultures. If recapping or removal of needles is performed, a mechanical device or one-handed technique must be employed. The location in the health care facility where recapping may occur and the reason for recapping must be documented in the health care facility's exposure control plan.

All contaminated sharps must be placed in sharps containers that are puncture resistant, visibly labeled or color-coded, and leakproof on the sides and bottom. Sharps containers must be readily accessible to the work area. The containers must be replaced routinely and not be allowed to overfill, because over-filling increases the risk of needle sticks. Disposable containers must be clos-able and have tight-fitting lids to prevent spilling during transport. Reusable sharps also require careful treatment. Sharps, including large bore needles, skin hooks, rasps, drill points, and saws pose a hazard to the surgical team. A safe work practice is to use a sharps zone on the sterile field. The scrub person identifies a small area on the surgical field to be the zone; the area may be a towel, a tray, or a small basin. Instead of passing sharps from hand to hand, they are placed in the zone by one person along with an audible announcement, i.e., "sharps up," and then retrieved from the zone by another. The practice precludes passing sharps from hand to hand and has substantially reduced the incidence of injuries in the OR.

At the completion of a procedure, contaminated, reusable sharps must be contained in a manner that eliminates or minimizes hazards until they are re-processed. The containers for reusable sharps must be puncture resistant, leak-proof on the sides and bottom, and labeled or color-coded. However, containers for reusable sharps are not required to be closable. Sharps containers are re-quired to be designed so that they may be emptied safely. Emptying may be as simple as turning the unit upside down. They may not be stored or processed in a manner that requires employees to reach their hand into the containers to re-trieve items. If retrieval is necessary, some type of instrument should be used. "Neither disposable or reusable sharps containers shall be opened, emptied, or cleaned manually, or handled in any manner which would expose employees to the risk of percutaneous injury" (OSHA, 1991).

REGULATED WASTE

OSHA requires regulated waste to be handled safely. OSHA's definition of regu-lated waste includes liquid or semiliquid blood or other potentially infectious materials; contaminated items that if compressed would release blood or other potentially infectious materials in a liquid or semiliquid state; items that are caked with dried blood or other potentially infectious materials and are capable of releasing these materials during handling; and pathologic and microbiologic waste containing blood or other potentially infectious materials. Other poten-tially infectious materials include body tissues and organs and all body fluids ex-cept sweat, tears, and saliva. OSHA does not consider urine, feces, or vomitus to present a potential bloodborne hazard, but personnel should still treat them as possible contaminants. Body fluids and specimens must be handled employing universal precautions. Safe handling of regulated waste requires containers that meet the same standards as sharps containers, except they do not have to be puncture resistant since they will not contain sharps.

INTERVENTIONS

Laundry

Fabrics used during surgery, disposable and reusable, must be properly handled to prevent the spread of infectious materials. Sheets, towels, blankets, patient gowns, surgical drapes, and protective clothing worn by the surgical team must be placed in a designated area or container for storage, washing, decontamina-tion, or disposal. The container must prevent indirect contamination of environ-mental surfaces or other people. Fabrics must not be sorted, rinsed, or handled unnecessarily in the area where they were used. Personnel handling the laundry must wear appropriate protective apparel.

Engineering Controls

Engineering controls refer to physical devices that reduce or remove hazards from the workplace. Included are items such as sharps disposal containers, self-resheathing syringes, needleless systems, phlebotomy devices, suction containers and liners, kickbuckets and liners, hoppers for disposal of filtered liquids, and splash guards on sinks. Engineering controls serve to reduce exposure in the workplace by either removing the hazard (hazard abatement) or isolating the personnel from exposure. In general, these controls act on the source of the hazard and eliminate or reduce the exposure without relying on people to take self-protective action, for example, by installing a protective shield. Engineering controls usually require maintenance or periodic replacement.

Work Practice Controls

Work practice controls refer to practices and procedures that reduce the likelihood of exposure to hazards by altering the manner in which a task is performed. Examples would be as follows: no two-handed recapping of needles; no food storage with potentially contaminated material; mandating handwashing after removing gloves; removing of PPE before leaving the immediate work area; using sharps containers appropriately. While work practice controls act on the source of the hazard, the protection they provide is based upon behavior rather than installation of a physical device.

Personal Protective Equipment: Gloves

Gloves must be worn whenever it can be reasonably anticipated that personnel may have hand contact with potentially infectious material, such as a patient's mucous membrane or nonintact skin. Glove types include disposable surgical gloves, exam gloves, and reusable utility gloves, i.e., the heavy duty rubber gloves used in housecleaning. Reusable gloves are permitted provided they can be disinfected and provided they exhibit no signs of deterioration and their ability to function as a barrier has not been compromised. Gloves must be changed as soon as possible when they become contaminated, torn, or punctured, and hands must be washed after gloves are removed. Although the OSHA standard does not require gloves to be changed between patients, changing gloves between patients is a standard infection control practice.

For people who are allergic to certain types of gloves such as those made from latex, or to glove powders or other glove lubricants, alternatives must be made available. Hypoallergenic gloves, glove liners, or powderless gloves must be readily accessible to employees who cannot wear the standard equipment. Gloves act as a primary barrier between hands and contact with potentially infectious materials. Double gloving during surgery has been proved to provide a greater level of protection to personnel. A 1991 study of 284 surgeons and first assistants recorded 51% hand contamination of individuals wearing single gloves compared with 7% hand contamination of those wearing double gloves (Quebbeman, 1992).

Although it is well recognized that gloves do not prevent needle stick injuries, some research suggests that gloves may provide some protection. This research, conducted by Dr. Julie Gerberding of San Francisco General Hospital, found that there was a significant (up to 50%) reduction in the amount of blood on a needle as it passed through a latex or vinyl glove. Because of the wipe-off effect of the material, the amount of inoculum that penetrates the skin is reduced. This research finding provides some evidence that gloves may afford protection from the risk of illness from a needle stick exposure (Gerberding, 1990).

Universal Precautions

Universal precautions require health care workers to treat all blood and certain body fluids as if they are known to be infected with a bloodborne pathogen. Body substance isolation (BSI) is another method of infection control in which *all* body fluids and substances are considered to be infectious. Since many patients have no idea they have a disease and many are nonsymptomatic, every patient should be treated as potentially infectious.

The operating room has been identified by OSHA as an area carrying a high potential for risk for bloodborne pathogens (Fig. 5–5). Studies have demonstrated that OR personnel are not only exposed but have frequent contact with blood and other potentially infectious materials (OPIM). Despite the risk, highly exposed health care workers have revealed a poor perception of the need to use universal precautions (Willy, 1990). This attitude must be corrected by the employer through educational programs and strictly enforced policies and procedures.

Some procedures carry especially high risk of blood contact (Table 5–5). Trauma, orthopedic and cardiac procedures, and cesarean sections have exceptionally high risks when compared with ophthalmologic and oral surgery. In a 1991 study of 684 operations, 293 personnel had blood contact events from just 28% of the procedures. Blood contact was defined as percutaneous, mucous membrane, or skin (intact or nonintact) exposure to blood. Eight of the procedures resulted in blood exposures to 63 personnel. Blood exposures were defined as percutaneous, mucous membrane, or nonintact skin contact with blood. Of the 684 procedures involved, 190 of them caused blood contact to one or more members of the surgical team. In all, 293 individuals reported blood contact. The longer the procedure, the more frequently contact events were recorded, with surgeons consistently experiencing the most blood exposures (Popejoy, 1991).

The likelihood of contamination of health care workers increases as the operative blood loss and length of the operation increases. However, the risk does not seem to alarm many health care workers, and compliance with universal precautions has been shown to be inconsistent. Improvement in adherence can be achieved by active infection control surveillance, continuous in-service training, and improved communication among health care workers (Hammond, 1990).

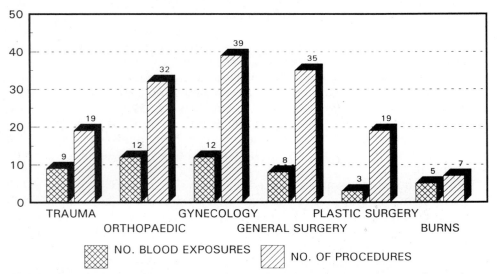

FIGURE 5–5. Documented Exposures to Blood in the Operating Room (151 Monitored Procedures) (From Willy, M. E. (1990). Adverse exposures and universal precaution practices among a group of highly exposed health professionals. *Infection Control Hospital Epidemiology, 11*(7), 351–356)

TABLE 5-5. **RISK OF BLOOD EXPOSURE EVENTS DURING SURGERY**

SERVICE	NUMBER PROCEDURES	NUMBER PEOPLE WITH EVENTS	NUMBER PEOPLE WITH EXPOSURES
Orthopedics	201	56	19
Gynecology	81	24	8
General Surgery	75	19	7
Otolaryngology	58	10	1
Pediatric Surgery	50	11	2
Neurosurgery	43	11	4
Trauma	39	19	6
Cardiothoracic	26	15	5
OB Cesarean Section	25	12	5
Urology	24	4	0
Plastic Surgery	23	7	1
Ophthalmology	22	0	0
Transplant	9	0	0
Burn	6	2	0
Oral Surgery	5	0	0

(From Popejoy, S. L., Fry, D. E. (1991). Blood contact and exposure in the operating room. *Surgery, Gynecology & Obstetrics, 172*(6), 480–483. By permission of *Surgery, Gynecology & Obstetrics*, now known as the *Journal of the American College of Surgeons*.)

Issues for Development

LITIGATION

Consumers of health care services have greater expectation of favorable outcomes than ever before, and they are more inclined to initiate legal action for perceived or real injury. Issues contributing to a patient's litigious attitude are actual injury, rapport deterioration, and unreasonable expectations. Although nurses should understand that patients have legal rights, there are support measures nurses can employ that improve the patient's understanding and willingness to accept less than desirable outcomes. Remember, a reassured patient is less likely to consider legal action because of care they received in the health care facility. Each facility needs to discuss actions nurses could initiate.

ANESTHETIC GASES

There is an unproven impression that the operation room team incurs health risks because of their exposure to waste anesthetic gases. Although studies have been done in the past, the results are inconclusive and the issue remains controversial. Previous studies have been flawed because some aspects have not been properly addressed. A proper study should answer the following questions:

- What are the long-term and short-term health risks of waste anesthesia gases to operating room personnel?
- What gases or mixtures of gases are dangerous to the OR staff?
- What duration of exposure causes a risk? Is there a minimum or maximum time before the dangerous level is reached?
- What is the concentration of gases that causes a risk? How is the level of waste gas measured? Is the gas level the same in all areas of the room?
- Where is the team member located during the administration of the gases? Do certain areas of the room have less risk than others?
- How frequently can staff be exposed before there is a risk? How many sequential days of exposure can be tolerated?

- What is the length of no-exposure time that must be achieved before a staff member no longer has a health risk?

REFERENCES

AHA. (1993). APIC call for end to confusing infectious waste regs. *Hospital Infection Control, 20*(5), 61–72.

Airway fires: reducing the risk during laser surgery. (1990). *Health Devices, 19*(4), 109–112.

American Dental Association. (1992). Guidelines for Teaching the Comprehensive Control of Pain and Anxiety in Dentistry.

Amos, R. J., et al. (1984). Prevention of nitrous oxide-induced megaloblastic changes in bone marrow using folinic acid. *British Journal of Anesthesia, 56*(2), 103–107.

ANSI. (1993). American National Standard for the Safe Use of Lasers, ANSI Z136.3, Orlando, FL: Laser Institute of America: 1–120.

AORN. (1990). Recommendations for electrosurgical fire safety. *Biomedical Safety and Standards, 20*(10), 18.

AORN. (1994a). Recommended Practices for Safe Care Through Identification of Potential Hazards in the Surgical Environment. *AORN Standards and Recommended Practices* (Denver: Association of Operating Room Nurses, Inc.), 171–176.

AORN. (1994b). Recommended Practices for Sponge, Sharp and Instrument Counts. *AORN Standards and Recommended Practices* (Denver: Association of Operating Room Nurses, Inc.), 239–244.

AORN. (1994c). Recommended Practices for Electrosurgery. *AORN Standards and Recommended Practices* (Denver: Association of Operating Room Nurses, Inc.), 141–147.

AORN. (1994d). Recommended Practices for Laser Safety in the Practice Setting. *AORN Standards and Recommended Practices* (Denver: Association of Operating Room Nurses, Inc.), 191–195.

AORN. (1994e). Recommended Practices for Reducing Radiological Exposure in the Practice Setting. *AORN Standards and Recommended Practices* (Denver: Association of Operating Room Nurses, Inc.), 219–225.

Atkinson, L. J. (1992). The healthcare team. In: Coon, N., ed. *Berry & Kohn's Operating Room Technique.* 7th ed. St. Louis: Mosby-Year Book. (p. 31).

Brodman, M. (1993). Operating room personnel morbidity from carbon dioxide laser use during preceptored surgery. *Morbidity From Laser Surgery, 81*(4), 607–609.

Charron, D. (1991). Nonionizing radiation. *Dimensions, 68*(2), 16–18.

Consumer Products Safety Commission. (1994). Standards for Flammability of Clothing Textiles, 16 CFR 1610, 546–563.

Farman, A. G. (1991). Concepts of radiation safety and protection: beyond BEIR V. *The Dental Assistant, 60*(1), 11.

Gardner, M. J., et al. (1990). Results of case-control study of leukaemia and lymphoma among young people near Sellafield nuclear plant in West Cumbria. *British Medical Journal, 300*(6722), 423–429.

Gerberding, J. L. (1990). Risk exposure of surgical personnel to patients' blood during surgery at San Francisco General Hospital. *The New England Journal of Medicine, 322*(25), 1788–1793.

Hall, J. R. (1991). Causes of fires in facilities that care for the sick. In: *The U.S. Fire Problem Overview Report Through 1989.* Quincy, MA: National Fire Protection Agency. (pp. 58–60).

Hammond, J. S., et al. (1990). HIV, trauma and infection control: universal precautions are universally ignored. *The Journal of Trauma, 30*(5), 555–561.

Hendrix R. (1992). Environmental risk of chlorofluorocarbon anesthetic agents. *The New England Journal of Medicine, 326*(24), 1640.

Joint Commission on Accreditation of Healthcare Organizations. (1995). *Accreditation Manual for Hospitals.* Vols I and II, Standards and Steering Guidelines. Oakbrook Terrace, IL: JCAHO.

Koch, F. A., Solomon, R. P., Nash, S. E. (1992). The safe medical devices act. *AORN Journal, 55*(2), 537–548.

Murphy, E. K. (1991). OR nursing law: liability for inaccurate counts. *AORN Journal, 53*(1), 157.

National Safety Council. (1991). Avoiding injury in the workplace. *Journal of Healthcare Material Management,* (6), 26–30.

Neel, J. V. (1991). Update on the genetic effects of ionizing radiation. *Journal of the American Medical Association, 267*(5), 698.

Newman, M. A., Kachuba, J. B. (1991). Protect the health of your health care worker. *Journal of Hospitals & Health Services Administration, 36*(4), 537–542.

Newman, M. A., Kachuba, J. B. (1992). Glutaraldehyde: a potential health risk to nurses. *Society of Gastroenterology Nurses and Associates, 14*(6), 296, 300.

Nezhat, C., et al. (1987). Smoke from laser surgery: is there a health hazard? *Lasers in Surgery and Medicine, 7*(4), 376–382.

Occupational Safety and Health Administration. (1991). 29 CFR 1910.1030: Occupational exposure to bloodborne pathogens: Final rule. Federal Register 56(235): 64004–64182.

Occupational Safety and Health Administration. (1993). Hazardous Waste Operations and Emergency Response, 29 CFR 1910. 1200, 385–420.

OR fire occurrence low, but resulting liability high. (1992). *Hospital Risk Management, 14*(9), 113–128.

Paper drapes and gowns a fire risk. (1992). *Hospital Digest, 70*(2), 44.

Patterson, P. (1993). OR exposure to electrosurgery smoke a concern. *OR Manager, 9*(6), 1–8.

Popejoy, S. L., Fry, D. E. (1991). Blood contact and exposure in the operating room. *Surgery, Gynecology & Obstetrics, 172*(6), 480–483.

Price, J. (1990). Laser fires cause patients' deaths. *The Washington Times*, October 4.

Quebbeman, E. J., et al. (1992). Double gloving protecting surgeons from blood contamination in the operating room. *Archives of Surgery, 127*, February, 213–216.

Regulated medical waste definitions and treatment: a collaborative document. (1993). *AORN Journal, 58*(1), 110–114.

Rupke, G. (1992). Vigilance, education are keys to overcoming laser safety complacency. *AORN Journal, 56*(3), 523–525.

Sass-Kortsak, A. M., et al. (1992). Exposure of operating room personnel to potentially harmful environmental agents. *American Industrial Hygiene Association Journal, 53*(3), 203–209.

Smalley, P. J. (1991). Clinical laser safety issues survey. *Journal of Laser Applications, 48*(1), 48–49.

Smith, G. L., et al. (1993). Ionizing radiation: are orthopaedic surgeons at risk? *Annals of the Royal College of Surgeons of England, 74*(5), 326–328.

Steelman, V. McG. (1992). Ethylene oxide, the importance of aeration. *AORN Journal, 55*(3), 773–775.

Stouffer, D. J. (1991). Fires in operating rooms: an unrecognized problem? *Inside Firehouse*, (12), 30–33.

Stouffer, D. J. (1992). Fires during surgery: two fatal incidents in Los Angeles. *Journal of Burn Care & Rehabilitation, 13*(1), 114–117.

Tokars, J. I., et al. (1992). Percutaneous injuries during surgical procedures. *Journal of American Medical Association, 267*(21), 2899–2904.

UCLA operating room fire. (1990). Los Angeles: LA City Fire Department, Bureau of Fire Prevention and Public Safety, 1–192.

Vidor, K. K., Puterbaugh, S., Willis, C. J. (1989). Fire safety training. *AORN Journal, 49*(4), 1045–1049.

Weisman, E. (1993). Buying PPE: consider employees' concerns. *Materials Management, 2*(5), 24–28.

Willy, M. E., et al. (1990). Adverse exposures and universal precaution practices among a group of highly exposed health professionals. *Infection Control Hospital Epidemiology, 11*(7), 351–356.

Wisniewski, P. M., et al. (1990). Studies on the transmission of viral disease via CO_2 laser plume and ejects. *Journal of Reproductive Medicine, 35*(12), 1120.

Woods, C., et al. (1992). Exposure of operating room personnel to nitrous oxide during pediatric anesthesia. *Canadian Journal of Anesthesia, 39*(7), 682–686.

Practice Scenario 1
Environmental Safety

by Theresa K. Kulb, RN, BSN, CNOR

Christian Sannds is a 32-year-old male admitted to the hospital for a laparoscopic cholecystectomy using the KTP laser. This procedure will be performed in the main operating room. Christian is in excellent health, is 6 feet tall, weighs 310 pounds, and plays starting lineman for a professional football team. Recently, Christian has developed a dry hacking cough, and he will have a chest x-ray exam after being put to sleep. Christian's hands and upper chest are raw and seeping with a small amount of blood from the rough game he played in last weekend. Christian is allergic to iodine and most varieties of soap.

PERIOPERATIVE INTERPRETATION

Using what you have just learned in this chapter, as an experienced perioperative nurse you would consider the following in the care of this patient.

1. Assessment
   - The patient's height and weight pose a potential problem in placing the patient correctly on the OR bed.
   - Knowing that the KTP laser will be used, laser safety is a primary concern.
   - The electrosurgical unit should be procured to be used if needed.
   - The use of fiber-optic cords presents a possible ignition source and must be considered for patient safety.
   - Based on the patient's allergy to iodine and soap, alcohol used as a prepping agent could provide a fuel for a fire along with the surgical drapes. The laser, electrosurgical unit, or fiber-optic cord could provide the ignition source.
   - Since the patient will be having a chest x-ray exam, precautionary measures will be necessary to protect the rest of the patient's body, and to limit exposure to the x-rays.
   - The patient's open lesions could provide a source of possible blood exposure for the staff.

NURSING DIAGNOSES

High risk for injury related to:
- patient's body size
- surgical positioning
- ionizing radiation

High risk for fire related to the use of:
- laser
- fiberoptic light cords
- electrosurgical unit
- gowns and drapes
- flammable fuel used for prepping

2. Planning
   - Review department policies on laser safety and test required equipment, such as the laser, prior to use and assure proper functioning.
   - Procure sufficient padding and support to prevent the patient's skin from coming into contact with nonpadded surfaces of the OR bed and to provide proper support for body parts extending beyond the OR bed.
   - Remind surgeon and anesthesiologist about patient's body size, the x-ray study ordered prior to start of surgery, and open areas on patient's hands and upper chest.
   - Position the patient preoperatively to allow the patient to verbalize any problems with the surgical position. Preserve the patient's privacy during positioning.
   - Obtain protective devices for x-rays, such as lead aprons and thyroid collars.

3. Implementation
   - Position the patient while awake assuring that all body parts are padded. Ask the patient if the position places any unnecessary strain on his back, hips, head, or feet.
   - Check all electrical equipment used for the case. Check biomedical engineering preventive maintenance dates, cords and plugs, and the cleanliness of the equipment. Record the equipment numbers on the intraoperative record.

- Monitor electrosurgical safety for pad placement, staff competency, and visual and audible safety alarms.
- Assure laser safety for patient and staff by:
  - covering exposed tissues
  - providing eye protection with appropriate goggles
  - providing high-filtration masks
  - checking for the presence of a fire extinguisher on the accessory cart
- Reduce the possibility of fire by monitoring ignition sources by:
  - allowing time for the alcohol prep to dry prior to draping the surgical site
  - assuring that the active electrosurgical electrode is stored in the safety holster when not in use
  - monitoring the placement of the fiberoptic light cord when disconnected from the telescope
- Control possible fire spread by checking for the presence of a fire blanket in the OR room prior to the beginning of the surgical procedure.
- Provide personal protective equipment and monitor the implementation of universal precautions for personal safety against bloodborne pathogens and body fluids.

4. Evaluation
  - Assess the patient's skin integrity for any bruises, lesions, or burns due to the surgical position.
  - Ask patient when awake if he has any discomfort in his back, hips, or neck.
  - Convey to the post-anesthesia care unit nurse: the patient's history, allergies, size, open skin areas on hands and upper chest, cough, and that a chest x-ray film was taken in surgery prior to the beginning of the surgical procedure.
  - Document in the medical record: the patient's position and positioning aids used, safety measures taken, specific nursing interventions, and successful achievement of patient outcomes.

Practice Scenario 2
Environmental Safety

by Edith M. Hill, RN, BSN, CNOR

Matt Robinson is 11 years old, admitted with a diagnosis of left slipped femoral epiphysis. He is 62 inches tall and weighs 140 pounds. Matt is scheduled to undergo a left hip Knowles pinning procedure. His previous medical history includes fever of unknown origin at age 14 months and tonsillectomy and adenoidectomy at age 5 years. He is allergic to penicillin, which causes hives and swelling. Matt lives at home with his parents and a 7-year-old brother. He is quiet and both parents are in attendance in the preanesthesia room. Upon interview Matt listens while his parents answer your questions. When asked a direct question he answers in brief sentences. He shows his apprehension by struggling to hold back tears. General anesthesia will be used.

PERIOPERATIVE INTERPRETATION

Using what you have just learned in this chapter, as an experienced perioperative nurse you would consider the following in the care of this patient.

1. Assessment
   - The patient's apprehension may result in non-compliance, which could jeopardize his safety.
   - The patient has a known allergy to penicillin, and antibiotics are commonly given to orthopedic patients.
   - The patient's size will possibly require the use of added padding and restraints.
   - The surgical procedure will require multiple x-ray studies with the C-arm.
   - The fracture table will be required for the procedure.
   - Draping the patient for surgery must provide for adequate wound exposure, facilitate C-arm movement, and allow for proper placement of equipment such as suction devices, electrosurgical electrodes, and power equipment.
   - Electrical safety measures are necessary to prevent injury to patients and coworkers.
   - Aseptic technique practices will minimize the risk of nosocomial infection.

- Universal precautions will be required to provide a safe environment for patients and for the health care team.
- Counting sharps, sponges, and instruments is necessary for patient safety.
- Safely transferring and transporting patients for surgery requires specific procedures identified by the facility and regulatory agencies.

NURSING DIAGNOSES

- High risk for injury related to
  - Patient's fear/anxiety and resultant non-compliance
  - Use of electrosurgical equipment
  - Transfer to OR bed
  - Positioning for surgery
  - Radiation exposure
  - Application of traction during surgery
  - Size of patient on the fracture table
- High risk for retention of foreign body related to surgery
- High risk for infection related to surgery

2. Planning
   - Have available antibiotics as ordered by physician. Avoid penicillin, penicillin-type antibiotics, and cephalosporins.
   - Procure available positioning aids, restraints, and draping materials so the nurse can remain with patient during intubation and positioning.
   - Notify the radiology department and technician when they will be needed in the operating room. Have available lead shields for patient and staff.
   - Position fracture table in room. Have all table attachments available. Check for proper functioning of all table parts.
   - Check for proper functioning of suction devices, electrical equipment and outlets, and electrical safety monitors. Ensure that appropriate personnel are knowledgeable in the use of electrical equipment.
   - Coordinate the availability of extra personnel to

assist in the movement of the patient from the stretcher/bed to the OR bed. Be sure that all personnel are aware of their specific roles.

3. Implementation
   - Allow patient to verbalize concerns, apprehension, anxiety. Reassure with a calm and professional approach. Explain the procedures to be done prior to implementation. Follow his cue. Move slowly, show him the monitoring equipment prior to placement, show him the fracture table and how he will lie on it before having him move onto the table. Repeat instructions as necessary. Provide as calm an atmosphere as possible to minimize his apprehension.
   - Document medications according to policy. Observe for any signs or symptoms of adverse reactions to the drug.
   - Position the patient on fracture table with affected limb in traction applied by orthopedic surgeon. Maintain traction and adjust as necessary. Restrain unaffected limb in stirrup or as instructed by surgeon. Knee stirrup is padded well to avoid neuromuscular or skeletal injury. Upper extremities are restrained in place and out of the way of the surgical procedure. Head supported on small pillow. Safety belt in place across patient's upper abdomen, avoiding restriction of breathing.
   - Assist the radiology technician with C-arm placement. Observe for any potential injury to the patient from the equipment. Drape patient with lead shield as appropriate: cover groin, trunk, neck. Assure that OR personnel use appropriate radiologic shielding.
   - Check for proper functioning of all room equipment. Assure that all room personnel are knowledgeable in proper functioning of room equipment and furniture. Check all electrical equipment for intact cords and plugs and proper function. Check date of most recent safety check. Properly ground equipment before use. Clean equipment as necessary following recommendations of manufacturer. Check alarms to be sure they are working properly. Avoid overlapping cords. Clean up spills as they occur. Call appropriate biomedical engineer/maintenance personnel for corrective measures.
   - Document on perioperative record position and aids used, antibiotics administered, radiologic exposure time and safety shields used for the patient, position of the dispersive grounding pad for the electrosurgical unit, and results of the counts.

4. Evaluation
   - Assess for areas of injury such as burns, pressure sores, reddened areas, alterations in skin integrity, impaired sensory and motor functions.
   - Convey to the post-anesthesia care unit nurse the patient's allergy to penicillin, his preoperative anxiety, and patient's responses to surgery and nursing interventions.

Chapter Six

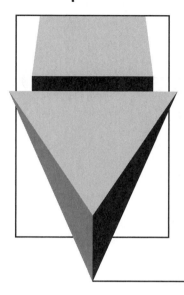

Planning Perioperative Patient Care

Susan V. M. Kleinbeck, RN, MS, CNOR

Prerequisite Knowledge   Prior to beginning the chapter, the learner should review the nursing process and its application in practice.

Chapter content correlates with several AORN *Standards and Recommended Practices*. These standards and recommended practices may be referred to as a prerequisite, or upon completion of the chapter as a refresher.

Standards of Perioperative Administrative Practice

Standards of Perioperative Clinical Practice

Standards of Perioperative Professional Performance

Patient Outcomes: Standards of Perioperative Care

Recommended Practice for Documentation of Perioperative Nursing Care

Learning Objectives

1. Describe the interrelationship between planning patient care and achievement of expected postoperative outcomes

2a. Apply the nursing process to the perioperative patient
2b. Identify preoperative and intraoperative strategies necessary for planning perioperative care

3. Recognize a variety of documentation styles appropriate to the perioperative setting

4. Distinguish preoperative teaching needs from the postoperative educational requirements of perioperative patients

Planning Patient Care

The focus of perioperative nursing is to minimize the patient's risks during surgery and to maximize the potential for an uneventful postoperative recovery. In today's climate of economic constraints and technologic advances, perioperative nurses need a flexible yet systematic process to meet these two objectives. The nursing process facilitates the continuity of care required for a safe transition from the preoperative holding room, to the intraoperative arena, and later into the post-anesthesia care unit.

The nursing process describes an adaptable, dynamic, problem-solving mechanism used by nurses to assess, plan, and complete the business of nursing care (Yura, 1988). The challenge for perioperative nurses is to design nursing actions necessary to meet both the routine surgical care requirements for all patients and the personal needs of the individual. A strategy that acknowledges both procedural requirements and individual needs will optimize the potential for a positive outcome immediately following surgery and a successful home recovery.

NURSING PROCESS, STANDARDS, AND COMPETENCY

The components of the nursing process—assessing, planning, implementing, and evaluating—are deeply integrated into the clinical practice of all specialties. Indeed, the nursing practice standards of care, the documentation requisites for most reviewing agencies, and the clinical competency statements listed by the Association of Operating Room Nurses (AORN, 1994) all parallel the steps of the nursing process. As illustrated in Table 6–1, *assessment* identifies the needs of the patient, *planning* outlines the interventions predicted to best meet those needs, *implementation* requires the activation or delegation of the planned care, and *evaluation* determines whether the selected interventions produced the desired result.

TABLE 6-1. COMPONENTS OF THE NURSING PROCESS RELATED TO THE STANDARDS OF CARE, CLINICAL COMPETENCIES FOR NURSES, AND THE PROCESS OF SURGICAL INTERVENTION BY THE PHYSICIAN

BASIC COM-PONENTS OF THE NURSING PROCESS	Assess				Plan	Implement	Evaluate
CYCLICAL THOUGHTS IN THE NURSING PROCESS	Assess person/ family	Analyze assessed data	Decide nursing diagnosis	Set goals based on diagnoses	Plan nursing actions	Implement the plan	Has goal [expected outcome] been achieved?
STANDARDS (STD) OF CLINICAL NURSING PRACTICE	Std 1 Assessment		Std 2 Diagnosis	Std 3 Identify outcomes	Std 4 Planning	Std 5 Implement	Std 6 Evaluate outcomes
CLINICAL COMPE-TENCY STATE-MENTS IN NURSING	Assessment skills		Diagnosis skills	Outcome-identifying skill	Planning skill	Skill in implementing nursing actions	Evaluation skills
SURGEON'S PROCESS	History, physical exam, x-ray studies, lab studies	Analyze assessed data	Decide medical diagnosis	Recommend surgery	Plan surgical technique	Excise pathology	Evaluate at 1-3 weeks in office

THE NURSING PROCESS IN PERIOPERATIVE NURSING

The four basic components of the nursing process also serve as the conceptual framework for perioperative nursing. *Perioperative* refers to the patient's experience before, during, and immediately after a surgical procedure. Although the nursing process is ongoing and cyclical through all three phases, the registered nurse who specializes in perioperative nursing generally assesses and plans for patient care preoperatively, implements the planned care during the surgical procedure, and evaluates the outcomes of the delivered care postoperatively. The model used to measure the quality of care delivered before, during, and after surgery is the *Standards of Perioperative Clinical Practice* (AORN, 1994).

The standards require the following:

- A systematic and continuous *assessment* that can be retrieved and communicated to others
- An analysis of the assessment with conclusions written as a *nursing diagnosis*
- Patient-oriented *goals* describing the *expected outcomes* predicted by the plan
- A written *plan* of nursing actions designed to achieve the desired patient outcomes
- A prescribed plan deliberately *implemented* or delegated to a qualified individual
- A systematic *evaluation* of the plan to determine if the expected outcomes were achieved by the patient.

The keywords of the nursing process are italicized to emphasize the integration of the concept into the standards of care. The standards stress the need for detailed information and a deliberate plan of action before any patient care begins. The perioperative nursing process is fundamental to implementation of quality care for surgical patients and to the professional practice of perioperative nurses.

Perioperative Implementation of the Nursing Process

Nurses constantly seek solutions to identified problems, devise approaches directed toward solution, and evaluate whether the solution was effective. Often clinical judgment occurs so rapidly that seasoned perioperative nurses are unaware of the event and frequently cannot explain to others the steps taken to accomplish the analysis (Benner, 1987). The nursing process for experienced perioperative nurses is like tying a bow; it's easier to do it than to explain the steps necessary to accomplish the task. For the benefit of the novice perioperative nurse, the steps of the nursing process are described in a linear fashion from preoperative assessment and plan, through intraoperative implementation, to postoperative evaluation. The novice is reminded that this linear representation in no way minimizes the "real world" nature of the concept.

PERIOPERATIVE ASSESSMENT

Assessment is divided into two parts: data collection and data organization. Data collection is the gathering of information through interview, physical examination, observation, consultation with family members or another health care professional, and reading of the medical record. Once information is collected, it is organized into logical patterns or clusters to facilitate valid decision making.

The Collection of Data

Data may be objective, that is, what can be seen, heard, smelled, or touched by anyone; or subjective, information that is spoken and subject to interpretation by the listener. Examples of objective data include pulse rate, breath sounds, skin color, and pulse oximetry reading. Subjective data are collected by interview or verbal consultation. Subjective data include a patient's account of the medical history (allergies reported), a description of pain following surgery, or a colleague's interpretation of the cause of an abnormal laboratory value.

MINIMUM ASSESSMENT RECOMMENDATIONS The *Standards of Clinical Practice* (AORN, 1994), agency policy, and clinical judgment determine the minimum amount of information it is necessary to collect. Objective data should include

---

STEPS OF ASSESSMENT

Data collection

  Interview

  Physical examination

  Observation

  Consultation

  Medical record

Data organization

Nursing diagnosis

CLASSIFICATION OF DATA

Objective data	Subjective data
Scheduling information	Understanding about procedure
Physical appearance	Past surgical history
Physical impairments	Appropriate preparation
Skin condition	Potential problem areas
Mental/emotional status	Personal concerns
Iatrogenics	
Laboratory values	
Legal/ethical documents	

- Scheduling information: medical diagnosis, proposed procedure, age, and anesthesia modality
- Physical appearance: weight, height, base-line vital signs, activity level
- Physical impairments: hearing, sight, speech, motor ability, neurosensory problems, pain, skeletal position limitations, drainage, bowel or bladder dysfunction
- Skin condition: intact, breaks, scars, dry/moist, rash, pale, reddened, bruises, jaundiced, edematous, ulcers
- Mental/emotional status: level of consciousness, responds to name, crying, tremor, anger, talkative, composed, calm, sad
- Iatrogenics (medically ordered devices/measures in use): oxygen, drains, catheters, tracheostomy, nasogastric tube, colostomy, pacemaker
- Laboratory values: on chart, significant abnormal values noted
- Legal/ethical documentation: consent signed? blood available? family in waiting room?

Much of this information can be gleaned from the medical record. A time-saving strategy is to delegate the search for data missing from the chart to a secretary while conducting the patient interview and physical examination.

The purpose of the interview is to verify critical elements noted on the chart (e.g., allergies and reactions) and to complete the data collection process. The skillful interviewer uses open-ended phrases and moves from broad general statements to specific targeted questions. Open-ended statements solicit views, opinions, thoughts, and feelings; in fact, it is impossible to answer an open-ended question with "yes" or "no." A broad open-ended question appropriate for beginning a preoperative interview would be as follows:

- "What do you understand the doctor is going to do today?" The patient's answer may be technical (". . . repair my inguinal herniorrhaphy") or colloquial (". . . fix my rupture"). The response to the open-ended question suggests the patient's level of understanding and will clue the nurse to any potential delays in the schedule ("I'm going to x-ray first and then to surgery").

Other general open-ended questions the perioperative nurse might incorporate into the interview are the following:

- What did you do to prepare for your surgery?
- What surgery experiences have you had prior to today?
- Do you have any problem areas we should know about? (e.g., bad back, bruises, diarrhea)

Some interview questions need to be very narrow, targeted to specific information.

- When did you last have anything to eat or drink?
- What medication did you take this morning?
- Who will be with you after surgery? (Tell them where to wait.)

Patients find it difficult to understand why so many professionals ask the same question. For example, "Do you have any allergies?" An explanatory phrase preceding the often heard question will change patient frustration to respectful cooperation. For example,

- I know many people have asked this question, but for your safety, I would like to confirm what is written on the chart . . . (e.g., concerning allergies and surgical site).

Closing an interview by asking if there are any questions often yields little response. Perhaps it is because patients are in a scary, stressful environment and find themselves unable to formulate an appropriate question. Asking if patients have concerns is a broader statement that permits both questions and unorganized thoughts to surface, such as "I just hope everything goes all right." The caring nurse's response might be "We are going to take care of you. Is there anything in particular that is worrying you?" (Parsons, 1993).

SYSTEMATIC FORMAT FOR DATA COLLECTION   To be sure a complete assessment of the patient's needs has been accomplished, an existing form that meets both professional and third party payer requirements is recommended. The assessment form permits collection of routine information as well as the individual variances that demand special attention by the nurse.

A common complaint heard from nurses is "There just isn't time to do a good assessment." Strategies to shorten time requirements include establishing a routine set of broad questions that will supply the minimum basic information. When abnormal values or patient responses indicate a possible problem, focus on that topic by asking specific narrow questions. Seasoned perioperative nurses complete a full preoperative assessment in about 5 minutes. The key to success is a systematic approach.

Taking the time to collect information preoperatively will often save time intraoperatively. The data collection before decision making is essential. Action based on inaccurate information is unsafe and unprofessional.

Data Organization

Organizing collected information into logical patterns or clusters prevents decision making based upon a single fact. For example, the observation of a patient trembling with her face turned toward the wall in the preoperative holding area could be interpreted as a sign of hypothermia, hyperthermia, or a fearful reaction to impending surgery. A response of "I'm so cold" immediately rules out fear as a cause, but leaves hypothermia or hyperthermia as remaining possible diagnoses. Further review of the medical record indicates a white blood cell (WBC) count of 28,000/mm and an oral temperature of 100.6°F. The pattern of muscular tremor, elevated WBC count, and low-grade fever suggests a diagnosis of actual infection accompanied by chills. Action based on one fragment of information would have been erroneous for the trembling patient. When nurses organize patterns of assessment information into concise health problem statements, a nursing diagnosis is formulated.

Nursing Diagnosis

The term nursing diagnosis is both a process and a label (Diomede, 1991). The diagnostic process remains constant across the professions of nursing, medicine, and dietetics. It is the area of responsibility that differs. Physicians diagnose medical problems requiring physician expertise. Nurses diagnose health responses

DIAGNOSTIC PROCESS

Analyze assessment data
Cluster into patterns
Label each pattern

List probable causes
Document selected label

treated by nursing expertise. For example, physicians diagnose and treat cancer; nurses diagnose and treat the patient's response to cancer. The process of systematically assessing, analyzing, and predicting a patient problem is based upon clinical judgment and reasoning skills. Diagnoses specific to nursing are defined and published biennially by The North American Nursing Diagnosis Association (NANDA). Nursing diagnoses provide a basis for selection of nursing interventions to achieve desired outcomes for which the nurse is accountable (Kleinbeck, 1994).

PERIOPERATIVE NURSING DIAGNOSES   In a research study of 179 patients designed to identify the most common perioperative nursing diagnoses, ten staff nurses were asked to check the nursing diagnoses applicable to their assigned patient and to write a statement that explained the reasons for the diagnosis selected (Kleinbeck, 1994). The check list, derived from an earlier study, included 33 nursing diagnoses from the NANDA-approved list (Kleinbeck, 1989).

The four most frequent nursing diagnoses identified by the perioperative staff nurses were risk of infection, risk of injury from burns, risk of injury from hemorrhage, and risk of injury from a foreign body. The loss of the ability by these patients to protect themselves from infection, burn, or foreign body was recognized by staff nurses in this study as requiring specific nursing actions. Clinically, the nurses observed patients unable to move a malpositioned extremity, retract from a skin-blistering surface, or protect themselves from other harmful stimuli. They labeled the observed patterns of signs as nursing diagnoses.

WRITING NURSING DIAGNOSES   The acronym PES, problem, etiology, and sign/symptom, describes the three parts of a nursing diagnosis. The diagnostic statement begins with a title that labels the health *problem* or life-style of concern to the nurse (e.g., high risk for infection). The label is followed by a probable cause or *etiology*. Because a cause-and-effect relationship is difficult to document, the connecting phrase between the problem and the etiology is "related to," (e.g., high risk for infection r/t incision of skin barrier). For example, in the perioperative nursing diagnosis study, staff nurses indicated as many as four different probable causes for a single diagnosed problem (Kleinbeck, 1994). The selection of from one to four etiology statements seems to indicate that there are a variety of signs, symptoms, or characteristics that influenced the selection of a particular diagnosis. For example, risk of infection had a total of 17 different etiology statements generated across 176 of the total 179 cases, whereas the risk of injury from a retained foreign body had nine etiology statements across 111 cases (Tables 6–2 to 6–4). A high risk of infection could be attributed to both a low white blood cell

THE PES OF NURSING DIAGNOSIS

*P*roblem statement
*E*tiology of problem
*S*igns, symptoms, or characteristics of the problem

TABLE 6-2. **INCIDENCE AND FREQUENCY OF PERIOPERATIVE NURSING DIAGNOSES IN PATIENTS UNDERGOING SURGERY IN A LARGE MEDICAL CENTER (N = 179)**

DIAGNOSTIC LABEL	FREQUENCY	%
Risk of infection	176	98.3
Risk of burn injury	144	80.4
Risk of hemorrhage	120	67.0
Risk of injury from foreign body	111	62.0
Anxiety	107	59.8
Impaired tissue integrity	103	57.5
Risk of embolus/clot	101	56.4
Impaired skin integrity	100	55.9
Pain	98	54.7
Impaired physical mobility	92	51.4
Altered breathing pattern	91	50.8
Risk of injury from fall	91	50.8
Risk of hypothermia	86	48.0
Altered urine elimination	86	48.0
Risk of injury from position	81	45.3
Fear	68	38.0
Inadequate nutrition	60	33.5
Powerlessness	54	30.2
Mucous membrane impairment	53	29.6
Decreased cardiac output	52	29.1
Self-concept (body image)	50	27.9
Risk of aspiration	49	27.4
Impaired verbal communication	49	27.4
Risk of excess fluids/electrolytes	39	21.8
Risk of fluid deficit	38	21.2
Risk of hyperthermia	37	20.7
Risk of trauma injury	37	20.7
Hypothermia	30	16.8
Fluid/electrolyte deficit	28	15.6
Nutrition, more than	24	13.4
Excess fluids/ electrolytes	19	10.6
Hyperthermia	9	5.0
Other	22	

TABLE 6-3. **REASONS FOR PERIOPERATIVE STAFF NURSE SELECTION OF THE NURSING DIAGNOSIS: HIGH RISK OF INFECTION**

RISK FACTORS	FREQUENCY
Open incision	96
Invasive procedure	46
Endogenous exposure	26
Immunosuppression	16
Re-operation	15
Active infection	15
Open traumatic wound	14
Diabetes present	7
Geriatric, frail, elderly	6
Obesity	6
Technique break	5
Other (skin shave, open wounds, long procedure, long length of hospital stay)	4

Of 179 patients, 176 received the nursing diagnosis of high risk for infection.

TABLE 6-4. **REASONS FOR PERIOPERATIVE STAFF NURSE SELECTION OF THE NURSING DIAGNOSIS: HIGH RISK OF INJURY FROM FOREIGN BODY**

RISK FACTORS	FREQUENCY
Needles used in wound	77
Sponges used in wound	75
Fragments (risk and actual wire, balloon, catheter)	15
Instruments in wound	13
Throat pack	4
Repositioning of patient	3
Patties or peanuts	3
Dirt/gravel from trauma	2
Lost protection from eyelid retraction, trachea open	2

Of 179 patients, 111 received the nursing diagnosis of high risk of injury from foreign body.

count (immunosuppression) and the risk of contamination during bowel surgery (exposure to endogenous *Escherichia coli*).

The *signs, symptoms, and/or characteristics* substantiating the diagnosis form the third part of the nursing diagnosis. In academia, students are required to attach the objective and subjective signs, symptoms, or characteristics to the diagnostic statement. In the clinical setting, perioperative nurses document the signs, symptoms, or characteristics on the agency assessment form. The rationale for this distinction is a principle of documentation — duplication of information is unnecessary and is discouraged. Thus, perioperative nurses are not required to document the assessed justification for a diagnosis adjacent to the diagnostic label. Examples of perioperative clinical nursing diagnoses are as follows:

- High risk for neuromuscular injury r/t lithotomy positioning
- Hypothermia r/t cool environment
- Fluid imbalance r/t NPO status.

Additional information concerning the appropriate method of formulating perioperative nursing diagnoses may be found in Seifert and Rothrock (1989) and Kleinbeck (1990).

PLANNING INTRAOPERATIVE CARE

Once patient data are collected and organized into identified problems and diagnostic statements, the perioperative nurse consciously plans a strategy for care.

Establishing Priority

In the planning sequence, patient, environment, equipment, and supply needs are prioritized according to the availability of assessment data. For example, scheduling information is frequently available hours or days before the perioperative nurse has the opportunity to assess the patient. Based upon knowledge of the patient's age, the procedure scheduled, and the surgeon's preferences, instrumentation and team membership needs can be anticipated. It is logical to prioritize intraoperative problems and begin planning based upon known information about the procedure rather than to wait for the remainder of patient data. Occasionally, the planning sequence is altered when all assessment information becomes available. Priority for patients scheduled for emergent surgery (e.g., airway management, control of hemorrhage) is based upon meeting survival physiologic needs first. Once a patient is stabilized, the problems can be ordered based upon a known framework, such as Maslow's hierarchy of needs (Maslow, 1970).

STEPS IN PLANNING INTRAOPERATIVE CARE

Prioritize problems   Select nurse interventions

                                           Preoperative communication
                                           Environment requirements
                                           Supplies and equipment
                                         Intraoperative patient needs

Only active nursing diagnoses are considered when the nurse prioritizes problems to be treated. Because preoperative nursing diagnoses often differ from intraoperative diagnoses, the problems of concern may change according to the patient's perioperative phase (Kleinbeck, 1989). Patients under general anesthesia do not have psychologic coping problems that require intervention. Neither is there a risk for injury from an electrocoagulation burn while the patient is in the preoperative holding area. The perioperative nurse can discontinue a preoperative diagnosis, anxiety r/t unknown diagnosis, while the patient is asleep and reactivate it once the patient is fully awake. Establishing priorities, doing first things first, requires analysis of the following:

- the known information
- the patient's physiologic survival needs
- the relevance of the nursing diagnosis or problem to the time of intervention.

Selection of Nurse Interventions

Nurses plan interventions in four general areas: content of preoperative communication, environmental preparation of the room, acquisition of supplies and equipment, and attention to the individual's intraoperative needs.

PREOPERATIVE COMMUNICATION Effective preoperative teaching is achieved through a structured program of content and methods. Teaching is not limited to just telling information. When time is limited to a few minutes, preoperative teaching becomes an opportunity to communicate to the patient and family the sequence of events to expect prior to anesthesia. Research summarized by Rothrock (1989) suggests inclusion of

- sensory perceptions (cold, sting of local anesthetic, sound of suction, noise in the post-anesthesia care unit)
- sequence of events (transport by stretcher, move to narrow bed, large lights, wake up in post-anesthesia care unit, cast on arm, see family in step-down unit)
- how to participate (tell us if your knee is out of position, hunch your back like a "mad cat" during spinal anesthesia).

Content of preoperative communication includes both the routine events common to all procedures and the specific experiences the person can expect.

ENVIRONMENTAL REQUIREMENTS Operating room conditions are evaluated daily prior to the first patient. Survey the room and plan to avoid the hazards possible during transportation or as a result of marginal operating room conditions (humidity, electrical exposure, ambient temperature, and air exchange rate). AORN's recommended practices for hazards in the surgical environment offer suggestions to minimize the risk for injury (AORN, 1994).

SUPPLIES AND EQUIPMENT Coordination of supplies and equipment for a surgical procedure is difficult in this day of frequent technologic change. Computerized equipment and specialized single-purpose supplies make planning for surgical procedures particularly difficult to learn. The introduction of unfamiliar equipment for evaluation further complicates this process. Many nurses new to the specialty find a quick review of anatomy and procedure sequence from a basic perioperative text such as *Alexander's Care of the Surgical Patient* (Meeker, 1990) useful in anticipating the needs of the surgeon during a procedure. If unfamiliar with breast surgery, for example, the nurse could read the text and find illustrations of gross anatomy, examples of abnormal mammograms, assessment and planning recommendations, common instrumentation, and brief descriptions of the operative procedures frequently performed. Although the supplies and equipment for a specific surgeon are not listed in the text, general knowledge about the procedure will promote understanding of the rationale for various requests.

The nurse must plan to identify and collect materials well before the admission of the patient to the operating room. Routine supplies and equipment for a scheduled procedure are listed on surgeon preference cards or online in computer files. Consulting the manufacturer's instructions for requested equipment can help the nurse in the planning process. The instructions will identify the essential component parts and recommend set-up procedures for the most effective operation. For example, fluid-bag heights and adjustments in pressure of the cataract emulsifier pulsating irrigator are clearly defined by the manufacturer. Some surgical suites conveniently attach the instructions directly to the equipment for easy access.

Facility policy, standards, and procedures also will affect planning for a scheduled procedure. If facility policy mandates that ambulatory surgery patients may arrive 1 hour before their scheduled procedure, the equipment plan for positioning will need to be deferred until a patient assessment can be completed. If an admissions office secretary reports a tall basketball player is scheduled for a procedure, it is not until the patient arrives that assessment furnishes sufficient information to plan positioning devices (how tall is tall?). Planning for essential supplies and equipment is complex and vital to a safe and successful patient outcome.

INTRAOPERATIVE PATIENT NEEDS Approximately 75% of nursing diagnoses occur repeatedly from one surgical patient to another (Kleinbeck, 1989). This research finding justifies standardized planning for common needs of most surgical patients. Nurses can anticipate that all patients will have some problems (e.g., high risk for infection, fluid imbalance, hypothermia) and that each patient will have a few specific needs (e.g., impaired skin integrity due to decubitus, impaired verbal communication, acute pain). A review of the *Recommended Practices for Perioperative Nursing* (AORN, 1994) is helpful when planning both routine technical care and individualized special care.

IMPLEMENTATION OF PLANNED INTERVENTIONS

Intellectual skill, interpersonal skill, and technical skill are integral to the implementation of nursing interventions (Pinnell, 1986). Whether the planned intervention is performed by the originating nurse, or delegated to a team member, each skill is necessary.

Preparation and Performance

Intellectual skills include cognition, reasoning, and memory. Application of intellectual skills represents the ability to use what has been learned in a new situation. Novice perioperative nurses exercise a great deal of intellectual skill as they integrate their nursing knowledge with a magnitude of new clinical demands. Intellect also permits the transfer of information learned in one specialty

---

STEPS IN IMPLEMENTATION OF PLAN

Preparation   Documentation
Performance

   Intellectual skill
   Interpersonal skill
   Technical skill
   Delegation

(lateral positioning for a thoracic procedure) to another specialty (lateral positioning for a renal procedure). The transfer of professional intellectual skills must be moderated by clinical judgment.

Interpersonal skill is integral to the helping relationship surgical patients expect during their stressful experience. Interpersonal refers to any communication, verbal or nonverbal, between two people. An individual who functions effectively in the helping relationship is understanding, genuine, respectful, sensitive, and nonjudgmental, as well as knowledgeable (Parsons, 1993). These traits facilitate both patient/nurse interaction and collegial teamwork.

Technical skill, the ability to perform complex tasks, is crucial to the perioperative nurse's role. Technical skills reflect the psychomotor domain of learning behavior. The ability to set up a sterile field with an array of instrumentation is a technical skill that is learned and retained in memory only with practice.

DELEGATION Decisions regarding whether to delegate perioperative nursing interventions require intellectual skill, technical skill, and awareness of team members' scope of practice. Five factors affecting the delegation decision are

- Potential for harm (Is there a potential that the intervention will cause harm to the patient?)
- Complexity of the activity (What intellectual and technical skills are required? Is the team member qualified?)
- Problem solving and innovation required (If a problem is encountered, will it require nonroutine problem solving to achieve a successful outcome?)
- Predictability of outcome (How predictable are the outcomes of the intervention?)
- Time parameters (Will delegating an activity increase or decrease the amount of time required by the nurse later?)

These factors, adapted from the American Association of Critical-Care Nurses (1990), offer guidelines when considering whether it is safe and efficient to delegate a nursing intervention.

SYSTEMATIC IMPLEMENTATION Systematic implementation of a plan expedites nursing actions and adheres to the principle of "Put it down, don't move it around." A target of systematic implementation is to touch each item only once. The systematic approach begins prior to admission of the patient to the operating room and proceeds in a chronologic fashion. For example, arrange equipment and room furniture to permit accessibility before supplies arrive. Sort sterile and nonsterile supplies according to the anticipated order of use. Open supplies such as suction tubing at the beginning of the procedure, while retaining closure sutures until the procedure is completed.

INTERVENTION PHILOSOPHY Intraoperative nursing actions are implemented for the benefit of the patient. Data indicate that the longer a wound is open, the greater the risk of infection; the shorter the length of anesthesia time, the greater the patient's potential for optimal outcome. Nurses who rush for supplies or equipment are racing because the longer the patient is in surgery, the greater the patient's risk of complications. A philosophy directed toward maximizing patient outcomes through expeditious interdisciplinary teamwork is the ideal approach to implementation of perioperative care.

Documentation

The implementation process concludes with documentation of the nursing actions completed and the patient's response. The AORN's recommended practice for documentation lists the minimum requirements for recordkeeping. Every facility has a standard format and written procedures outlined for recording the movement of the patient through all three phases of the perioperative experience. Documentation of charges, implants, diagnostic testing, and professional care may be by computer or written entry. Should the nurse desire to document an event not detailed on the standard form, it is appropriate to write an intraoperative note on the nurses notes section of the perioperative record or on the medical record progress notes. Evaluation of the patient's experience before, during, and immediately after surgery is dependent on the accuracy of documentation.

EVALUATION OF THE DELIVERED CARE

Evaluation answers the questions "Is the patient progressing toward achievement of the expected outcomes?" and "Are modifications necessary for this patient or the next similar patient for which I care?" Evaluation is completed by reassessment. For example, during the review of a patient's chart, the nurse observes documentation of an allergy to iodine. The nursing diagnosis is possible allergy to the iodophor prepping solution. The plan is to interview the patient to clarify the source of allergy and previous reaction. During the interview, the nurse learns that the patient's allergy is to ". . . the paint they put on your skin in the doctor's office." The diagnosis is changed to actual iodophor allergy. A plan to have an alternative prepping solution is recorded on the chart. The site is cleansed with chlorhexidine. The skin is reassessed postoperatively to verify the expected outcome of no allergic response to the prepping solution.

Although evaluation of the patient's response occurs on a repetitive basis, perioperative nurses generally evaluate the delivered care after the surgical dressing has been applied. The criteria for excellence against which patient outcomes are measured are the *Patient Outcomes: Standards of Perioperative Care* (AORN, 1994). At the end of the surgical procedure, the nurse reassesses the patient to determine whether the implemented plan achieved:

- freedom from signs or symptoms of infection
- skin integrity equivalent to preoperative status
- absence of any injury from positioning, extraneous objects, or chemical, physical, and electrical hazard
- homeostatic balance in fluid and electrolytes
- sufficient patient awareness of the physiologic and psychologic responses to surgery to enable the patient to participate in the rehabilitation process.

The purpose of postoperative outcome evaluation is to maintain the standard of care. Retrospective evaluation (chart review, patient/family interview) of the documented care of several patients over a fixed period of time will verify that the quality of care is being monitored and maintained.

Documentation of Perioperative Nursing Care

Documentation is the recording of the nursing process in the medical record. Perioperative documentation includes the following:

DOCUMENTATION

Minimum requirements	Criteria
Assessment	Legal
Nursing diagnosis/problem	Logical
Professional actions	Complete
Patient response	Retrievable
	Confidential
	Systematic

- identifying factors that distinguish one patient from all others
- assessing biopsychosocial data associated with surgery and postoperative recovery
- listing patient problems (by clinical standards, written in nursing diagnosis format)
- chronicling the patient's perioperative experience
- documenting nursing activity (interventions) before, during, and immediately following surgery
- listing of other members of the interdisciplinary team
- evaluating actual patient outcomes resulting from nursing activity (generally listed under evaluation of care).

Documentation may be in any style and divided into any series of facility forms, as long as it is logically communicated and retrievable.

Patient information is considered confidential data protected by the Privacy Act of 1974 and governed by both federal and state statutes. Data from the medical record may be used for legal purposes to substantiate or dispute an allegation; to communicate patient information across disciplines; as a resource for demonstrating nurse accountability and quality of care; and in statistical or cost analyses for research, teaching, or reimbursement. Indeed, the maxim "If it wasn't documented, it wasn't done" becomes particularly crucial when one realizes the multiple uses of perioperative nursing documentation. The volume of documented information required, however, makes it imperative that team members avoid duplication of information. For example, base-line vital signs do not need to be on a graph and included in the admission data. To maintain the integrity of documentation, professionals will

- sign full name with title once on each chart page
- allow no blank spaces, crowded entries, or skipped lines
- write legibly in ink using objective, clear language
- place quotation marks around patient's exact words
- accurately record only observed data, not hearsay
- include patient's response to any intervention
- follow facility policy and procedure (e.g., use only facility-approved abbreviations).

DOCUMENTATION FORMATS

Facility policies, procedures, and standards dictate the format and style of nursing documentation. There are five general classifications of documentation formats. The oldest and least desirable is the traditional source-oriented format. It is a chronologic narration of events in an open space often labeled nurse's notes. The primary disadvantage of narrative charting is the absence of consistency and completeness, for example, "IV started, tolerated procedure well." Narrative

> If it wasn't documented, it wasn't done.

notes, however, are useful as an adjunct or a supplement to systematic styles of documentation.

Systematic formats of documentation include problem-oriented medical records (data base, problem list, initial plan, interdisciplinary progress notes), focus charting (data, action, response), SOAPing (Subjective and Objective assessment, Analysis, Plan), and the PIE method (Problem, Implementation, Evaluation). Each of these formats is described in the AORN booklet, *Perioperative Nursing Documentation* (Watson, 1990). A format common in perioperative settings is a combination flow record. The routine items are recorded on a serial flow sheet by checking a box or writing a few words, and the individualized items are documented in the nursing notes section. A systematic, step-by-step format saves time and prevents the busy professional from forgetting to write essential fragments of information during the documentation process. This is particularly helpful when the format is computerized.

PERIOPERATIVE FORMS Forms required for recording the patient's perioperative experience vary among facilities. Generally speaking, there is a preoperative checklist to ensure appropriate preparation of the patient, an assessment form for base-line data, an operating room record listing both preoperative and intraoperative events, and a method of recording the immediate postoperative course of the patient. Evaluation of patient outcomes following surgery may be located on the operating room record or on a separate postoperative document. The perioperative patient care document is complete when patient outcomes have been identified.

Perioperative Patient Education

Positive, cost-relevant effects have been obtained from preoperative and postoperative teaching across a wide range of patients, surgical providers, and health care facility settings. Devine and Cook (1986) found statistically reliable positive effects on surgical patients' recovery, pain, psychologic well-being, and satisfaction with care when psychoeducational interventions were implemented. Empirical evidence suggests what perioperative nurses understand: Perioperative patient education reduces anxiety, minimizes the extent of postoperative discomfort, and returns patients to productivity more quickly. In addition, Hinshaw (1983) reported safer, more individualized perioperative care for patients and more nurse satisfaction with the care delivered when a structured preoperative education program was in place.

The trend toward hospital admissions the morning of surgery and the shift away from inpatient surgery has reduced the time nurses spend with preoperative patients. In 1982, outpatient surgery constituted 18% of the surgery schedule (AHA, 1992). Depending on geographic location and health care facility size, 60% to 100% of surgical procedures in 1992 were performed on an outpatient basis. Perioperative nurses now see patients 1 to 2 hours before the surgery, rather than 24 hours before. The insertion of preoperative teaching into the perioperative experience, even when it must be abbreviated, is valid. Creativity in the development of perioperative education programs that honor economy of time and resources is essential if patients are to receive the benefits demonstrated by research.

> ## PERIOPERATIVE EDUCATION
>
> Assess patient ability
> Define content material
> Select variety of methods
> Document patient response

STRUCTURED PROGRAM OF PERIOPERATIVE EDUCATION

Telling does not equate with teaching; therefore, telling cannot be the sole component of a perioperative education program. Perioperative education is concerned with the ability of the patient to learn and the content of instructions. Ability is influenced by willingness (motivation), previous life experiences, and intelligence available to respond to instruction. Instruction refers to the content and methods by which the information is delivered.

The Ability to Learn

Physiologic responses to stress can reduce a patient's attention span and reduce the ability to learn. Personal control is a factor that modifies reactions to stressful experiences (Redman, 1993). One approach to enhancing personal control is to increase the patient's ability to anticipate experiences by providing a description of the impending experience.

In a series of research studies, preparatory information that focused on sensory elements of the surgical experience was associated with the patient's rapid resumption of usual activities. Sensory content was described from the patient's perspective, rather than how or where a procedure would be done from the providers' perspective. The information included when events would occur; how long they would last; and what would be heard, smelled, seen, tasted, or felt during the event (Johnson, 1985). The level or intensity of the sensation (e.g., how bad a taste might be) was not included in the instruction because perceptions vary among individuals.

Personal control strategies may not benefit persons with high situational anxiety. Indeed, highly anxious patients may request to be spared information beyond that which is necessary for informed surgical consent.

Intellect remains constant or improves in adulthood (Sundeen, 1989). Assessment of an individual's ability to understand new information is estimated by the choice of words a patient uses to respond to an interview. If an individual employs technical words as a part of a response, then the nurse reciprocates. If the terminology is limited to simply two- or three-syllable words, the nurse responds in a similar manner. The objective is to give the same basic content to all patients, but at a level each individual can understand.

THE INFLUENCE OF AGE ON LEARNING   The care of children is a perioperative subspecialty that requires information beyond what is offered in this chapter. However, the novice nurse should understand that cognitive learning is based upon developmental age. Play is particularly beneficial in reducing anxiety and in preparing children for surgery. Children will attend to perioperative information for longer periods of time when participating in projects, coloring in a book with pictures of surgical events, dressing up as a doctor, or "operating" on a doll.

The meaningfulness of material is an important factor in the motivation of people beyond childhood to learn. Indeed, adults are more motivated to learn something that they consider important. Adults value accuracy more than speed; hence, a slow delivery of brief content is more beneficial than a speedy delivery of much information. Another strategy to help adults learn is for the instructor to organize the new material they are about to receive (Redman, 1993). The nurse could say

> "I am going to tell you
>> What will happen to you in the next hour
>> How your family will be informed during that hour
>> What you can expect to feel when you wake up
>> How you can help yourself when you go home
> First, what will happen to you . . . ."

Providing a mental filing system for patients to categorize information increases retention of the material.

Adults also like strong emotional support. Research findings suggest preoperative teaching that offers emotional support and anxiety-reducing measures is more effective than an approach limited exclusively to information. A combination of both methods appears to be superior. Direct eye contact during instruction, assurance that the patient will not be left alone, and concentrating exclusively on the patient for a few focused moments, all transmit emotional support.

LIFE EXPERIENCES   Chronic disease requires multiple encounters with the health care system. Those who have had a previous surgical experience are generally familiar with the system and may have heard the standard preoperative dialog several times. The best approach with the experienced patient is to ask "What do you expect to happen today?" "Can you describe your last visit?" These broad open-ended questions will validate the patient's experience and allow the nurse to assess the extent and accuracy of the patient's knowledge. Conversely, the novice patient will not have a history against which to compare the new experiences in the surgical facility. One strategy to use with novice patient learners is to make an audiotape recording of the teaching session and then give the tape to the patients to replay as they wait.

Content of Teaching Program

The content of a perioperative education program will vary according to the patient's needs and the routine of a particular health care facility. For example, the expense of obtaining care for an illness causes indigent patients to underutilize health care facilities, thereby receiving less knowledge about health promotion in general. As a group, they need the most health information and are the least likely to receive it from appropriate sources. Often indigent patients receive information from their neighbors and peers — people who are also lacking in accurate health information. It may be impossible for a member of this group to eat a balanced diet to promote wound healing. Rather than instructing these patients to eat a specific diet, the nurse would need to identify the usual meal pattern and recommend the food choices that proximate a balanced diet. All health care

---

STEPS IN PREOPERATIVE TEACHING PROGRAM

Assess current knowledge	Include emotional support
Instruct	Document content and response
Sequence of events	
Clarify expectations	
Include sensory content	
Demonstrate special care	
Obtain return demonstration	

POSTOPERATIVE INSTRUCTIONS

Inpatient

    Turn, deep breathe
    Exercise muscles
    Drink fluids (if permitted)
    Expect to go home to finish recovery
      process

Outpatient

    How to get in/out of car
    Rest when tired
    Physical care
    Limitations with time frames
    Suggestions for progression
    Demonstrate how to implement
      surgeon's orders
    Obtain return demonstration
  Document content and response

strategies need to include the patient and family as participants in the planning process. This is particularly true when making self-care recommendations to indigent patients.

Although all surgical patients may be concerned about the course of their disease and surgical treatment, they differ in their needs for postoperative recovery information. Inpatients are able to consult with nurses on a 24-hour basis. Nurses are available to help them get in and out of bed, dietitians prepare the appropriate diet, and all their basic needs are met. Immediate access to professional nursing care affects the content of perioperative instruction. Inpatients, for example, do not need to be taught by perioperative nurses how to change their dressings. Outpatients, on the other hand, do not have the benefit of extended nursing care following surgery. These patients feel particularly vulnerable when they leave the facility to go home.

Postoperative education for outpatients should include physical care ("shower tomorrow; you don't have to eat but be sure to drink plenty of fluids"), type and length of limitations ("don't drive your car for 24 hours"), suggestions for progressive activity ("walk in the house today and increase the distance tomorrow as your energy permits"), recommendation to "rest when you feel tired," and how to get in and out of a car. Because these patients will not have immediate access to nurses to answer their questions, instructions should also be written, home-oriented, and as specific as possible. The patient going home after an endoscopic inguinal herniorrhaphy should be told "not to lift anything heavier than your shoes" rather than "not to lift anything heavy."

A return demonstration is essential when outpatients are expected to manage their own care (e.g., crutch walking, dressing change, discontinuing an indwelling urinary catheter). Postoperative outpatients describe feeling little "squiggles" or "twitches," which are alarming. Explaining that isolated occasional tugs close to the surgical area are a part of the normal process of healing prevents sudden increases in anxiety.

Methods of Teaching

Employing visual and touch augmentation increases the retention of oral instructions. Pamphlets, videotapes, and the handling of appliances such as drains are examples of ways of adding sight and sound to the presentation of information. Structured group teaching of both preoperative and postoperative information has been successful. Patients learn from their peers' questions, and group teaching offers more economical use of the nurse/educator's time. Teaching is a two-way interaction that can be initiated by telephone or interactive video. Creative solutions to the problem of minimal teaching access by the nurse include media technologies as well as printed material.

Patients benefit from structured preoperative and postoperative education. However, designed perioperative educational programs may not be written into a facility procedure. Recall that nursing students learn preoperative teaching from the surgical unit's perspective. Policies supporting the validity of perioperative teaching and a procedure outlining the basic educational content for each phase are recommended. Systematic teaching and postoperative instructions complete the overall goal of perioperative nursing to offer quality care to surgical patients.

Summary

Perioperative nurses assess, plan, implement, evaluate, document, and teach patients. Each of these components of the perioperative patient care process requires intellectual skill, interpersonal skill, and technical skill to execute. In an effort to minimize patients' risks, all components of the perioperative nursing process must be completed under constrained time limits. Systematic implementation following the principles outlined in the *Standards and Recommended Practices* (AORN, 1994) will expedite patients' progress through the operating room and maximize their opportunity for successful recovery.

ISSUES FOR FUTURE DEVELOPMENT

1. *Interdisciplinary valuing of the assessment and preoperative teaching process.* Most patients can move through the perioperative experience without catastrophic effects if the registered nurse is denied access to the patient preoperatively. The assumption justifying this behavior is that all patients are alike and that professional nursing care is dependent on physician direction. However, people do vary and both the public and the legal system prohibit blind obedience to medical direction without evaluating the effect on patient safety. People should not be reduced to the scheduled "gallbladder" or "knee." Research indicates patient benefits and nurse satisfaction increase when nursing assessment and teaching are incorporated into perioperative practice. Strategies to aid the perioperative nurse in articulating a rationale for consuming 5 to 10 minutes of the limited preoperative preparation time for assessment and teaching are needed. Management strategies to economically implement the nursing process in the surgical suite are needed.

2. *A taxonomy of perioperative nursing diagnoses.* Research designed to define a taxonomy of perioperative diagnoses is recommended. The listing of diagnoses with associated interventions could be entered into a computerized data base. The nurse then could indicate the perioperative nursing diagnoses appropriate for a patient and the interventions implemented during a procedure. Hard copy for documentation and evaluation purposes could be printed out in the post-anesthesia care unit, signed by the nurse, and attached to the medical record.

3. *Plan now to incorporate advanced media technology in patient care.* An average of 75% of surgical procedures will be performed in an outpatient/ambulatory basis by the turn of the century. Perioperative nurses will complete preoperative teaching in the patient's home using video telecommunications. Community tours of the surgical suite utilizing virtual reality may become commonplace. Strategies need to be developed now to prepare

perioperative nurses to begin and end the perioperative cycle of care in the community.

REFERENCES

American Association of Critical-Care Nurses. (1990). *Delegation of Nursing and Nonnursing Activities in Critical Care: A Framework for Decision.* Aliso Viejo, CA: The Association.

American Hospital Association. (1992). *Ambulatory Surgery: Ambulatory Care Trendlines 1980–1990, 1.* Chicago, IL: American Hospital Association.

Association of Operating Room Nurses. (1994). *AORN Standards and Recommended Practices.* Denver: Association of Operating Room Nurses, Inc.

Benner, P., Tanner, C. (1986). How expert nurses use intuition. *American Journal of Nursing, 87,* 23–31.

Devine, E. C., Cook, T. D. (1986). Clinical and cost-saving effects of psychoeducational interventions with surgical patients: a meta-analysis. *Research in Nursing & Health, 9,* 89–105.

Diomede, B. (1991). *Perioperative Nursing Process.* Denver: Association of Operating Room Nurses, Inc.

Hinshaw, A. S. (1983). The use of predictive modeling to test nursing practice outcomes. *Nursing Research, 32,* 35–42.

Johnson, J. E., Christman, N. J., Stitt, C. (1985). Personal control interventions: short- and long-term effects on surgical patients. *Research in Nursing & Health, 8,* 131–145.

Kleinbeck, S. V. M. (1994). Staff nurses explore perioperative nursing diagnoses. In: Carroll-Johnson, R., Paquette, M. eds. *Classification of Nursing Diagnoses, Proceedings of the Tenth Conference: NANDA.* Philadelphia: J.B. Lippincott Company (pp 246–249).

Kleinbeck, S. V. M. (1990). Introduction to the nursing process. In: Rothrock, J. C., ed. *Perioperative Nursing Care Planning.* St. Louis: Mosby (pp 3–12).

Kleinbeck, S. V. M. (1989). Developing nursing diagnoses for a perioperative care plan. *AORN Journal, 49,* 1613–1625.

Maslow, A. (1970). *Motivation and Personality.* New York: Harper & Row.

Meeker, M., Rothrock, J. (1990). *Alexander's Care of the Patient in Surgery.* St. Louis: Mosby.

Parsons, E. C., Kee, C. C., Gray, C. P. (1993). Perioperative nurse caring behaviors. *AORN Journal, 57,* 1106–1114.

Pinnell, N. N., deMeneses, M. (1986). *The Nursing Process.* Norwalk, Conn: Appleton-Century-Crofts.

Privacy Act of 1974, 5 U.S.C. Section 552A, 552A note, 1988.

Redman, B. K. (1993). *The Process of Patient Teaching.* 7th ed. St. Louis: Mosby–Year Book.

Rothrock, J. C. (1990). *Perioperative Nursing Care Planning.* St. Louis: Mosby.

Rothrock, J. C. (1989). Perioperative nursing research, I: Preoperative psychoeducational interventions. *AORN Journal, 49,* 597–619.

Seifert, P. C., Rothrock, J. C. (1989). Perioperative assessment tool. In: Guzzetta, C. E., Bunton, S. H., Prinkey, L. A., Sherer, A. P., Seifert, P. C., eds. *Clinical Assessment for Use with Nursing Diagnoses.* St. Louis: Mosby (pp 198–222).

Sundeen, S. J., Stuart, G. W., Rankin, E. A., Cohen, S. A. (1989). *Nurse-Client Interaction.* St. Louis: Mosby.

Watson, D. S., Groah, L., Murphy, R. N., Woolery, L. (1990). *Perioperative Nursing Documentation.* Denver: Association of Operating Room Nurses, Inc.

Yura, H., Walsh, M. B. (1988). *The Nursing Process.* 5th ed. Norfolk, Conn: Appleton & Lange.

Practice Scenario 1
Patient Care Planning

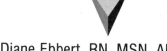

by Diane Ebbert, RN, MSN, ARNP, CNOR

SCENARIO

Sandy Parsons is a 36-year-old female admitted to the ambulatory surgery unit for a biopsy of her left breast. She is 5 feet 3 inches tall, weighs 135 pounds, and has no known allergies. Her vital signs include blood pressure 150/90, pulse 90, and respirations 20. She discovered a breast mass 2 weeks ago during her monthly self-exam. The mass is nontender, fixed, and located in the upper outer quadrant of her left breast. Her past medical history is noncontributory. Her family history is positive for breast cancer in her mother. Sandy is single and lives alone. Her family and two sisters live 100 miles away. She recently moved to this area and is still getting acquainted. She has smoked one pack of cigarettes a day for the past 15 years. She loves coffee and drinks at least eight cups a day. She states she is "quite nervous this morning" and is glad that her mother has come to stay with her for several days. She asks many questions. She states that she is "hoping for the best, but probably has some tough choices to make." She has requested local anesthesia with intravenous sedation.

PERIOPERATIVE INTERPRETATION

Using what you have just learned in this chapter, as an experienced perioperative nurse you would consider the following in the care of this patient.

1. Assessment
   - Based upon the perioperative assessment, you know that the patient has a maternal history of breast cancer and a smoking history, which places her at high risk for breast cancer.
   - The description of the lesion as being fixed and in the upper outer quadrant strongly suggests malignancy.
   - Anxiety is evidenced by her statement and her blood pressure and pulse readings.
   - The daily caffeine intake may predispose her to some withdrawal effects of decreased caffeine intake due to the NPO status.

- The smoking history is significant and could compromise her respiratory effort.
- Being awake during the procedure because of the choice of anesthesia may add to her anxiety level.

NURSING DIAGNOSES

Anxiety related to the surgical procedure and possible diagnosis of cancer
Sensory/perceptual alterations related to local anesthesia with intravenous sedation
High risk for ineffective breathing pattern related to sedation, surgical draping, and smoking history

2. Planning
   - Plan to procure all supplies on surgeon's preference card prior to patient's entering the room to assure being able to remain with the patient to provide emotional support.
   - Since an anesthesiologist will not be present, validate the availability and functioning of the cardiac, blood pressure, and pulse oximetry equipment.
   - Check with the surgeon regarding the required intravenous sedation and review the drug sheet for maximum allowable dose, adverse reactions, and nursing considerations.

3. Implementation
   - Provide the patient with the opportunity to verbalize concerns and questions, and provide explanations for all intraoperative activities prior to their initiation. Distract the patient with conversation during the intraoperative phase.
   - Provide for patient privacy during the prepping and draping of the patient.
   - Provide for patient comfort by warming the prepping solutions with consideration of the manufacturer's guidelines and using warm bath blankets to cover the patient.
   - Control extraneous noise and traffic in the room to reduce the stimuli that patient is exposed to.

- Position the ether screen to keep the drapes off the patient's face and to restrict the patient's view of the surgical procedure.
- Assess the patient's vital signs every 15 minutes along with oxygen saturation via pulse oximetry. Provide oxygen via nasal cannula at 2 ml/minute or per physician order.
- If the surgeon sends the specimen for a frozen section, mark on the pathology sheet that the patient is under local anesthesia so the pathologist is aware of this when the report is called back to the operating room.
- Document the intraoperative nursing activities, including the intravenous sedation ordered, amount given with patient response, oxygen administered, and amount of local anesthesia used.

Assure that the physician cosigns the verbal order for the medication and the oxygen administered.

4. Evaluation
- Convey to the postoperative ambulatory surgery nurse the patient's preoperative anxiety level, family history for breast cancer and current diagnosis, smoking history, local anesthesia and sedation administered, and current status.
- Evaluate the patient's postoperative anxiety level through verbal feedback and blood pressure and pulse readings.
- Evaluate the patient's breathing effectiveness through the vital signs and oxygen saturation levels.

Practice Scenario 2
Patient Care Planning

by Shirley Hazen, RN, MN, CNOR

SCENARIO

Joyce Strong is a 38-year-old female who is 5 feet 9 inches tall and weighs 185 pounds. Ms. Strong is scheduled to have a vaginal hysterectomy. The patient's history indicated that she has been healthy until 8 months ago when her menstrual periods began to last 9 days with heavy bleeding and severe cramping. Ms. Strong is tearful, stating that she and her husband have only been married 4 years and had hoped to have a child. As a result of a skiing accident, Ms. Strong has difficulty with flexion and extension of her right knee. The preoperative laboratory values were hemoglobin = 12 and hematocrit = 34. Allergies include sensitivity to iodine. Ms. Strong asks how many people would be seeing her with her legs in stirrups.

PERIOPERATIVE INTERPRETATION

Using what you have just learned in this chapter, as an experienced perioperative nurse you would consider the following in the care of this patient.

1. Assessment
   - The surgical procedure requires the patient to be placed in the lithotomy position. The patient's limited range of motion in the right knee necessitates additional planning.
   - The patient's weight may require additional padding for the stirrups.
   - The hematocrit value is slightly below normal, and the patient may require blood replacement during surgery.
   - The patient's expression of loss in not being able to have a child indicates the grieving process.
   - Allergy to iodine will require a replacement surgical prepping solution.
   - The patient's question regarding the number of people who will see her in stirrups indicates concern for exposure while in the surgical position.

NURSING DIAGNOSES

Anxiety related to surgical outcome and sterility

Loss of dignity related to surgical position and exposure during surgery

High risk for neuromuscular injury related to lithotomy position, limited range of motion in right knee, and body weight

2. Planning
   - Review physician's preference card; obtain lithotomy positioning devices and padding.
   - Accomplish as much preparation as possible prior to the patient's entering the operating room so that the nurse can remain with the patient during induction and positioning.
   - Arrange for additional personnel to assist in placing Ms. Strong into the lithotomy position.
   - Check the status of blood units ordered for the patient.

3. Implementation
   - Place towels over the windows into the operating room and control traffic into the room to provide privacy for the patient.
   - Explain perioperative activities to the patient as initiated.
   - With Ms. Strong awake and using the covering sheet as a drape, simultaneously place the patient's legs in the lithotomy stirrups. Assess any discomfort or strain in the hip or knee joints. Place additional padding to protect the patient's skin from coming in contact with the metal edges of the stirrups.
   - Assess peripheral pulses prior to and after placement in the stirrups to assure optimum circulation in the lithotomy position.
   - Position towel/pad under the patient's buttocks prior to initiation of the surgical skin prep. Remove the towel/pad after the prep.
   - Place a pillow under the knees following removal from the lithotomy position.

- Document on the perioperative record the skin prep used, emotional support given to the patient, comfort and positioning measures implemented, and patient responses.

4. Evaluation
   - At the completion of the surgical procedure, assess the patient's skin integrity for any redness or bruises related to the surgical position and skin prep used.

- Convey to the post-anesthesia care unit nurse the patient's preoperative anxiety, hematocrit level, sensitivity to iodine, right knee limitation, and positioning aids used.
- Request the post-anesthesia care unit nurse to evaluate the patient's statements about discomfort in right knee related to the surgical position.

Chapter Seven

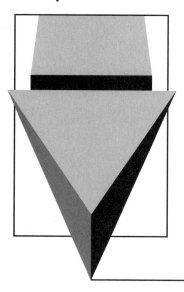

Anesthesia and Perioperative Nursing Care

Karen Zaglaniczny, CRNA, PhD • Sandra Maree, CRNA, MEd

Prerequisite Knowledge   Prior to beginning this chapter, the learner should review pharmacology and human physiology. Chapter content correlates with several AORN recommended practices. These recommended practices may be considered a prerequisite prior to beginning the chapter or a refresher upon completion of the chapter.

Recommended Practices for Anesthesia Equipment — Cleaning and Processing

Recommended Practices for Documentation of Perioperative Nursing Care

Recommended Practices for Monitoring the Patient Receiving Intravenous Conscious Sedation

Recommended Practices for Monitoring the Patient Receiving Local Anesthesia

Learning Objectives

1. Describe the anesthetic approach to the care of the surgical patient.

2. State the rationale for specific monitoring devices used during anesthesia.

3. List one anesthetic agent used for
   • inhalation
   • induction
   • neuromuscular blocking
   • local anesthesia.

4. Describe malignant hyperthermia and its treatment protocol.

Surgical anesthesia as we know it today had its beginning in 1846 when William Morton, a Boston dentist, demonstrated the use of ether as a surgical anesthetic. Following the painless surgery using ether anesthesia, an eminent surgeon attending the demonstration remarked "I have seen something today that will go around the world." Within a month, ether was used in other cities in the United States and in Great Britain and was soon established as legitimate (Smith, 1985).

Anesthesia today is a complex process that has become highly refined. Advances in pharmacology, technology, monitoring standards, equipment, education, and risk management initiatives have contributed to more positive patient outcomes. The purpose of this chapter is to describe the anesthesia process today, highlight technologic advances, identify potential complications associated with anesthesia, and define nursing responsibilities. It is hoped that a broader understanding of professional roles in the operating room will enhance collaboration among team players, efficiency, team spirit, and patient outcomes. Anesthesia care is provided by nurses, certified registered nurse anesthetists (CRNA), physicians, and anesthesiologists. The role of each provider varies from hospital to hospital.

Anesthesia Care

Like all of nursing, professional goals for anesthesiologists and nurse anesthetists include provision of consistent, safe care. Anesthesia care, like nursing, is based upon four principles: assessment, planning, implementation, and evaluation. Anesthesia practice is guided by professional standards, which describe the practitioner's role in providing quality anesthesia care.

employers to inform employees of the existence of potential hazards in the work site. Federally enforceable, this law requires employers to have a written communication program to educate employees regarding hazardous chemicals. Each year, some health care facilities are found to be in substantial noncompliance with this mandate for three major reasons:

1. Lack of appropriate training in the handling of hazardous substances
2. Lack of chemical/hazard inventory and paperwork
3. Lack of a written hazard communication program

To achieve and maintain compliance, health care facilities must develop a hazards communication program. The program requires health care facilities to

- Conduct a chemical inventory; include the method of disposal and spill procedures; maintain an inventory in the materials management office.
- Identify chemicals listed as carcinogenic by OSHA or NIOSH; delete them or substitute where possible.
- Establish a labeling system for all containers, including refill bottles; the label must describe the hazard.
- Maintain a master set of material safety data sheets (MSDS). The emergency room, nursing, and safety offices should have copies. Each health care unit should have a list of hazardous products used in its respective department.
- Ensure employee notification of new hazardous products when the products are introduced.
- Mandate annual employee training for hazard communication. Training must include a review of employee rights; location of MSDS; instructions for reading the MSDS; evaluation of the training method for educating employees; and a system for reporting and documenting the training.
- Develop a written hazard communication policy.

Each health care facility is also required to have a management system for the required material safety data sheets (MSDS). An MSDS is mandated for each hazardous chemical. Its purpose is to inform employees about chemical hazards and about how to protect themselves. The MSDSs are supplied by the manufacturer to buyers who must in turn educate their employees. The employer must identify and list hazardous chemicals; ensure that labeling includes precautions or special handling instructions; signs and symptoms of toxic exposure; and first aid treatment for exposure. Waste anesthesia gases are included in the category of hazardous chemicals.

Each MSDS has nine sections that must be filled out.

1. Material information—include manufacturer's name, location, and phone number; identify the chemical by its generic and brand or trade name.
2. Hazardous ingredients—list all the hazardous ingredients by name and percentage by weight and exposure limits.
3. Physical data—describe the chemical characterizations.
4. Fire and explosion hazard data—classify how easily the product will burn or explode and explain how to extinguish any fire.
5. Emergency and first aid data—explain how to respond to accidental exposure according to the route of entry (eyes, skin, inhalation, or ingestion); include signs and symptoms of exposure.
6. Reactivity data—identify the stability of the product and list what products will not mix safely with the chemical.
7. Spill or leak procedures—describe proper cleanup of spills, including personal protective equipment (PPE) for employees and approved method of disposal.
8. Special protection information—list the type of PPE to wear when using the chemical, appropriate ventilation, and other necessary precautions.
9. Special precautions—list information related to shelf life and storage; identify any special handling requirements.

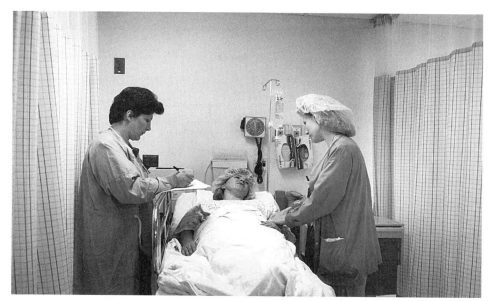

FIGURE 7-1. Preoperative Patient Preparation

ASSESSMENT

Anesthesia care begins with a thorough and complete preanesthetic assessment (Fig. 7-1). The overall goal of preoperative assessment is to reduce perioperative morbidity and mortality. Specific objectives include familiarity with coexisting medical conditions, past and present surgical history, review of physical examination with emphasis on areas that may be associated with anesthetic complications, and laboratory tests pertinent to medical history or contemplated surgical procedure. Information to be elicited during the preoperative visit and interview is listed in Table 7-1.

Pertinent points of the physical examination include auscultation of heart and lung sounds, blood pressure range, peripheral pulse assessment, and venous access assessment. Physical examination also includes assessment for neurologic dysfunction, cyanosis, and mouth and airway. Neck flexion, mouth opening, temporomandibular joint mobility, and visibility of the uvula and dentition are important points for airway assessment. Height, weight, and pertinent laboratory data are noted. Laboratory tests are ordered according to findings on history and physical examination and according to institutional policy. Fewer tests are routinely ordered today than formerly, and most are ordered only for a specific indication.

Perioperative nurses can assist with the anesthesia assessment by informing the anesthesia provider of pertinent information gained from the nursing assessment. Patient statements regarding a history of asthma, previous anesthesia problems in themselves or in their family, and abnormal laboratory data are of special interest to the anesthesia provider.

TABLE 7-1. **INFORMATION NEEDED FOR PREANESTHETIC ASSESSMENT**

General state of health
Previous anesthetic history
Current drug use
History of allergy
Menstrual or obstetric history
General organ system review

TABLE 7-2. **ASA PHYSICAL STATUS CLASSIFICATION**

ASA 1	A normal healthy patient
ASA 2	A patient with mild systemic disease usually well controlled (hypertension, mild diabetes, chronic bronchitis)
ASA 3	A patient with a severe systemic disease that limits activity (angina, chronic obstructive pulmonary disease, prior myocardial infarction) but is not incapacitating
ASA 4	A patient with a severe disease that is a constant threat to life (heart failure, renal failure)
ASA 5	A moribund patient not expected to survive 24 hours with or without operation (ruptured aneurysm, head trauma with intracranial hypertension)

An E is added for emergence operations.

PLAN

Following patient assessment, a patient-specific plan for anesthesia care is formulated. Such a plan includes strategies for preoperative, intraoperative, and postoperative care. Informed consent for the planned anesthetic intervention is then obtained from the patient or legal guardian, and questions are invited. Obtaining informed consent involves discussing the anesthesia plan and alternatives and potential complications in terms understandable to the layperson. Risks associated with the anesthetic procedure are disclosed.

A preoperative notation is made in the progress notes or on a separate preanesthesia form. It includes date and time of interview, proposed procedure, relevant findings on history, physical and laboratory examinations, and identification of the American Society of Anesthesiologists' (ASA) Physical Status Classification (Table 7-2). The room is prepared for surgery, and equipment is carefully checked. The anesthesia plan is then skillfully implemented, and the plan of care is adjusted as needed to adapt to the patient's response to anesthesia and surgical stimulation. The OR nursing considerations for preoperative care are listed in Table 7-3.

Patients are counseled about food and fluid intake during the preoperative interview. The practice for safely preparing patients for anesthesia traditionally included fasting for at least 6 hours preoperatively. This practice was based upon fear of vomiting or regurgitation during general anesthesia with development of aspiration pneumonitis. Even a small volume of acidic material can cause severe pneumonitis. The critical pH has been accepted as 2.5, and the volume of gastric content considered to place a patient at risk is thought to be 0.4 ml/kg (Teabeaut, 1952; Roberts, 1974). Evaluation of NPO status began in Britain and has spread. In 1977, Hester and Heath showed no correlation between starvation time and gastric pH or volume (Hester, 1977). Later Miller showed that an overnight fast did not guarantee an empty stomach, and a light breakfast 2 to 3 hours before surgery did not alter gastric volume or pH (Miller, 1983). Moderate amounts of clear liquids are emptied almost completely from the stomach in healthy patients in 2 to 3 hours (Shevde, 1991; McGrady, 1988). Based on these studies, it seems safe to

TABLE 7-3. **PREOPERATIVE NURSING CONSIDERATIONS**

1. Complete Patient Assessment
    Physical needs
    Psychologic needs
    Medical and surgical history
    Previous surgeries
    Completion of required documents, including consent and laboratory data
2. Determine Readiness and Mode of Transport to OR
3. Assess Health Care Team Availability
    Surgeon
    Anesthesiologist/Anesthetist
    Scrub person
    Circulating nurse

TABLE 7–4. **GOALS OF PREMEDICATION**

Relief of anxiety
Sedation
Amnesia
Analgesia
Antiemetic
Aspiration prophylaxis
Dry secretions

permit clear liquid ingestion until 2 to 3 hours before surgery in healthy, compliant patients. These guidelines do not apply to solids (Kallar, 1993).

Preoperative medication consists of pharmacologic preparation as necessary and psychologic support. Goals for pharmacologic premedication are listed in Table 7–4. Premedication also facilitates induction of anesthesia and reduces anesthetic requirements. Determinants of drug choice and dose for premedication are based on age, weight, ASA physical status, level of anxiety, drug allergies, and previous tolerance to depressant drugs. Choices are also made according to whether the procedure is being done on an inpatient or outpatient basis and whether the procedure is elective or of an emergency nature. Timing of drug administration is as important as drug selection.

Opioids are given today as premedication when there is a need for analgesia. Side effects of opioid premedication include ventilatory depression, nausea and vomiting, delayed gastric emptying, pruritus, and cholidochoduodenal sphincter spasm. Although butyrophenones such as droperidol possess good antiemetic effects, they can result in dysphoria and unexpected patient refusal of surgery. Benzodiazepines such as diazepam (Valium), lorazepam (Ativan), and midazolam (Versed) work well as premedicants because of their antianxiety effects. Versed is especially good since it has a rapid onset, brief duration, and is usually not painful following intramuscular or intravenous injection.

The inclusion of anticholinergics such as atropine, scopolamine, and glycopyrrolate as part of premedication is not a routine practice today. These drugs are sometimes given if there is a need to reduce airway secretions or to prevent vagolytic activity. Prevention or treatment of reflex bradycardia is best accomplished by intravenous administration of atropine near the time of the initiating event.

Aspiration pneumonitis, although uncommon, is a significant and potentially preventable complication of anesthesia. Although 40% to 80% of patients scheduled for elective surgery may be at risk for aspiration pneumonitis based upon gastric pH and volume, the current reported incidence is 1.4 to 6 per 10,000. The incidence is higher in infants, the elderly, and patients with high ASA physical classification (Olsson, 1986). Patient conditions contributing to aspiration include a history suggesting delayed gastric emptying such as obesity, diabetes, peptic ulcer disease, stress or pain, trauma, and narcotic premedication. Risk is also higher than average in esophageal, upper abdominal, and emergency laparoscopic surgery (Blitt, 1970; Carlsson, 1981). The presence of an incompetent lower esophageal sphincter also places the patient at risk. Although presence of a hiatus hernia by itself does not imply increased risk, patients may be at greater risk if they have symptoms of reflux (Cohen, 1971). Obese, obstetric, and ambulatory surgical patients as well as the very old and very young are also at greater risk for aspiration (Vaughan, 1975; Hall, 1940; Mendelson, 1946; Ong, 1978; Cote, 1982).

A number of pharmacologic adjuncts have been recommended to reduce the risk of aspiration. They include anticholinergics, antacids, H_2 receptor antagonists, and gastrokinetics.

Anticholinergics such as atropine and glycopyrrolate may decrease gastric secretion, but the effect is not reliable in doses used for premedication (Manchikanti, 1984a). These drugs may also relax the lower esophageal sphincter and make regurgitation more likely (Cotton, 1981).

Antacids (sodium citrate, (Bicitra) 15 to 30 ml) when administered 15 to 30 minutes before induction of anesthesia raise gastric pH above 2.5 in nearly all patients. Efficacy may depend on patient movement and complete mixing of the antacid with gastric fluid. The effect on gastric fluid pH is immediate, but gastric volume may be increased. The duration of effect is variable and may depend on gastric emptying (Morgan, 1984). A disadvantage of antacids includes the potential for emesis. Clear antacids are preferred today because of concern for pulmonary damage if particulate matter is aspirated (Gibbs, 1979).

H_2 receptor antagonists such as cimetidine increase gastric fluid pH by blocking histamine-induced secretion of gastric fluid with a high hydrogen content. Gastric fluid volume is not influenced.

Cimetidine (Tagamet) is an example of a competitive histamine H_2 receptor antagonist that blocks the effects of histamine, pentagastrin, and acetylcholine on gastric acid secretion. The oral, IV, or IM dose is 300 mg (7.5 mg/kg). Onset after oral or IV dose is less than 45 minutes. Duration is 4 to 4.5 hours following an IV dose and 6 to 8 hours following an oral dose. A variety of regimens have been shown to be effective preoperatively in most patients: cimetidine 300 mg orally at bedtime followed by 300 mg orally or intramuscularly the morning of surgery (Weber, 1979); single oral dose of 300 to 600 mg given 1 to 2 hours before surgery or 200 mg given intravenously 1 hour before surgery (Salemenpera, 1980). The most reliable risk reduction is with cimetidine at bedtime and cimetidine and metoclopramide the morning of surgery (Manchikanti, 1984b).

Rapid intravenous administration of cimetidine may produce bradycardia, hypotension, or heart block. It may also produce increased airway resistance in patients with asthma secondary to loss of H_2 receptor-mediated bronchodilation with unopposed H_1 receptor bronchoconstriction. This drug may be associated with confusion and agitation, especially in the elderly.

Ranitidine (Zantac) is also a histamine H_2 receptor antagonist. It has no side effects, is longer acting, and has an efficacy at least comparable to that of cimetidine. The oral dose is 150 mg. Ranitidine has an onset of less than 30 minutes and a duration of 8 to 12 hours. The intravenous dose of 50 mg has an onset of less than 15 minutes and a duration of 6 to 8 hours. Intravenous ranitidine at doses of 40 to 100 mg given 1 hour before surgery has been shown to be effective (Maile, 1983).

Metoclopramide (Reglan) is a gastrokinetic drug that increases gastric emptying, increases tone of the lower esophageal sphincter, and acts as an antiemetic (Cotton, 1981). Gastric fluid pH is not altered. Extrapyramidal side effects are due to central antidopaminergic effects. Metoclopramide administered orally has an onset of 30 to 60 minutes, but onset is 3 to 5 minutes when it is given intravenously. A combination of metoclopramide and an H_2 antagonist may be the most reliable approach for reducing gastric volume and elevating pH.

Whereas the routine use of antacids, H_2 receptor antagonists, and gastrokinetics is recommended in patients at risk for aspiration pneumonitis, it has not been proven that prophylaxis changes morbidity or mortality in otherwise healthy patients receiving elective surgery. A rapid sequence induction with cricoid pressure is equally important in the prevention of aspiration pneumonitis.

The planning phase of the nursing process corresponds to the development of an anesthesia plan. A collaborative approach to the plan of care enhances the quality of care provided to the patient. The perioperative nurse should address with the anesthesia provider special concerns regarding the intraoperative position, projected need for blood replacement, and anesthesia method chosen for the patient. An astute perioperative nurse alerts the anesthesia provider of the fact that the surgical consent is unsigned and does not give the patient any sedative. Thorough planning on the nurse's part to coordinate the preoperative collection of all supplies allows the nurse to remain with the patient during the induction.

IMPLEMENTATION

Anesthesia choices involving anesthesia personnel include monitored anesthesia care (MAC), regional anesthesia, general anesthesia, and a combination of general and regional techniques. With all of these techniques, the patient's physiologic condition is monitored according to accepted standards and patient needs.

Monitored anesthesia care (MAC) refers to instances in which an anesthesia provider has been called to provide specific anesthesia services to a patient undergoing a planned procedure. The patient may receive local anesthesia and oxygen, is monitored, and receives medications as needed. During MAC cases, the anesthetist provides sedation and analgesia. Midazolam, fentanyl, alfentanil, and propofol are often used for MAC cases. Optimal management during MAC cases depends on the highly specialized skill of anesthesia providers. The American Association of Nurse Anesthetists believes that the safe administration of conscious sedation requires the sole attention of a professional who is educated in the specialty of anesthesia and skilled in the administration of sedation, monitored anesthesia care, and regional and general anesthesia. The American Nurses Association (ANA) position statement provides guidelines for IV conscious sedation (Table 7–5).

Regional anesthesia with local anesthetics may be a helpful alternative to general anesthesia in some patients. Common regional techniques consist of peripheral nerve blocks and spinal, epidural, or caudal anesthesia. Room preparation, monitoring, and immediate availability of resuscitative equipment and medications are similar to those of general anesthesia cases. OR nursing considerations for regional anesthesia are listed in Table 7–6.

Spinal and epidural anesthesia (Fig. 7–2) are the two most popular regional anesthetic procedures in surgery, obstetrics, and postoperative analgesia. Advantages of these techniques include inhibition of most surgically induced endocrine and metabolic changes, reduction of intraoperative blood loss, and reduction of thromboembolic complications. Absolute contraindications to either block are patient refusal, infection at the puncture site, uncorrected hypovolemia, and coagulation abnormalities. Relative contraindications include bacteremia, neurologic disorders, and minidose heparin.

Spinal anesthesia consists of injection of local anesthetic drugs into the subarachnoid space. Lidocaine, tetracaine, and bupivacaine are selected most often, according to the site of surgery, desired intensity of motor block, and duration of surgery. Determinants of the dose of local anesthetic include baricity of the local anesthetic solution (hyperbaric, isobaric, hypobaric), shape of the spinal canal, and position of the patient. Addition to the local anesthetic solution of vasoconstrictors such as epinephrine, 200 to 250 mcg, or phenylephrine, 2 to 5 mg, prolongs the spinal anesthesia by localized vasconstriction.

Physiologic effects of spinal anesthesia include blockade of the sympathetic nervous system, intercostal muscle paralysis, and renal, hepatic, and gastrointestinal effects. Cardiovascular effects of spinal anesthesia include bradycardia, venodilation, and decreased blood pressure due to decreased venous return and decreased cardiac output. Intercostal muscle paralysis interferes with the ability to cough and clear secretions. Both renal blood flow and hepatic blood flow are reduced parallel to blood pressure. Sympathetic blockade of the gastrointestinal tract leaves vagal tone intact and results in a contracted bowel and may possibly contribute to increased peristalsis and nausea. Nausea and vomiting during spi-

TABLE 7–5. **ANA POSITION STATEMENT ON THE ROLE OF THE RN IN THE MANAGEMENT OF PATIENTS RECEIVING IV CONSCIOUS SEDATION FOR SHORT-TERM THERAPEUTIC, DIAGNOSTIC, OR SURGICAL PROCEDURES**

A. Definition of IV Conscious Sedation

Intravenous conscious sedation is produced by the administration of pharmacologic agents. A patient under conscious sedation has a depressed level of consciousness, but retains the ability to independently and continuously maintain a patent airway and respond appropriately to physical stimulation and/or verbal command.

B. Management and Monitoring

It is within the scope of practice of a registered nurse to manage the care of patients receiving IV conscious sedation during therapeutic, diagnostic, or surgical procedures provided the following criteria are met:

1. Administration of IV conscious sedation medications by nonanesthetist RNs is allowed by state laws and institutional policy, procedures, and protocol.
2. A qualified anesthesia provider or attending physician selects and orders the medications to achieve IV conscious sedation.
3. Guidelines for patient monitoring, drug administration, and protocols for dealing with potential complications or emergency situations are available and have been developed in accordance with accepted standards of anesthesia practice.
4. The registered nurse managing the care of the patient receiving IV conscious sedation shall have no other responsibilities that would leave the patient unattended or compromise continuous monitoring.
5. The registered nurse managing the care of patients receiving IV conscious sedation is able to:
   a. Demonstrate the acquired knowledge of anatomy, physiology, pharmacology, cardiac arrhythmia recognition, and complications related to IV conscious sedation and medications.
   b. Assess total patient care requirements during IV conscious sedation and recovery. Physiologic measurements should include, but not be limited to, respiratory rate, oxygen saturation, blood pressure, cardiac rate and rhythm, and patient's level of consciousness.
   c. Understand the principles of oxygen delivery, respiratory physiology, transport and uptake, and demonstrate the ability to use oxygen delivery devices.
   d. Anticipate and recognize potential complications of IV conscious sedation in relation to the type of medication being administered.
   e. Possess the requisite knowledge and skills to assess, diagnose, and intervene in the event of complications or undesired outcomes and to institute nursing interventions in compliance with orders (including standing orders) or institutional protocols or guidelines.
   f. Demonstrate skill in airway management resuscitation.
   g. Demonstrate knowledge of the legal ramifications of administering IV conscious sedation and/or monitoring patients receiving IV conscious sedation, including the RNs responsibility and liability in the event of an untoward reaction or life-threatening complication.
6. The institution or practice setting has in place an educational/competency validation mechanism that includes a process for evaluating and documenting the individuals' demonstration of the knowledge, skills, and abilities related to the management of patients receiving IV conscious sedation. Evaluation and documenting of competence occurs on a periodic basis according to institutional policy.

C. Additional Guidelines

1. Intravenous access must be continuously maintained in the patient receiving IV conscious sedation.
2. All patients receiving IV conscious sedation will be continuously monitored throughout the procedure as well as the recovery phase by physiologic measurements including, but not limited to, respiratory rate, oxygen saturation, blood pressure, cardiac rate and rhythm, and patient's level of consciousness.
3. Supplemental oxygen will be immediately available to all patients receiving IV conscious sedation and administered per order (including standing orders).
4. An emergency cart with a defibrillator must be immediately accessible to every location where IV conscious sedation is administered. Suction and a positive pressure breathing device, oxygen, and appropriate airways must be in each room where IV conscious sedation is administered.
5. Provisions must be in place for backup personnel who are experts in airway management, emergency intubation, and advanced cardiopulmonary resuscitation if complications arise.

November, 1991, ANA Position Statement, Washington, D.C.

nal anesthesia may also be due to hypotension, cerebral ischemia, or medication for sedation.

Major complications associated with spinal anesthesia include hypotension, spinal or postdural puncture headache, extensive spread of spinal, backache, major neurologic injury, and infection. Adequate hydration before spinal anesthesia or positioning to encourage venous return is often all that is needed to prevent or manage hypotension. A vasopressor, such as ephedrine (Ectasule), 5 to 10 mg IV, may be necessary to restore normotension.

Postdural puncture headache (spinal headache) is due to decreased cerebrospinal fluid pressure due to leakage of cerebrospinal fluid through the needle hole in the dura. It may be prevented by utilizing a small-gauge needle and is

TABLE 7-6. **PERIOPERATIVE NURSING CONSIDERATIONS FOR REGIONAL ANESTHESIA**

Type and dose of local anesthetic
Patient position
Onset and duration of regional block
Physiologic response
    Blood pressure and heart rate
    Pain relief
Monitoring equipment and data
Use of adjunct drugs for sedation
Environmental aspects
    Warm comfortable operating room
    Awake/sedated patient aware of noise, voices, radio

treated with analgesics, bed rest, hydration, caffeine infusion, or epidural blood patch. An epidural blood patch consists of aseptic placement of 10 to 20 ml of autologous blood into the epidural space. This treatment is usually reserved for headaches that last longer than 24 hours.

Extensive spread of spinal anesthesia or total spinal is marked by agitation, hypotension, nausea, absent intercostal muscle function, and inaudible voice secondary to inadequate air movement. Management includes ventilation of the lungs with oxygen and support of blood pressure.

Epidural anesthesia consists of placement of local anesthetic into the epidural space (Fig. 7-3). Determinants of the quality of epidural anesthesia are local anesthetic selected; dose, volume, and concentration of drug injected; and site of injection. Addition of epinephrine 1:200,000, reduces systemic absorption, especially if lidocaine is given. Sympathetic nervous system block sufficient to cause hypotension is more gradual in onset with epidural anesthesia. Major complications associated with epidural anesthesia include hypotension, accidental subdural or subarachnoid injection, dural puncture with headache, and

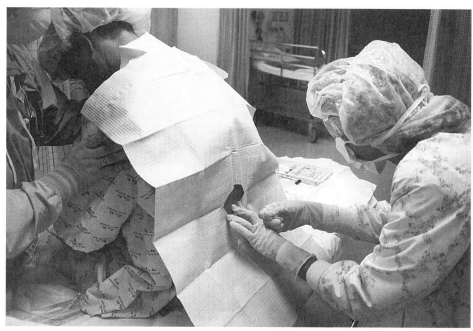

FIGURE 7-2. Administration of Regional Anesthetic

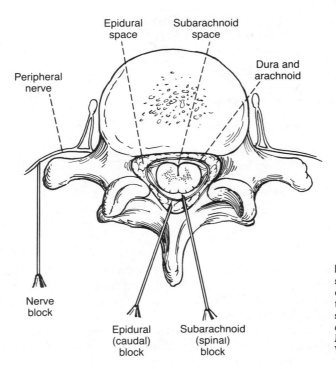

Epidural
space

Subarachnoid
space

Dura and
arachnoid

Peripheral
nerve

Nerve
block

Epidural
(caudal)
block

Subarachnoid
(spinal)
block

FIGURE 7–3. Cross section of the spinal cord showing spinal and epidural injection sites for anesthesia (From Black, J. M., Matassarin-Jacobs, E. (1993) *Luckmann and Sorensen's Medical-Surgical Nursing.* 4th ed. Philadelphia: W.B. Saunders Company. p. 423.)

neural damage due to epidural hematoma in patients with coagulopathy. Toxicity of local anesthetics owing to intravascular injection or systemic absorption of large amounts of drug are also complications of this technique.

Caudal anesthesia is produced by injection of local anesthetic through a needle introduced through the sacral hiatus into the sacral canal (Fig. 7–4). A larger dose of local anesthetic is required because of the large volume of the sacral canal. This is a popular technique for anesthesia and postoperative analgesia in children.

General anesthesia consists of three major phases: induction, maintenance, and emergence. Induction may be accomplished by the IV, IM, rectal, or respiratory routes (Fig. 7–5). The most commonly used induction agents are ultrashort-acting barbiturates, ketamine, etomidate, or benzodiazepines. Potent inhalation agents can be administered for induction by mask, which is a common technique in children. Mask anesthesia, or anesthesia without the endotracheal tube, is sometimes chosen for short, uncomplicated, peripheral procedures. Endotracheal anesthesia is indicated when surgery involves a major body cavity, risk of aspiration, difficult airway management, awkward positioning, head or neck procedures, and long procedures. Neuromuscular blocking agents are given to facilitate endotracheal intubation after the ability to ventilate is established.

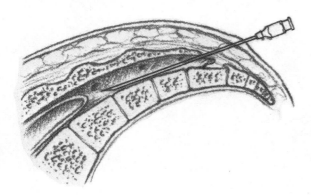

FIGURE 7–4. Position of the needle for caudal anesthesia common in obstetric patients (From Nealon, T. F. (1994) *Fundamental Skills in Surgery.* 4th ed. Philadelphia: W.B. Saunders Company. p. 94.)

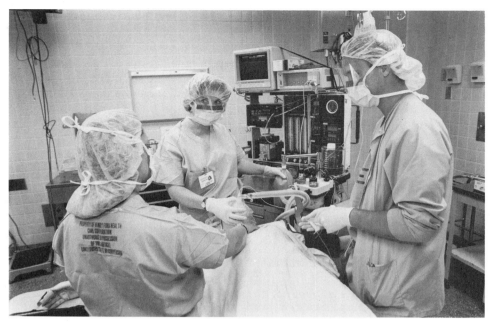

FIGURE 7–5. Induction of General Anesthesia

Patients with a full stomach at risk for aspiration are intubated awake, or a rapid-sequence induction is administered. In a rapid-sequence induction the patient is preoxygenated and induced with thiopental or ketamine. Cricoid pressure or the Sellick maneuver (Fig. 7–6) is applied as the patient loses consciousness. When the neck is extended, firm pressure of the cricoid cartilage compresses the esophagus against the cervical vertebrae and prevents passive reflux

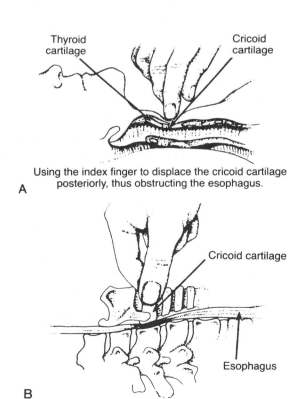

FIGURE 7–6. Sellick Maneuver (Reprinted with permission from Ethicon (1978). *Nursing Care of the Patient in the OR.* 2nd ed. Somerville, NJ: Ethicon. p. 23.)

of fluid into the oropharynx. Cricoid pressure should be maintained by an assistant until the endotracheal cuff is inflated and breath sounds are heard bilaterally. Paralysis for rapid-sequence induction is usually accomplished by the administration of succinylcholine, which is given immediately after thiopental. The patient is not ventilated by mask with this technique.

Once general anesthesia has been induced, it can be maintained by a number of methods such as an inhalation, total intravenous, or N_2O-narcotic-relaxant technique. Neuromuscular blockade is provided as needed. At the end of the procedure, anesthesia is discontinued, components are reversed, and emergence is begun (Fig. 7–7). Extubation of the trachea is generally best accomplished when the patient maintains adequate spontaneous ventilation and responds to verbal commands. The peripheral nerve stimulator, head lifting, and hand squeezing are convenient ways to assess the adequacy of reversal of neuromuscular blockade.

Extubation is delayed until the patient is fully awake for the following conditions: hemodynamic instability, bleeding, tracheal or maxillofacial surgery, difficulty with mask ventilation, full stomach, or glottic edema. Extubation in deep anesthesia is done in asthmatics and in patients in whom coughing and straining are to be avoided. OR nursing considerations for general anesthesia are listed in Table 7–7.

Fluid and electrolyte balance are important goals for good patient outcome. Perioperative management of a patient's fluid balance includes preoperative evaluation and intraoperative maintenance and replacement of losses. Preoperative evaluation includes mental status, input and output history, supine and sitting blood pressure, heart rate, skin turgor, and urinary output. Concentration of constituents in extracellular fluid compartments is determined by total-body water content and measured by serum sodium concentration and serum osmolarity. The composition of extracellular fluid is determined by test results of the electrolytes.

Fluid administration intraoperatively is aimed at maintenance of normal body-fluid composition. Deficit, maintenance, and third-space losses must all be

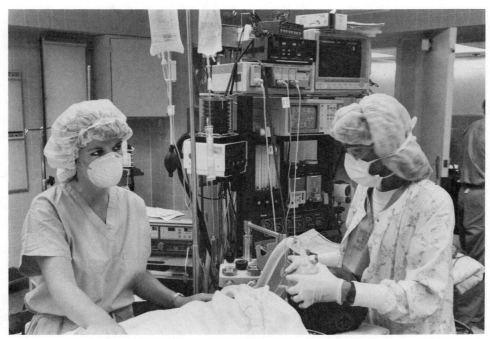

FIGURE 7–7. Emergence from General Anesthesia

TABLE 7–7. **PERIOPERATIVE NURSING CONSIDERATIONS FOR GENERAL ANESTHESIA**

Induction
    Assist with monitoring devices
    Help during airway management
Maintenance
    Obtain fluid and blood products
    Acquire drugs if needed
    Send blood specimens to the laboratory
    Monitor blood loss (sponges and suction)
    Monitor urine output if Foley catheter is
      present
Emergence
    Assist with extubation and airway control
    Avoid or help prevent shivering
    Facilitate transport

replaced. This is generally done with crystalloids or colloids. Major blood loss requires blood replacement.

Significant blood loss is replaced with red blood cells or whole blood. Treatment of deficient oxygen-carrying capacity or anemia is best with red blood cells, whereas acute blood loss is best treated with whole blood. Disadvantages to packed cells for acute blood loss are also infusion rates, inadequate volume replacement, and deficiency of coagulation factors. Reconstitution with saline overcomes the problems of slow infusion and inadequate volume. Coagulation factors may be obtained from fresh frozen plasma and platelets from platelet concentrates.

During the implementation of anesthesia, the perioperative nurse should remain with the patient during the induction to offer emotional support and to assist the anesthesia provider as necessary. The immediate access to suction during the induction of general anesthesia is very important to prevent aspiration. During spinal anesthesia placement, the nurse can assist with positioning the patient to facilitate the placement of the spinal needle (Fig. 7–8). During the beginning of an extremity anesthesia block, the circulating nurse can assist the anesthesia provider in applying the tourniquet and supporting the patient's arm. All intraoperative activities, such as patient positioning and preparation of the skin, should be coordinated through the anesthesia provider for the patient's safety.

EVALUATION

The anesthesia process begins with assessment, planning, and implementation, and it requires a maintained vigilance for untoward identifiable reactions and a well thought out plan of action for optimal patient outcome. Airway complications or emergencies, cardiovascular compromise, and hypermetabolic states are examples of complications that require immediate action.

The fundamental responsibility of anesthesia providers is to maintain adequate gas exchange. Gas exchange requires a patent airway and prevention or management of respiratory complications, such as laryngospasm, bronchospasm, or central and peripheral respiratory depression.

More than 85% of all respiratory-related closed malpractice claims involve a brain-damaged or dead patient. Inability to manage difficult airways is estimated to be responsible for as many as 30% of deaths attributable to anesthesia (Caplan, 1980). Disorders commonly associated with airway difficulty include congenital facial and upper airway deformities, maxillofacial and airway trauma, airway

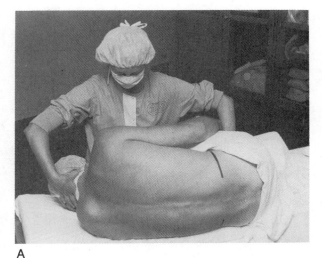

A

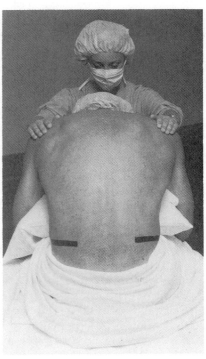

B

FIGURE 7–8. Positioning for Spinal Needle in General Anesthesia. *A*, Lateral decubitus positioning (forehead-to-knees). *B*, Sitting position, in which the assistant provides the patient a foot rest and a pillow and prevents the patient from slumping to either side. (From Miller, R. D. 1990). *Anesthesia.* 4th ed. New York: Churchill Livingstone. p. 1514.)

tumors and abscesses, face and neck fibrosis surgically induced deformities, and disorders that require cervical spine immobility. Anatomic causes of airway difficulty include a small mouth, large tongue, short neck, and inability to extend the neck at the atlanto-occipital joint. Successful management of a difficult airway begins with recognition of the potential problem. If there is a good possibility that intubation and ventilation by mask will be difficult, the airway should be secured while the patient is awake. If the patient is anesthetized and can be ventilated, it is best to proceed by mask or to awaken the patient. Transtracheal jet ventilation or the laryngeal mask airway may be used in patients who cannot be ventilated or intubated (Benumof, 1989).

Airway or respiratory complications may also result from laryngospasm or bronchospasm. Laryngospasm is reflex closure of the vocal cords that may occur in anesthetized patients when the vocal cords are irritated by secretions or when unintubated patients experience painful stimulus. Partial laryngospasm is characterized by a high-pitched crowing noise, whereas total laryngospasm results in no gas exchange. Treatment includes a head-tilt-jaw thrust, positive pressure on the airway with 100% oxygen, or succinylcholine.

Bronchospasm is defined as reflex bronchiolar constriction that is centrally mediated, as in asthma, or as a local response to airway irritation. Anaphylactoid drug reactions and transfusion reactions may also cause bronchospasm. Signs and symptoms include wheezing, dyspnea, decreased chest wall compliance, tachycardia, and decreased oxygen saturation. In full bronchospasm, gas exchange does not occur. Management includes administration of drugs that result in bronchodilation.

The etiology, recognition, and management of cardiovascular instability is beyond the scope of this chapter. Common problems leading to cardiovascular compromise include hemorrhagic, septic, or cardiogenic shock; cardiac tamponade; or serious dysrhythmias. Management is specific to the cause, urgent, and often requires participation of the entire operating room team.

The conclusion of anesthesia and extubation is as critical a period for complications as the induction phase. The perioperative nurse should remain by the patient's side to assist the anesthesia provider as necessary. Transfer from the operating room bed to the stretcher is done in coordination with the anesthesia provider. The perioperative nurse can help by communicating to the receiving unit, the post-anesthesia care unit or ambulatory surgery unit, specific equipment that will be needed in the immediate post-anesthesia period for the patient. Having this equipment, such as a ventilator, set up in advance will facilitate the care upon the patient's arrival.

Monitoring the Anesthetized Patient

The term *monitor* can be defined as that which warns, advises, or cautions. Since all anesthetic agents depress physiologic function, it is essential that all patients be monitored throughout the perioperative period. The degree of monitoring is dependent upon medical compromise, contemplated surgery, and skill and judgment of the anesthetist. The challenge is to match appropriate monitors with various patients and surgical procedures; to recognize abnormal parameters early; to provide aggressive corrective therapy; and to insure compliance with practice standards. Routine monitors are listed in Table 7-8. Everything done in anesthesia carries some risk for the patient. A reduction in risk is directly related to greater safety during the perioperative period and forms the rational basis for monitoring. It has been estimated that over 80% of anesthetic deaths are due to human error and, in most cases, are predictable. When the most common errors are listed (breathing circuit disconnect, breathing system leak, breathing system misconnection, loss of oxygen supply), it is striking how many of these errors could have been eliminated by monitoring and vigilance (Cooper, 1984; Cooper, 1978).

Patients are monitored intraoperatively from two perspectives: one looks at function and the other at substrate delivery and utilization. Under functional

TABLE 7-8. **MONITORING TECHNIQUES**

Electrocardiogram
Capnography (end tidal carbon dioxide)
Blood pressure
Temperature
Pulse oximetry

monitoring, the focus is on indicators of metabolic activity in cells in the brain, heart, liver, and kidneys. Since it is not possible to easily and routinely monitor cellular activity, the next best indicator is clinical assessment of the electrical activity of cells. Assessment of renal function by urinary output, muscular function by twitch response on peripheral nerve stimulation, cerebral function by pupillary size and reactivity, and level of consciousness by electroencephalogram are examples of functional monitoring. The electrocardiogram denotes electrical activity of the heart, and patterns of respiration suggest normal or abnormal respiratory function.

Substrate monitoring looks for information about the supply of substrate the patient is receiving. This involves organ perfusion, which is indirectly monitored by blood pressure and heart rate, and oxygen delivery, which is assessed by oxygen analyzers on the anesthesia machine. Substrate utilization may be assessed by pulse oximetry or capnography.

Before 1985, there were no minimal intraoperative monitoring standards available in the United States. In 1985, the Department of Anesthesia at Harvard Medical School adopted minimal monitoring standards for its nine component hospitals. These standards included

1. Presence of anesthesia personnel throughout the conduct of all general and regional anesthesia and monitored anesthesia care
2. Blood pressure and heart rate monitoring every 5 minutes
3. Continuous display of EKG from beginning of anesthesia until the patient is prepared to leave the location
4. Continuous monitoring of ventilation (palpation or observation of the breathing bag, auscultation of breath sounds or monitoring of respiratory gases) and circulation (palpation of pulse, auscultation of heart sounds, monitoring of intra-arterial tracings or pulse oximetry)
5. Breathing-circuit disconnect monitors
6. Oxygen analyzer on anesthesia machine
7. Means readily available to monitor patient temperature.

These standards are applied to the administration of preplanned anesthesia in all anesthetizing locations.

In emergency circumstances, life-threatening measures come first with attention turning to monitoring standards as soon as possible. Minimal standards may be exceeded at any time based on the judgment of involved anesthesia personnel. Although these standards would encourage high quality patient care, implementation cannot guarantee any specific patient outcome (Eichhorn, 1986).

Although the Harvard standards stopped short of mandating pulse oximetry, capnography, or temperature monitoring on all patients, they were a step in the right direction. They were endorsed by the American Association of Nurse Anesthetists (AANA) shortly after their introduction. Minimal monitoring standards were adopted by the AANA in 1990 and revised in 1992.

Essential monitors for all cases include the alert clinician, precordial or esophageal stethoscope, blood pressure and EKG monitors, oxygen analyzer; oximetry, capnography, and temperature monitors (see Table 7–8). In cases involving neuromuscular blocking drugs, a peripheral nerve stimulator is used to assess residual effects or recovery from drug effects.

The EKG is essential for detection of cardiac arrhythmias (leads I, II) and myocardial ischemia (lead V). It may also be helpful in the detection of electrolyte abnormalities and calculation of heart rate. Detection and management of myocardial ischemia are vital, because perioperative ischemia can result in postoperative myocardial infarction.

Pulse oximetry and capnography have rapidly emerged as monitoring standards in operating rooms in the United States. Pulse oximetry provides a noninvasive, continuous measurement of oxygen saturation of hemoglobin (SaO_2) and detects arterial hypoxemia in anesthetized, recovering, or critically ill patients. Normal values are greater than 90%. Cyanosis and bradycardia are late indicators of hypoxia and may not occur until the SaO_2 is 72%. Hypoxia can occur at any time during the procedure, and there is no relationship to duration of the case (Cote, 1988). Many factors can interfere with pulse oximetry, including external light, hypothermia, hypotension, and hemoglobinopathy. The pulse oximeter can assist in early detection of significant respiratory events.

Capnography (CO_2 waveform and end tidal CO_2 readout) serves as a quick check for endotracheal rather than esophageal intubation and is valuable in early detection of hypermetabolic states such as malignant hyperthermia. It provides a useful guide for adjustments in respiratory rate or volume and is a rapid detector of decreased pulmonary blood flow. When pulmonary blood flow is decreased (reduced cardiac output, pulmonary embolus), less CO_2 is carried to the lungs, and end tidal CO_2 decreases.

Renal function during surgery is monitored by a urinary catheter. The primary reason for monitoring renal function is to evaluate extracellular fluid volume and adequacy of cardiac output as reflected by renal blood flow. A urinary catheter is in place when procedures are long or when fluid or volume status are subject to substantial changes perioperatively.

Specialized Monitors

More specialized monitors are occasionally needed for optimal patient care (Fig. 7–9). Many of these monitors are invasive, and complications associated with them are well documented. Although useful in some patients, they are not completely accurate or reliable. They add to, but do not replace, the senses, clinical assessment, and judgment of the anesthesia provider.

Direct arterial blood pressure monitoring was developed in response to the need to monitor blood pressure during the nonpulsatile flow of cardiopulmonary

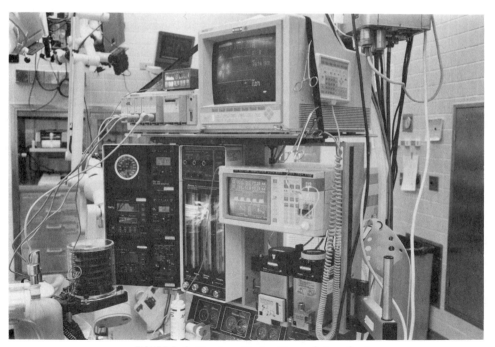

FIGURE 7–9. Monitors During General Anesthesia

bypass. Current indications for invasive monitoring are cardiac surgery with cardiopulmonary bypass, induced hypotension, expected wide fluctuations in blood pressure, major surgery involving coronary or myocardial disease, and cases that require repeated blood sampling. Advantages include continuous monitoring and immediate detection of serious hemodynamic alterations and the ability to monitor lower blood pressures. Examination of the arterial waveform may allow estimation of left ventricular function, stroke volume, systemic vascular resistance, and volume.

Measurement of central venous pressure (CVP) is an important adjunct to clinical management when combined with other observations. Catheters in the central circulation are used for measurement of CVP, rapid infusion of fluids, parenteral alimentation, insertion of transvenous pacemaker, and for patients at high risk for venous air embolus. Complications include infection, air embolus, arterial puncture, pneumothorax, and thoracic duct injury. The CVP monitor reflects how well the right heart handles the volume presented to it.

Pulmonary artery catheters measure the filling pressure of the left heart. Additionally they are useful for measuring cardiac output and systemic vascular resistance. Although they have been recommended for management of patients with poor left ventricular function, valvular heart disease, or recent myocardial infarction, and for management of patients in shock, their use remains controversial in some cases. Dysrhythmias are the most common complication associated with the use of pulmonary artery catheters. The most catastrophic complication is pulmonary artery perforation and hemorrhage.

Anesthesia Pharmacology Today: An Overview

Anesthesia is a term denoting loss of sensation with or without loss of consciousness. The anesthetic state can be produced by sedatives, local anesthetics, or global or site-specific general anesthetics.

General anesthesia is generally divided into the four components listed in Table 7–9. About 50 years ago, one agent, such as ether, provided the anesthetic state. Today a combination of agents from different pharmacodynamic classes are administered. This approach builds upon the best pharmacologic characteristics of each drug, reduces drug requirements, and enhances patient safety.

Patient safety and comfort and excellent operating conditions are also anesthetic goals. Anesthetic requirements change according to surgical stimulation and during general anesthesia. Agents must be carefully titrated according to monitored parameters and surgical and individual patient needs. In 1937, A. E. Guedel published a synthesis of clinical observations of ether anesthesia, which were divided into four stages of general anesthesia: analgesia and amnesia, delirium, anesthesia, and respiratory paralysis (Guedel, 1937). Anesthesia today is often accomplished with several drugs. Potent inhaled anesthetics, opioids, intravenous agents, and muscle relaxants preclude simple definitions of depth. An approach to anesthetic depth that emphasizes the type of noxious stimuli and the

TABLE 7–9. **COMPONENTS OF GENERAL ANESTHESIA**

Hypnosis	Unconsciousness
Analgesia	Insensibility to pain
Amnesia	Loss of memory
Muscle relaxation	Relaxation or paralysis of skeletal muscle

TABLE 7–10. **ASSESSMENT OF ANESTHETIC DEPTH**

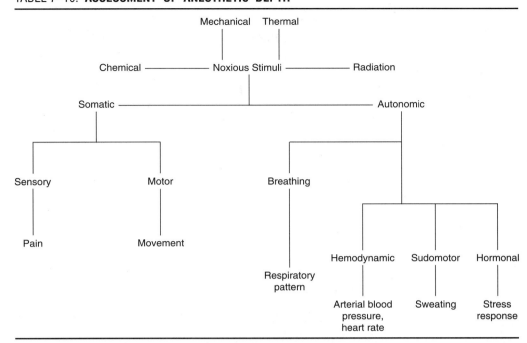

Adapted from Prys-Roberts, C. (1987). Anaesthesia: a practical or impossible construct. *British Journal of Anaesthesia, 59,* (11), 1341–1346.

specific class of drug that eliminates that response is the concept most appropriate regarding anesthetic depth for current clinical practice. Anesthetic depth today is better monitored by the body's response to noxious stimuli (Table 7–10).

Somatic responses to noxious stimuli include both sensory and motor activity. Sensory input obtained through the central nervous system can originate from somatic or visceral tissue. The patient must be conscious to perceive pain. Low concentrations of inhaled or intravenously administered anesthetics can eliminate recall of pain but still allow movement. The concentration of anesthetics required to eliminate somatic motor responses is higher than that needed to induce unconsciousness and eliminate perception of pain. The motor response of the respiratory system to noxious stimuli can involve an increase in tidal volume and frequency of breathing.

Autonomic responses to noxious stimuli consist of hemodynamic, sudomotor, and hormonal responses. Hemodynamic responses include increased sympathoadrenal activity with elevated arterial blood pressure and heart rate.

The *sudomotor* response includes sweating, and the *hormonal* response consists of elevation of the stress hormones, which is very difficult to completely eliminate. Pain relief, muscle relaxation, and suppression of autonomic activity can be achieved by anesthetic drugs. Some drugs achieve all these end points, whereas others achieve only one or two. A feature common to most anesthetics is the suppression of sensory perception and the production of unconsciousness.

Modern anesthesia is produced by global or site-specific agents. Global agents produce generalized depression of the central nervous system, and site-specific agents act through interaction at specific sites in the central or peripheral nervous systems. A balanced anesthetic technique consists of the use of several drugs, each of which address one or more of the four components of anesthesia (Table 7–11).

TABLE 7–11. **COMPONENTS OF ANESTHESIA**

	HYPNOSIS	ANALGESIA	AMNESIA	RELAXATION
GLOBAL AGENTS				
Volatile agents	+++	+/−	+	+
Propofol	+++	0	+	+/−
Thiopental	+++	−	+	0
Nitrous oxide	+	+	+	0
SITE-SPECIFIC AGENTS				
Opioids	+/−	+++	0	−
Midazolam	+	0	+++	0
Muscle relaxants	0	0	0	+++

+++ = primary effect
+ = weaker effect
+/− = doubtful effect
0 = no effect
− = antagonist effect

Inhalation Agents

The role of inhalation agents in general anesthesia is changing with increased administration of site- or receptor-specific agents. The inhaled agents are nitrous oxide (N_2O) and the halogenated hydrocarbons—fluothane (Halothane), enflurane (Ethrane), isoflurane (Forane), and desflurane (Suprane). Anesthetic effect is achieved by inhalation of the agent, uptake by the blood, and delivery to the target sites within the nervous system. Anesthetic requirements for inhalation anesthetics are judged by the *minimum alveolar concentration*. This concentration is an indication of anesthetic potency. It is the minimum alveolar concentration of inhaled anesthetic at 1 atmosphere that prevents movement in 50% of subjects in response to painful stimulus (Merkel, 1963).

Although the minimum alveolar concentration can serve as a guideline for required concentration of inhalation agent, it is influenced by various physiologic and pharmacologic factors. These influences are lessened by increased age, hypothermia, ethanol intoxication, and pregnancy. Combinations of N_2O with the other inhaled anesthetics have additive effects on the minimum alveolar concentration. This same concentration is decreased when other central nervous system depressants, such as opioids and benzodiazepines, are given (Saidman, 1964). The minimum alveolar concentration is increased by hyperthermia, chronic ethanol abuse, and increased levels of central nervous system neurotransmitters; it is unaffected by duration of anesthesia or gender.

All inhalation agents affect organ systems. Inhaled agents target central nervous system tissue and produce dose-related depression of the central nervous system. Cortical function is depressed at lower concentrations than medullary or spinal cord function. All agents result in cerebrovascular dilatation and thus elevate cerebral blood flow. These increases are dose dependent.

Halothane and *Ethrane* dilate both resistance (arterioles) and capacitance (venules) blood vessels and tend to reduce arterial blood pressure. Both drugs have negative inotropic and chronotropic effects on the heart, and both reduce myocardial oxygen consumption. Downward displacement of normal cardiac pacemaker activity encourages nodal rhythms. Halothane sensitizes the myocardium to the arrhythmogenic effects of catecholamines and epinephrine and norepinephrine.

Isoflurane is less of a myocardial depressant but more of a vasodilator and thus produces decreased blood pressure secondary to decreased systemic vascular resistance.

Suprane does not cause coronary steal or sensitize the heart to arrhythmias to the same extent as Halothane (Helman, 1992). It has less cardiac depression effect alone than with N_2O, but it does decrease systemic vascular resistance and blood pressure as does Forane.

All volatile anesthetics produce a moderate increase in $PaCO_2$ of 20%, reflecting an increase in respiratory rate insufficient to offset the reduction in tidal volume. Respiratory depression has a direct effect on the medullary ventilatory center and peripheral effects on intercostal muscles. These drugs are bronchodilators, and most inhibit hypoxic pulmonary vasoconstriction (HPV) in a dose-dependent manner. The latter effect may increase intrapulmonary shunting and reduce PaO_2.

Direct or indirect effects of these drugs on the renal and hepatic systems are considerations in the selection of these agents. Cardiovascular, endocrine, and nervous system changes associated with these agents are associated with moderate reduction in renal or hepatic blood flow and slight changes in function. Direct organ toxicity associated with these volatile agents is the result of biodegradation with the release of toxic products. Halothane, which undergoes 20% biodegradation, has resulted in hepatic dysfunction. One type of hepatic dysfunction is characterized by transient elevations in serum levels of liver transaminase enzymes and the other type by fulminant hepatic failure. Enflurane is slowly metabolized (12%) by the hepatic mixed-function oxidase system, and biotransformation releases fluoride ions, which are occasionally nephrotoxic (Mazze, 1977). Forane's level of metabolism is below 1% and is not associated with viscerotoxicity (Mazze, 1974). Likewise, Suprane has 10 times lower metabolism than Forane and produces no viscerotoxicity (Sutton, 1991). There are no significant increases in serum inorganic fluoride concentrations or urinary excretion rates after exposure to Suprane.

All inhalation agents have muscle relaxant effects and result in potentiation of neuromuscular blocking drugs. All serve as pharmacologic triggers for the pharmacogenetic disease, malignant hyperthermia. They are contraindicated in patients susceptible to malignant hyperthermia. The advantages and disadvantages of these agents are listed in Table 7–12.

TABLE 7–12. INHALATION ANESTHETICS

AGENT	MAJOR ADVANTAGES	SIDE EFFECTS; DISADVANTAGES
Nitrous oxide (N_2O)	Amnesia, analgesia rapid onset	Low potency, diffusion hypoxia, expansion in closed gas spaces; postoperative nausea and vomiting
Halothane (Fluothane)	Decreased $CMRO_2$; good induction agent for children; bronchodilator; uterine relaxant	Increased CBF, decreased blood pressure, heart rate, arrhythmias; respiratory depression, apnea; nausea, vomiting, ileus; hepatic dysfunction; trigger for malignant hyperthermia
Enflurane (Ethrane)	Decreased $CMRO_2$; bronchodilator; less myocardial sensitization to catecholamines; no coronary steal; uterine relaxant	Increased CBF; seizure activity on EEG; hypotension, arrhythmias; respiratory depression, apnea; nausea, vomiting; occasional renal dysfunction; trigger for malignant hyperthermia
Isoflurane (Forane)	Decreased $CMRO_2$; uterine relaxation; no organ toxicity; less myocardial sensitization to catecholamines	Trigger for malignant hyperthermia; coronary steal, hypotension, tachycardia; apnea or respiratory depression; nausea, vomiting, ileus
Desflurane (Suprane)	Decreased $CMRO_2$; uterine relaxation; rapid induction and emergence; no organ toxicity	Increased CBF; coughing; excitation during inhalation induction; trigger for malignant hyperthermia; hypertension, arrhythmias; respiratory depression, apnea; nausea, vomiting, ileus.

$CMRO_2$ = Cerebral metabolic oxygen consumption rate
CBF = Cerebral blood flow

Intravenous Induction Agents

BARBITURATES

Intravenous anesthesia as we know it today had its beginning in 1934 when John Lundy introduced thiopental sodium (Pentothal). While Pentothal remains a popular choice for induction of general anesthesia, other useful barbiturates include thiamylal (Surital) and methohexital (Brevital). The advantages and disadvantages of these agents are listed in Table 7–13.

Sodium pentothal is an ultrashort-acting thiobarbiturate that depresses the central nervous system and induces hypnosis and anesthesia but not analgesia. Recovery after a short dose is rapid, but high lipid solubility and slow elimination result in cumulative drug effects after repeated bolus injection or infusion. The drug produces some anterograde amnesia, and airway reflexes are heightened. It is associated with respiratory depression and hemodynamic effects include a decrease in systemic vascular resistance, arterial pressure, cardiac output, and coronary perfusion pressure. Histamine release can occur.

Pentothal is given for the induction of anesthesia and the supplementation of regional anesthesia, as an anticonvulsant, and as an agent for reduction of elevated intracranial pressure. Pentothal's onset of action following intravenous administration is 10 to 15 seconds with a peak effect in 30 seconds and a duration of action of 5 to 15 minutes. Pentothal potentiates the depressant effects of narcotics, sedative hypnotics, alcohol, and volatile anesthetics on the central nervous and circulatory systems. Pentothal can be associated with a number of side effects (Becker, 1978; Brown, 1968; Burn, 1960; Etter, 1980; Hirshman, 1985; Homer, 1985; Nussmeier, 1986).

Thiamylal is indistinguishable from thiopental as an intravenous induction agent. Both undergo maximal brain uptake within 30 seconds, accounting for the rapid onset of central nervous system depression. Prompt awakening reflects redistribution of the drug from the brain to inactive tissue. Thiamylal, like Pentothal, can evoke histamine release, and hemodynamic effects are similar.

Brevital depresses the sensory cortex; decreases motor activity; alters cerebellar function; and produces dose-dependent drowsiness, sedation, and hypnosis. It does not produce analgesia and has no muscle relaxant properties. In elderly patients and children and in the presence of acute or chronic pain, Brevital may induce excitement. Premedication with opioids reduces incidences of excitatory phenomena. Induction may be associated with involuntary muscle movements and respiratory depression. Cardiovascular effects are secondary to a decrease in myocardial contractility and peripheral vasodilation. Adverse reactions associated with Brevital are rare but may include arrhythmias, laryngospasm, bronchospasm, prolonged somnolence, nausea, hiccups, and shivering

TABLE 7–13. INTRAVENOUS AGENTS FOR INDUCTION OR MAINTENANCE

AGENTS	ADVANTAGES	DISADVANTAGES
Sodium Thiopental (Pentothal)	• Rapid induction • Cerebral vasoconstrictor	• Decreased blood pressure, increased heart rate • Venodilation • Laryngeal reflexes not depressed • Contraindicated with porphyria • Hypotension with hypovolemia • Vasospasm with intra-arterial injection; tissue necrosis with subcutaneous administration • No skeletal muscle relaxation • Shivering • Anaphylaxis • Laryngospasm; bronchospasm
Methohexital (Brevital)	• Most rapid induction	• Involuntary muscle movement • Seizures

(Hudson, 1983). Brevital is generally associated with a more rapid recovery of consciousness, making it useful for outpatient procedures.

Nonbarbiturate Induction and Maintenance Drugs

Several intravenous drugs have gained popularity as intravenous induction and maintenance drugs. The advantages and disadvantages are listed in Table 7 – 14.

Ketamine (Ketalar) is a phencyclidine derivative that produces rapid-acting dissociative anesthesia, which is characterized by normal or slightly enhanced skeletal muscle tone, respiratory stimulation, and occasionally a transient and mild respiratory depression. Anesthesia with ketamine resembles a cataleptic state in which the eyes remain open with a slow nystagmic gaze, and although wakefulness may appear to be present, the patient is noncommunicative (Reich, 1989; White, 1982). Salivary secretions are increased, but its bronchial smooth-muscle relaxant effects make ketamine as effective as inhalation agents in preventing bronchospasm. Central sympathetic stimulation and neuronal release and inhibition of reuptake of catecholamines lead to an increase in systemic and pulmonary artery pressure, heart rate, and cardiac output (Takeshita, 1972; Baraka, 1973). These properties make it extremely valuable as an induction agent in patients with hemodynamic compromise such as hypovolemia or cardiac tamponade.

A major disadvantage of ketamine is in emergence reactions such as dreaming, hallucinations, or confusion. These reactions are more common in 15- to 65-year-old patients and in patients in whom large doses are given rapidly. The incidence of these reactions is reduced when benzodiazepines or droperidol are provided as premedication (Fine, 1973). Increased salivary secretions can cause laryngospasm, especially in children. This can be attenuated by the preoperative administration of an anticholinergic.

Etomidate (Amidate) is a nonbarbiturate hypnotic without analgesic activity. Therapeutic doses have minimal effect on myocardial metabolism, cardiac

TABLE 7 – 14. **NONBARBITURATE INDUCTION AND MAINTENANCE AGENTS**

AGENTS	ADVANTAGES	DISADVANTAGES
Etomidate (Amidate)	Minimal changes blood pressure, heart rate Respiratory stability No histamine release No emergency reaction	Myoclonic movement Pain with injection Transient adrenocortical depression
Diazepam (Valium)	Less depression of ventilation Minimal change in heart rate Anticonvulsant properties	Thrombophlebitis
Lorazepam (Ativan)	Long duration of action	
Midazolam (Versed)	Low incidence thrombophlebitis	
Ketamine (Ketalar)	Profound analgesia Bronchodilator Hemodynamic support	Increased skeletal muscle tone Increased blood pressure and heart rate Increased cerebral blood flow and metabolic oxygen requirements Increased intracranial pressure Increased salivary gland secretion Emergence reaction; delirium, hallucinations
Propofol (Diprivan)	Hypnosis Rapid induction Clearheaded, rapid recovery Less nausea, vomiting	Hypotension, tachycardia or bradycardia Clonic myoclonic movement on emergence Pain on injection Sexual illusions

output, or peripheral or pulmonary circulation. Etomidate reduces intraocular and intracranial pressure (Owen, 1984). Principal adverse side effects include myoclonic movements, adrenal suppression, and pain on injection. Myoclonic movements occur in about one third of patients during induction, but this effect can be reduced by premedication with a benzodiazepine or opioid (Laughlin, 1985; Holdcroft, 1976). Adrenocortical suppression can occur after a single-induction dose of drug and may last 4 to 8 hours (Frager, 1984; Wagner, 1984). Pain on injection is reduced if the drug is given in large veins. Cardiovascular and respiratory stability associated with this drug make it extremely attractive as an induction agent. Etomidate's onset of action is 30 to 60 seconds; it peaks in 1 minute; and its duration of action is 3 to 10 minutes.

Propofol (Diprivan) is a newer intravenous induction and maintenance agent introduced into clinical practice in the United States in 1989. It exists as oil at room temperature. This gives it a white milky appearance. It has no antimicrobial properties, and guidelines for handling include strict aseptic technique, single-patient use, and use of the drug within 6 hours of opening the vial (Sebel, 1989). Anaphylaxis has been occasionally associated with this drug (Leon-Casasola, 1992; Laxenaire, 1992).

Propofol is a hypnotic agent that produces rapid induction of anesthesia with minimal excitatory activity. Onset of action is within 40 seconds, and duration of action is 5 to 10 minutes. Propofol undergoes extensive distribution and rapid elimination. In fact, clearance exceeds the capacity of hepatic blood flow suggesting extrahepatic mechanisms for clearance. Compared with thiopental, recovery is more rapid and there is less nausea and vomiting. It appears to be associated with reduced levels of nausea and vomiting in high risk patients and may possess a direct antiemetic effect (Martin, 1993; Weir, 1993; Borgeat, 1992).

Induction doses of propofol are associated with apnea and hypotension secondary to slight myocardial depression and a decrease in systemic vascular resistance with minimal change in heart rate. Venodilation contributes to the hypotension, and a 15% to 30% decrease in systolic, diastolic, and mean arterial blood pressure can occur (Muzi, 1992). This is especially likely in elderly, hypovolemic, and high risk patients who have received other central nervous system depressants, such as narcotics. Propofol can be used for induction of anesthesia by bolus injection or rapid infusion.

Propofol has been associated with pain on injection, which can be minimized by injecting in a large vein and by mixing IV lidocaine (0.1 mg/kg) with the induction dose of propofol. In some cases, up to 20 mg of lidocaine is added (King, 1992). Lidocaine can be injected before propofol (Gehan, 1991). Various arrhythmias have been reported with propofol, and several cases of addiction are known (Follette, 1992). There have been rare reports of seizures and opisthotonos after propofol. This activity is unique in that it more commonly occurs postoperatively (DeFriez, 1992). The incidence of severe postoperative myoclonus requiring intervention is low. Sexual illusions and disinhibition have also been reported with propofol sedation. This points out the potential danger of legal action. To avoid implications of misconduct, it is advisable to have a third party in the room at all times (Kent, 1992).

BENZODIAZEPINES

Benzodiazepines interact with receptors in the central nervous system producing favorable pharmacologic effects for the surgical patient. These effects include production of anterograde amnesia, minimal depression of the cardiovascular system or ventilation, anticonvulsion, and sedation. Mechanism of action of benzodiazepines includes interaction with the benzodiazepine receptor with modulation of the gamma-aminobutyric acid (GABA) receptor in the central nervous system. Modulation at the GABA receptor increases chloride conductance and leads to hyperpolarization of the postsynaptic membrane (Mohler, 1977; Mohler, 1988). The advantages and disadvantages are listed in Table 7–15.

Diazepam (Valium) is the standard with which all benzodiazepines are compared. This drug has calming effects. It has no autonomic nervous system blocking effects and minimal respiratory or circulatory depression in the absence of other central nervous system depressant drugs. Diazepam is useful as a premedication; as an adjunct to general (sedative, hypnotic, amnesia) or regional anesthesia (anticonvulsant); and as a treatment for acute alcohol withdrawal and panic attacks.

Lorazepam (Ativan) is a longer-acting benzodiazepine that produces dose-related sedation, relief of preoperative anxiety, and amnesia (Frager, 1976). It produces minimal depressant effects on ventilation and circulation in the absence of other central nervous system depressants.

Midazolam (Versed) is a short-acting benzodiazepine that also possesses antianxiety, sedative, amnestic, anticonvulsant, and skeletal-muscle relaxant properties. This benzodiazepine depresses ventilation and decreases peripheral vascular resistance, and blood pressure, especially in the presence of opioids or hypovolemia. Compared with Diazepam it has a more rapid onset, a greater amnestic action, and a sedative potency 3 to 4 times greater. (Reeves, 1985). Midazolam is water soluble, does not require solubilizing preparations, and is less irritating to the vein. It can be given by mouth and is very useful as a premedicant in pediatric patients. This benzodiazepine can also be given for induction of anesthesia and may be administered to supplement opioids or inhaled anesthetics during maintenance of anesthesia (Gamble, 1981; Jensen, 1982). Table 7–15 lists the pharmacologic characteristics of the benzodiazepines.

Some patients demonstrate unusual sensitivity to benzodiazepines. In the past, unwanted pharmacologic effects could be reversed only with nonspecific drugs such as aminophylline or physostigmine (Caldwell, 1982; Wangler, 1985). In 1989, *flumazenil* (Romazicon) was introduced into clinical practice as the first benzodiazepine receptor antagonist. Doses and plasma levels required to reverse agonist activity depend on the particular benzodiazepine used and the residual plasma level of the drug. Flumazenil reverses sedation, respiratory depression, and psychomotor effects of benzodiazepines; but hypoventilation and amnesia may not be fully reversed (Mora, 1989). Flumazenil, unlike naloxone, is remarkably free of cardiovascular effects. Antagonism is not followed by acute anxiety, hypertension, tachycardia, or neuroendocrine evidence of a stress response in postoperative patients (White, 1989; Kaukinsen, 1990). Resedation may occur

TABLE 7–15. **BENZODIAZEPINES**

DRUG	ONSET IV	PO	DURATION IV	PO	ADVANTAGES	DISADVANTAGES
Diazepam (Valium)	<2 min	15–60 min	15 min	120 min	Amnesia; sedation hypnosis; skeletal muscle relaxant; anticonvulsant activity	Circulatory and respiratory effects potentiated by other CNS depressants; thrombophlebitis; resedation in 6–8 hours
Lorazepam (Ativan)	1–5 min	60–360 min	360 min	1440 min	Amnesia; sedation; hypnosis; long acting	Unpredictable blood level—CNS response; circulatory-respiratory depression when combined with other CNS depressants
Midazolam (Versed)	1–5 min	5–10 min	120 min	360 min	Amnesia; sedation; hypnosis, rapid onset; no venous irritation; predictable blood level—CNS response	Increased sensitivity in patients with COPD; hypotension in elderly or hypovolemic patients; potentiates respiratory and circulatory effects of other CNS depressants

CNS = Central nervous system
COPD = Chronic obstructive pulmonary disease

and is more common with longer-acting drugs (diazepam, lorazepam), large doses of benzodiazepines (midazolam 20 mg), procedures lasting longer than 60 minutes, and with neuromuscular blocking drugs (Whitwam, 1990). Flumazenil can produce withdrawal symptoms in the presence of physical dependence on benzodiazepines and can be associated with seizures in patients receiving tricyclic antidepressants (Spivey, 1992).

Opioid Agonist, Agonist-Antagonist, Antagonist

Opioid is an inclusive term that describes all drugs, both natural and synthetic, that bind to morphine or opioid receptors. Opioid receptors are classified as MU-1, MU-2, delta, kappa, and sigma. Drug interaction at MU-1 receptors provides supraspinal analgesia; and MU-2 receptor interaction is associated with respiratory depression, decreased heart rate, physical dependence, and euphoria. Delta receptor stimulation is associated with modulation of MU receptor activity. Kappa receptor stimulation leads to analgesia, sedation, respiratory depression, and miosis. Dysphoria, hypertonia, tachycardia, and tachypnea are effects of sigma receptor stimulation. Some agents are receptor agonist, some agonist-antagonist, and others antagonist (Vaught, 1982). An advantage of agonist-antagonist agents is that analgesia is achieved with less respiratory depression. Narcotic antagonists reverse all pharmacologic effects of opioids. Table 7–16 lists the indications, onset, duration, and side effects of these drugs.

Morphine sulfate is an alkaloid of opium that primarily affects the central nervous system and organs containing smooth muscle. It produces analgesia, drowsiness, euphoria, and dose-related depression of respiration. It may cause hypotension secondary to histamine release and a reduction in peripheral resistance. Histamine release also causes pruritus and can initiate bronchospasm. It is given as an epidural or a spinal analgesia and as a postoperative analgesic.

Meperidine (Demerol) is a synthetic opioid approximately one tenth as potent as morphine. It has a more rapid onset and shorter duration of action. This opioid may produce orthostatic hypotension at therapeutic doses and direct myocardial depression at high doses. Perioperatively, it is limited to premedication and postoperative analgesia.

Fentanyl (Sublimaze) is a potent opioid agonist with an analgesic potency 75 to 125 times greater than morphine. It is more lipid soluble and, therefore, has a rapid onset and short duration of action. Cardiovascular stability is maintained, but in high doses, fentanyl can cause bradycardia and chest wall rigidity. Respiratory depression is dose dependent, potentiated by other central nervous system depressants, and may last longer than analgesia. Fentanyl is widely administered in anesthesia for analgesia, induction, and supplementation of other agents. Fentanyl is administered for spinal and epidural as well as patient-controlled analgesia.

Alfentanil (Alfenta) is a potent opioid analgesic with a rapid onset and short duration of action. Small doses provide analgesia; larger doses provide induction and maintenance of anesthesia. Induction doses produce respiratory depression and hypotension secondary to vasodilation. Alfentanil is associated with more hypotension and bradycardia than is fentanyl or sufentanil.

Sufentanil (Sufenta) is also given for analgesia as well as induction and maintenance of anesthesia. This drug has 5 to 7 times the analgesia potency of fentanyl. Most pharmacologic effects are similar to those of fentanyl.

Opioid agonist-antagonists bind to MU receptors where they produce limited or no response. Additionally, they provide partial agonist action at delta and kappa receptors. Antagonist properties attenuate the efficacy of subsequently administered opioid agonists. Advantages of these drugs are their ability to pro-

TABLE 7–16. **OPIOID AGONIST, AGONIST-ANTAGONIST, ANTAGONIST**

DRUG	INDICATION	ONSET	DURATION	SIDE EFFECTS
Agonist				
Morphine	Analgesia Premedication	Immediate	2–7 hrs	Histamine release with hypotension, bronchospasm Nausea, vomiting Neonatal depression Bradycardia Urinary retention Biliary tract spasm Pruritus Chest wall rigidity
Meperidine (Demerol)	Premedication Analgesia	< 1 min	2–4 hrs	Cerebral irritation plus seizures with large doses Severe, fatal reactions with MAO inhibitors Aggravates adverse effects of isoniazid Biliary tract spasm Chest wall rigidity Pruritus Orthostatic hypotension
Fentanyl	Analgesia Anesthesia	30 sec	30–60 min	Hypotension, bradycardia Nausea, vomiting Delayed gastric emptying Biliary tract spasm Muscle rigidity Neonatal respiratory depression
Alfentanil	Analgesia Anesthesia	1–2 min	10–15 min	Bradycardia, hypotension Nausea, vomiting Biliary tract spasm Delayed gastric emptying
Agonist				
Sufentanil	Analgesia Anesthesia	Immediate	2–4 hrs	Hypotension, bradycardia Nausea, vomiting Delayed gastric emptying Muscle rigidity
Agonist/Antagonist				
Butorphanol tartrate (Stadol)	Analgesia	1–5 min	2–4 hrs	Hypertension, hypotension Hallucinations Nausea, vomiting Withdrawal in opioid-dependent patient
Nalbuphine (Nubain)	Analgesia Anesthesia	2–3 min	3–6 hrs	Hypertension, hypotension, tachycardia or bradycardia Dyspepsia Urinary urgency Pruritus Bronchospasm Withdrawal in opioid-dependent patient
Antagonist				
Naloxone (Narcan)	Reversal of narcotic	1–2 min	1–4 hrs	Tachycardia, hypertension, depression, hypotension, arrhythmia Pulmonary edema Reversal of analgesia Seizures Nausea, vomiting Sweating

duce analgesia with limited respiratory depression. They are sometimes used in the postanesthesia care unit to reverse respiratory depression of narcotics without eliminating analgesia (Bailey, 1987).

Butorphanol (Stadol) is a synthetic opioid agonist-antagonist with an analgesic potency 3.5 to 7 times that of morphine or 30 to 40 times that of meperidine. Analgesic doses increase blood pressure, pulmonary artery pressure, and cardiac output. Analgesia is not adequate for surgery.

Nalbuphine (Nubain) is also classified as an opioid agonist-antagonist. It is equal in potency as an analgesic to morphine and is one fourth as potent as nalorphine as an antagonist. Nalbuphine has been administered to reverse ventilatory depression following high-dose fentanyl anesthesia (Moldenhauer, 1985).

Minor changes in the structure of an opioid agonist can convert the drug into an antagonist at one or more receptor sites. *Naloxone* (Narcan) is such a drug. Narcan is a pure opioid antagonist with no agonist activity. By competitive inhibition at MU, delta, and kappa receptor sites, it prevents or reverses the effects of opioids and reverses respiratory depression, sedation, and hypotension (Longnecker, 1973; Kripke, 1976). Reversal of narcotic depression is achieved at IV, IM, or SC doses of 10 to 40 mcg/kg. This dose is repeated at 2- to 3-minute intervals until a maximum of 10 mg is given. The drug should be administered slowly at the lowest possible dose. Reversal of analgesia can be associated with increased activity of the sympathetic nervous system. Tachycardia, hypertension, cardiac arrhythmias, and pulmonary edema have been associated with naloxone (Axar, 1979; Flacke, 1977). Nausea and vomiting are related to the dose and speed of injection.

Neuromuscular Blocking Drugs

Neuromuscular blocking drugs interact at the myoneural junction and interfere with physiologic events in that area. Although they promote patient safety and optimize surgical conditions, they are not anesthetics. They produce no anesthesia effect but do cause paralysis of skeletal muscle. Indiscriminate use of these agents contributes to intraoperative awareness and recall under general anesthesia.

Neuromuscular blocking drugs or muscle relaxants are classified according to mechanism of action (depolarizing, nondepolarizing) and length of action (short, intermediate, long). Depolarizing agents such as succinylcholine consist of two molecules of acetylcholine, the normal neurotransmitter at the myoneural junction. The drug attaches to cholinergic receptors on skeletal muscle, causes sustained opening of transmembrane potentials and persistent depolarization, thus blocking action potentials and producing skeletal-muscle paralysis. Succinylcholine is hydrolyzed by plasma cholinesterase (pseudocholinesterase), and enzyme found in the liver. It has a rapid onset and short duration of action and is a short-acting muscle relaxant.

Nondepolarizing muscle relaxants bind to cholinergic receptors on skeletal muscle and prevent acetylcholine from activating sodium channels. Depolarization cannot occur, action potentials are not generated, and skeletal-muscle relaxation does occur. Diffusion of the relaxant away from the receptor or buildup of acetylcholine restores neuromuscular transmission. All relaxants today except succinylcholine are nondepolarizing drugs. As shown in Table 7-17, they are either intermediate-acting or long-acting drugs. Side effects associated with these drugs are often due to histamine release or stimulation of the autonomic nervous system.

Succinylcholine (Anectine, Quelicin), a short-acting depolarizing agent, has no effect on consciousness, pain, or smooth muscle. It increases intraocular (IOP), intragastric (IGP), and lower esophageal pressure (LEP) and may cause histamine release (Miller, 1977; Miller, 1968). Succinylcholine may stimulate adrenergic receptors, resulting in elevation of systemic blood pressure, heart rate, or cardiac muscarinic receptors leading to bradycardia. It is a trigger for malignant hyperthermia and may lead to life-threatening hyperkalemia in patients with severe burns, trauma, paraplegia, spinal cord injuries, or degenerative neuromuscular diseases (Cooperman, 1970; Kohlschutter, 1976). Prolonged respiratory paralysis may occur in patients with low plasma levels of pseudocholinesterase (severe liver disease, burns, cancer, pregnancy, atypical pseudocholinesterase) or when large doses are given over a prolonged period of time. The major advantage of succinylcholine is its rapid onset of action and short duration.

Mivacurium chloride (Mivacron) is a short-acting nondepolarizing muscle

TABLE 7–17. NEUROMUSCULAR BLOCKING DRUGS

TYPE	ONSET	DURATION	SIDE EFFECTS
Ultra-short Acting			
Succinylcholine	1 min	4–6 min	Hypertension, tachycardia, bradycardia, arrhythmia Hyperkalemia Increased intraocular pressure, intracranial pressure Increased intragastric pressure, increased lower esophageal sphincter pressure Muscle pain Phase II block Prolonged effect due to atypical pseudocholinesterase Trigger malignant hyperthermia
Intermediate Acting			
Mivacurium	2–3 min	6–10 min	Histamine release with vasodilation, hypotension, tachycardia, bradycardia Bronchospasm; laryngospasm Prolonged effect in patients with low plasma pseudocholinesterase
Atracurium	2–2.5 min	20–35 min	Slight histamine release with larger doses Bronchospasm
Vecuronium	2.5–3 min	25–40 min	No histamine release or significant hemodynamic changes
Rocuronium	60–90 sec	30–90 min	No significant hemodynamic changes
Long Acting			
d-Tubocurarine	3–5 min	30–40 min	Hypotension Tachycardia Bronchospasm Potentiation by inhalation agents and some antibiotics
Pancuronium	3–5 min	45–60 min	Hypertension Tachycardia
Metocurine	3–5 min	30–40 min	Weak histamine release
Pipecuronium	3 min	45–120 min	Histamine release rare No clinically significant hemodynamic effects
Doxacurium	4 min	30–160 min	Histamine release rare No clinically significant hemodynamic effects

relaxant. It is metabolized by plasma cholinesterase, and its duration of action is a third that of atracurium (Tracrium). Side effects are rare at recommended doses, but higher doses may be associated with elevation of plasma histamine, decreased blood pressure, and increased heart rate. Prolonged neuromuscular blockade may occur in patients with low plasma pseudocholinesterase (Savarese, 1988).

D-Tubocurarine chloride is an older long-acting nondepolarizing muscle relaxant. Hypotension associated with its use is due to autonomic ganglionic blockade and histamine release. Repeated doses may have a cumulative effect. Effects of D-tubocurarine are potentiated by volatile anesthetics and reversed by anticholinesterase drugs. Histamine-releasing properties suggest that the drug be given cautiously in patients with a history of bronchial asthma or allergy.

Metocurine iodide (Metubine) is similar to tubocurarine but it does not produce ganglionic blockade at autonomic ganglia and is less likely to cause histamine release. Repeated doses may be accompanied by cumulative effects (Savarese, 1977).

Atracurium besylate (Tracrium), vecuronium bromide (Norcuron), and rocuronium (Zemuron) are newer, intermediate-acting nondepolarizing muscle relaxants. Since atracurium undergoes rapid metabolism by Hoffman elimination and ester hydrolysis, repeated doses or continuous infusion have fewer cumulative effects than other muscle relaxants. Histamine release and hemodynamic changes are minimal when recommended doses are given slowly. Higher doses, rapidly administered, may cause histamine release with vasodilation, flushing, hypotension, tachycardia, or bronchospasm (Basta, 1982).

Vecuronium is similar to pancuronium but is one third more potent and has a shorter activity and more rapid recovery (Cronnelly, 1983; Fahey, 1987). The time to onset and duration of effect is increased with higher doses, but there is no histamine release and no clinically significant hemodynamic changes due to histamine (Basta, 1982).

Rocuronium (Zemuron) is similar to vecuronium, but it has a more rapid onset. It can be used for rapid sequence inductions in place of succinylcholine.

Pancuronium bromide (Pavulon) is a long-acting nondepolarizing neuromuscular blocking drug. Increased heart rate may result from vagolytic actions on the heart. Increased arterial blood pressure and cardiac output may occur owing to activation of the sympathetic nervous system and inhibition of catecholamine reuptake. Histamine release is rare.

Pipecuronium bromide (Arduan) and *doxacurium chloride* (Nuromax) are newer long-acting nondepolarizing muscle relaxants. Time of onset and duration of action of pipecuronium are similar to those of pancuronium (Pavulon) (Larijani, 1987). Doxacurium is 2.5 to 3 times more potent than pancuronium, but time to onset and duration are similar at comparable doses. Histamine release is rare with both drugs and there are no clinically significant hemodynamic effects (Basta, 1988).

Residual neuromuscular blockade associated with nondepolarizing muscle relaxants is generally reversed with anticholinesterase drugs (edrophonium, neostigmine, pyridostigmine) at the end of surgery. Anticholinesterase drugs inhibit acetylcholinesterase, the enzyme that metabolizes acetylcholine. This permits the accumulation of acetylcholine at the neuromuscular junction, which by mass action causes displacement of the nondepolarizing relaxant from receptors on skeletal muscle. Acetylcholine also stimulates muscarinic receptors on cardiac and smooth muscle and glands, causing bradycardia, bronchoconstriction, increased peristalsis, and secretions. These effects are prevented or attenuated by prior or simultaneous intravenous administration of an anticholinergic (atropine, glycopyrrolate).

Local Anesthetics

Local anesthetics block conduction in nerves by impairing propagation of the action potential in axons. These drugs act at specific receptor sites in the nerve membrane and inhibit passage of sodium ions through ion-selective sodium channels (Butterworth, 1990). Threshold potential is not reached, and the nerve impulse or action potential is not propagated. Conduction block in peripheral nerves progresses in the following order: peripheral vasodilation, skin temperature elevation, loss of pain and temperature sensation, loss of proprioception, loss of touch and pressure sensation, and motor paralysis.

Local anesthetics are subdivided into two classes: aminoesters and aminoamides. Examples of aminoesters are 2-chloroprocaine, procaine, and tetracaine. They are cleared from the plasma by plasma and liver cholinesterase. Aminoamides include lidocaine, prilocaine, mepivacaine, bupivacaine, and etidocaine. Aminoamides are cleared by hepatic metabolism.

The amount of local anesthetic that reaches a nerve depends on the proximity of injection to the nerve. The rapidity and extent of diffusion depends on the concentration of local anesthetic injected and its lipid solubility. Systemic absorption influences the amount of local anesthetic remaining at the injection site and the duration of anesthesia. The addition of epinephrine to the local anesthetic mixture slows systemic absorption of the drug and prolongs its anesthetic effect. Epinephrine also increases the intensity of the block and reduces surgical bleeding.

The principal side effects related to local anesthetics are allergic reactions and systemic toxicity. Allergic reactions are rare but when they occur can be life-threatening. Aminoesters are more allergenic than aminoamides because of the metabolite para-aminobenzoic acid (PABA). Parabens are present in multidose local anesthetic solutions, and the patient previously exposed to parabens may be sensitized and develop an allergic reaction unrelated to the local anesthetic. Local reactions may include erythema, urticaria, edema, and dermatitis. Systemic reactions include generalized erythema, urticaria, edema, bronchoconstriction, and hypotension. Treatment is symptomatic and supportive. Cutaneous reactions may respond to diphenhydramine (Benadryl 0.2 to 0.5 mg/kg IV), and more severe reactions may require a systemic glucocorticoid such as methylprednisolone (Solu-Medrol). Bronchoconstriction is treated with epinephrine 0.3 mg subcutaneously, and hypotension is managed with fluids and vasopressor (phenylephrine) or inotropic (dopamine) drugs.

Systemic toxicity of a local anesthetic is due to an excess plasma concentration of the drug. Determinants of local anesthetic blood levels include total dose of local anesthetic, vascularity of the injection site, addition of vasoconstrictors to the solution, local tissue binding, and tissue perfusion. Systemic absorption is greatest following injection for intercostal nerve block, intermediate for epidural block, and least for brachial plexus block (Covino, 1976). Addition of epinephrine reduces systemic absorption by one third. The most common mechanism for excessive plasma concentration of local anesthetic is accidental intravascular injection.

Systemic toxicity of local anesthetics involves the central nervous system and the cardiovascular system. Central nervous system manifestations of toxicity include numbness of tongue, lightheadedness, visual disturbances, muscular twitching, seizures, and coma. Central nervous system toxicity is increased by hypercarbia and decreased by barbiturates, benzodiazepines, and inhaled anesthetics. Cardiovascular system toxicity can produce decreased myocardial contractility, vasodilation, and dysrhythmias. Cardiovascular toxicity of local anesthetics is increased by acidosis, hypoxia, pregnancy, and hyperkalemia.

A small test dose of the local anesthetic with 15 mcg of epinephrine is often given in an attempt to detect intravascular injection. Intravascular injection can be detected by a 20% increase in heart rate associated with the test dose. Severe systemic toxicity is treated with oxygen. Seizures are controlled with diazepam 0.1 to 0.3 mg/kg, thiopental 0.5 to 2 mg/kg, or succinylcholine 0.2 to 0.5 mg/kg. Cardiovascular instability is treated with antiarrhythmics, inotropes, or vasopressors.

As illustrated in Table 7–18, regional anesthesia is classified according to site of placement of local anesthetic. Choice of local anesthetic depends on the anticipated duration of surgery, regional technique selected, surgical needs, and potential for systemic toxicity.

DOCUMENTATION

The anesthesia process is not complete without proper documentation. Documentation reflects the standards of practice and includes all anesthetic interventions and patient responses. Accurate recording facilitates comprehensive patient care, provides information for retrospective review and research data, and establishes a medical-legal record. The format for anesthesia documentation is facility specific.

EMERGENCE/POSTANESTHESIA CARE

At the end of the procedure, the patient's status is assessed, and a determination is made as to the safety of transferring responsibility of care to other qualified individuals. All essential information regarding the patient's condition is reported to those assuming responsibility for the care of the patient. Evaluation of anes-

TABLE 7-18. **LOCAL ANESTHETICS**

AGENT	CONCENTRATION (%)	USUAL ONSET	USUAL DURATION (h)	MAXIMUM SINGLE DOSE (mg)	MISCELLANEOUS
Procaine	0.5-1	Fast	0.5-1.0	1000	
Chloroprocaine	0.5-1	Fast	0.5-1.0	1000	Lowest systemic toxicity
Lidocaine	0.5-1	Fast	1-2	500	
Mepivacaine	0.5-1	Fast	.5-3	500	
Bupivacaine	0.25-0.5	Slow	4-12	200	Exaggerated cardiotoxicity with IV injection
PERIPHERAL NERVE BLOCK					
Chloroprocaine	2-3	Fast	.5-1	1000 + epi	
Procaine	1-2	Slow	.5-1	1000	
Lidocaine	1-2	Fast	1-3	500 + epi	
Prilocaine	1.5-2	Fast	1.5-3	600	Methemoglobinemia possible over 600 mg
Mepivacaine	1-2	Fast	2-3	500 + epi	
Bupivacaine	0.25-0.5	Slow	4-12	200 + epi	
Etidocaine	.5-1.0	Fast	3-12	300 + epi	
IV REGIONAL ANESTHESIA					
Lidocaine	0.25-.5			500	
Prilocaine	0.25-.5			600	Least toxic amide
SPINAL ANESTHESIA					
Procaine	10	Moderate	.5-1.0	200	
Tetracaine	0.5	Fast	2-4	20	
Lidocaine	5	Fast	0.5-1.5	100	
Bupivacaine	0.5-0.75	Fast	2-4	20	
EPIDURAL ANESTHESIA					
Chloroprocaine	2-3	Fast	0.5-1.5	1000 + epi	
Lidocaine	1-2	Fast	1-2	500 + epi	
Prilocaine	1-3	Fast	1-2.5	600	
Mepivacaine	1-2	Fast	1.0-2.5	500 + epi	
Bupivacaine	0.25-0.75	Moderate	2-4	200 + epi	
Etidocaine	1-1.5	Fast	2-4	300 + epi	

epi = epinephrine

thesia outcomes is made through postoperative interviews. This is often done by telephone in outpatient surgical facilities.

SAFETY PRECAUTIONS

Anesthesia care consists of appropriate safety precautions for patients and health care providers. Safety precautions and controls as established within the institution should be adhered to in order to minimize the hazards of electricity, fire, and explosion in areas where anesthesia is provided. All equipment should be checked, and the anesthesia machine should be maintained and checked according to guidelines. Occupational exposure to waste anesthetic gases is of concern to all who work in an operating room environment.

Epidemiologic surveys over the last few decades have suggested that chronic exposure to anesthetic waste gases may lead to reproductive hazards or neurologic toxicity. Although these studies did not prove a cause-and-effect relationship, they led to practice changes in the operating room. Equipment maintenance programs, monitoring for gas leaks, changes in anesthetic practices, and scavenging of waste anesthetic gases are now universally practiced. These efforts have resulted in a 10-fold reduction in exposure to waste anesthetic gases when compared with levels present years ago. Routine scavenging and control measures to keep concentrations of nitrous oxide below 25 ppm and concentrations of halogenated agents below 5 ppm are recommended by the National Institute of Occupational Safety and Health (Brodsky, 1992).

Malignant Hyperthermia

Malignant hyperthermia (MH) is a life-threatening disorder of skeletal muscle believed to be due to decreased calcium reuptake by the sarcoplasmic reticulum with increased resting intracellular calcium levels. It is a pharmacogenetic disorder, which very often is initiated by a pharmacologic trigger in a patient with genetic susceptibility (Gronert, 1980). Approximately 50% of children of MH-susceptible parents are potentially at risk. The incidence of MH is estimated to be 1 : 15,000 in children and 1 : 50,000 in adults. At one time the mortality was 70% but this has now decreased to 10% with early recognition and treatment with dantrolene.

Classic MH most often occurs in the operating room, but it can also occur within a few hours in recovery. Succinylcholine may accelerate the onset, but in some cases a volatile anesthetic plus succinylcholine is necessary to trigger the response. Some patients have multiple exposures to triggering agents before they develop MH.

Typical manifestations of this syndrome include hypercarbia, tachycardia, tachypnea, hyperthermia, hypertension, cardiac dysrhythmias, acidosis, hypoxemia, hyperkalemia, skeletal-muscle rigidity, and myoglobinuria. Management includes discontinuation of all inhalation agents and changing of anesthesia circuit and soda lime; hyperventilation of the lungs with 100% O_2; administration of sodium bicarbonate 1 to 2 mEq/kg with additional doses guided by frequent monitoring of arterial blood gases; administration of dantrolene 2.5 mg/kg up to 10 mg/kg; surface, nasogastric, intravenous, wound, and rectal cooling; treatment of ventricular arrhythmias; maintenance of urinary output; and monitoring of arterial blood gases, electrolytes, and coagulation. The patient should be observed for disseminated intravascular coagulopathy and monitored in the intensive care unit for 24 hours.

Patients known to be susceptible to MH should receive dantrolene 2.5 mg/kg IV 15 to 30 minutes before induction of anesthesia. This drug inhibits the release of calcium from the sarcoplasmic reticulum and prevents, attenuates, or reverses the metabolic and biochemical changes associated with MH crisis. A vapor-free anesthesia machine and full minimal monitoring, inclusive of temperature and capnography, should be used. Nontriggering anesthetics should be given. Known triggers are volatile anesthetics and succinylcholine. Safe drugs include nitrous oxide, barbiturates, opioids, benzodiazepines, amide and ester local anesthetics, and nondepolarizing muscle relaxants.

Issues for Future Development

Advances in the pharmacologic and technologic aspects of anesthesia practice will continue to be implemented in the care of patients. The challenge for the perioperative nurse is to stay current with the pharmacologic agents used, their action, and any adverse reactions. In addition, as the acuity of the surgical patient cared for in all settings increases and as the use of invasive monitoring increases, the perioperative nurse needs to learn how to interpret the results of this monitoring along with basic electrocardiogram interpretation.

Summary

Anesthesia is a complex process that includes an art and a science. A topic of enormous breadth is briefly summarized in this chapter. Components of anesthesia, an overview of commonly used anesthetic drugs, standards of practice, and severe complications have been reviewed. Tremendous advances have taken place in the field since 1846 when Morton demonstrated the use of ether, and new agents and technology are expected to be introduced. The ever changing nature of this specialty mandates a commitment to lifelong education by the anesthetist and the anesthesiologist. Patients benefit when each member of the operating room team has an appreciation for all practitioners' goals and concerns. Collaboration and team spirit are essential components for optimal patient outcomes.

REFERENCES

Axar, I, Turndorf, H. (1979). Severe hypertension and multiple atrial premature contractions following naloxone administration. *Anesthesia & Analgesia, 58,* 524–525.

Bailey, P. L., et al. (1987). Antagonism of postoperative opioid-induced respiratory depression: nalbuphine versus naloxone. *Anesthesia & Analgesia, 66,* 1109–1114.

Baraka, A., Harrison, T., Kachachi, T. (1973). Catecholamine levels after ketamine anesthesia in man. *Anesthesia & Analgesia, 52,* 198–200.

Basta, S. J., et al. (1988a). Clinical pharmacology of doxacurium chloride: a new long-acting nondepolarizing muscle relaxant. *Anesthesiology, 69,* 478–486.

Basta, S. J., et al. (1988b). Vecuronium does not alter serum histamine within the clinical dose range. *Anesthesiology, 59,* A273.

Basta, S. J., et al. (1982). Clinical pharmacology of atracurium besylate; a new nondepolarizing muscle relaxant. *Anesthesia & Analgesia, 61,* 723–729.

Becker, K. E., Tonnesen, A. S. (1978). Cardiovascular effects of plasma levels of thiopental necessary for anesthesia. *Anesthesiology, 49,* 198–208.

Benumof, J. L. (1991). Management of the difficult adult airway. *Anesthesiology, 75,* 1087–1110.

Benumof, J. L., Scheller, M. S. (1989). The importance of transtracheal jet ventilation in the management of the difficult airway. *Anesthesiology, 71,* 769–778.

Blitt, C. D., et al. (1970). 'Silent' regurgitation and aspiration during general anesthesia. *Anesthesia & Analgesia, 49,* 707–713.

Borgeat, A., et al. (1992). Subhypnotic doses of propofol possess direct antiemetic properties. *Anesthesia & Analgesia, 74,* 539–541.

Brodsky, J. B., Maze, M. (1992). Injury to the anesthetist. In: Benumof, J. L., Saidman, L. J., eds. *Anesthesia and Perioperative Complications.* St. Louis: Mosby-Year Book. (pp. 572–575).

Brown, S. S., Lyons, S. M., Dundee, J. W. (1968). Intra-arterial barbiturates: a study of some factors leading to intravascular thrombosis. *British Journal of Anesthesia, 40,* 13–19.

Burn, J. H. (1960). Why thiopentone injected into an artery may cause gangrene. *British Medical Journal, 2,* 414–416.

Butterworth, J. F., Strichartz, G. R. (1990). Molecular mechanism of local anesthesia: a review. *Anesthesiology, 72,* 722–734.

Caldwell, C. B., Gross, J. B. (1982). Physostigmine reversal of midazolam-induced sedation. *Anesthesiology, 57,* 125–127.

Caplan, R. A., et al. (1980). Adverse respiratory events in anesthesia: a closed claims analysis. *Anesthesiology, 72,* 828–833.

Carlsson, C., Islander, G. (1981). Silent gastropharyngeal regurgitation during anesthesia. *Anesthesia & Analgesia, 60,* 655–657.

Cohen, S., Harris, L. D. (1971). Does hiatus hernia affect competence of the gastroesophageal sphincter? *New England Journal of Medicine, 284,* 1053–1056.

Cooper, J. B., Newbourn, R. S., Kitz, R. J. (1984). An analysis of major errors in equipment failures in anesthesia management: considerations for prevention and detection. *Anesthesiology, 60,* 34–42.

Cooper, J. B., et al. (1978). Preventable anesthesia mishaps. *Anesthesiology, 49,* 399–406.

Cooperman, L. H., Strobel, G. E., Kennell, E. M. (1970). Massive hyperkalemia after administration of succinylcholine. *Anesthesiology, 32,* 161–164.

Cote, C. J., Goldstein, A. E., Coté, M. A. (1988). A single-blind study of pulse oximetry in children. *Anesthesiology, 68,* 184–188.

Cote, C. J., et al. (1982). Assessment of risk factors related to the acid aspiration syndrome in pediatric patients: gastric pH and residual volume. *Anesthesiology, 56,* 70–72.

Cotton, B. R., Smith, G. (1981). Single and combined effects of atropine and metoclopramide on the lower esophageal sphincter pressure. *British Journal of Anaesthesia, 53,* 869–874.

Covino, B. G., Vassallo, H. L. (1976). *Local anesthetics: mechanisms of actions and clinical uses.* New York: Grune and Stratton.

Cronnelly, R., et al. (1983). Pharmacokinetics and pharmacodynamics of vecuronium and pancuronium in anesthetized humans. *Anesthesiology, 48*, 405–408.

DeFriez, C. B., Wong, H. C. (1992). Seizures and opisthotonos after propofol anesthesia. *Anesthesia & Analgesia, 30*, 630–632.

Eichhorn, J. G., et al. (1986). Standards for patient monitoring during anesthesia at Harvard Medical School. *JAMA, 256*, 1017–1020.

Etter, M. S., Helrich, M., Mackenzie, C. F. (1980). Immunoglobulin E fluctuations in thiopental anaphylaxis. *Anesthesiology, 52*, 181–183.

Fahey, M. R., et al. (1987). Clinical pharmacology of atracurium besylate: a new depolarizing muscle relaxant. *Anesthesiology, 55*, 6–11.

Fine, J., Firestone, S. C. (1973). Sensory disturbances following ketamine anesthesia: recurrent hallucinations. *Anesthesia & Analgesia, 52*, 428–430.

Flacke, J. W., Flacke, W. E., Williams, G. P. (1977). Acute pulmonary edema following naloxone reversal of high-dose morphine anesthesia. *Anesthesiology, 47*, 376–378.

Follette, J. W., Farley, W. J. (1992). Anesthesiologist addicted to propofol. *Anesthesiology, 77*, 817–818.

Frager, R. J., et al. (1984). Effects of etomidate on hormonal responses to surgical stress. *Anesthesiology, 61*, 652–656.

Frager, R. J., Caldwell, N. (1976). Lorazepam premedication: lack of recall and relief of anxiety. *Anesthesia & Analgesia, 55*, 792–796.

Gamble, JA, et al. (1981). Evaluation of midazolam as an intravenous induction agent. *Anesthesia, 36*, 868–873.

Gehan, G, et al. (1991). Optimal dose of lignocaine for preventing pain on injection of propofol. *British Journal of Anaesthesia, 66*, 206–210.

Gibbs, CP, et al. (1979). Antacid pulmonary aspiration in the dog. *Anesthesiology, 51*, 380–385.

Gronert, GA. (1980). Malignant hyperthermia. *Anesthesiology, 53*, 395–423.

Guedel, AE. (1937). *Inhalation Anesthesia, a Fundamental Guide.* New York: Macmillan Publishing Co.

Hall, C. C. (1940). Aspiration pneumonitis: an obstetric hazard. *JAMA, 114*, 728–733.

Helman, J. D., et al. (1992). A comparison of desflurane and sufentanil in patients undergoing coronary artery surgery. *Anesthesiology, 77*, 47–62.

Hester, J. B., Heath, M. L. (1977). Pulmonary acid aspiration syndrome: should prophylaxis be routine? *British Journal of Anaesthesia, 49*, 595–599.

Hirshman, C. A., et al. (1985). Thiobarbiturate-induced histamine release in human skin mast cell. *Anesthesiology, 63*, 353–356.

Hirshman, C. A., et al. (1979). Ketamine block of bronchospasm in experimental canine asthma. *British Journal of Anaesthesia, 51*, 713–718.

Holdcroft, A., et al. (1976). Effect of dose and premedication on induction complications with etomidate. *British Journal of Anaesthesia, 48*, 199–205.

Homer, T. D., Stanski, D.R. (1985). The effect of increasing age on thiopental disposition and anesthetic requirements. *Anesthesiology, 62*, 714–724.

Hudson, R. J., Stanski, D. R., Burch, P. G. (1983). Pharmacokinetics of methohexital and thiopental in surgical patients. *Anesthesiology, 59*, 215–219.

Jensen, S., Schou-Olesen, Huttel, M. S. (1982). Use of midazolam as an induction agent: comparison with thiopental. *British Journal of Anesthesia, 54*, 605–607.

Kallar, S. K., Everett, L. L. (1993). Potential risks and preventive measures for pulmonary aspiration: new concepts in preoperative fasting guidelines. *Anesthesia & Analgesia, 77*, 171–182.

Kaukinen, S., Kataja, J. Kaukinen, L. (1990). Antagonism of benzodiazepine–fentanyl anesthesia with flumazenil. *Canadian Journal of Anaesthesia, 37*, 40–45.

Kent, E. A., et al. (1992). Sexual illusions and propofol sedation. *Anesthesiology, 77*, 1037–1038.

King, S. Y., et al. (1992). Lidocaine for the prevention of pain due to injection of propofol. *Anesthesia & Analgesia, 74*, 246–249.

Kohlschutter, B., Bauer, H., Roth, F. (1976). Suxamethonium-induced hyperkalemia in patients with severe intra-abdominal infections. *British Journal of Anesthesia, 48*, 557–562.

Kripke, B. J., et al. (1976). Naloxone antagonism after narcotic supplemented anesthesia. *Anesthesia & Analgesia, 55*, 800–805.

Larijani, G. E., et al. (1987). Vecuronium does not alter serum histamine within the clinical dose range. *Anesthesia & Analgesia, 68*, 734–759.

Laughlin, T. P., Newberry, L. A. (1985). Prolonged myoclonus after etomidate anesthesia. *Anesthesia & Analgesia, 64*, 80–82.

Laxenaire, M. C., et al. (1992). Life-threatening anaphylactoid reactions to propofol (Diprivan). *Anesthesiology, 77*, 275–280.

Leon-Casasola, O., Weiss, A., Lema, M. J. (1992). Anaphylaxis due to propofol. *Anesthesiology, 77*, 275–280.

Longnecker, D.E., Grazis, P. A., Eggers, G. W. N. (1973). Naloxone for antagonism of morphine-induced respiratory depression. *Anesthesia & Analgesia, 52*, 447–453.

Maile, C. J. D., Francis, R. N. (1983). Preoperative ranitidine: effect of a single intravenous dose on pH and volume of gastric aspirate. *Anesthesiology, 38*, 324–326.

Manchikanti, L., Roush, J. R. (1984a). Effect of preanesthetic glycopyrrolate and cimetidine on gastric fluid pH and volume in outpatients. *Anesthesia & Analgesia, 63*, 40–46.

Manchikanti, L., Marrero, T. C., Roush, J. R. (1984b). Preanesthetic cimetidine and metoclopramide for acid aspiration prophylaxis in elective surgery. *Anesthesiology, 61*, 48–54.

Martin, T. M., Nicolson, S., Burgas, M. S. (1993). Propofol anesthesia reduces emesis and airway obstruction in pediatric outpatients. *Anesthesia & Analgesia, 76*, 144–148.

Mazze, R. I., Calverley, R. K., Smith, N. T. (1977). Inorganic fluoride nephrotoxicity: prolonged enflurane and halothane anesthesia in volunteers. *Anesthesiology*, *46*, 265–271.

Mazze, R. I., Cousins, M. J., Barr, G. A. (1974). Renal effects and metabolism of isoflurane in man. *Anesthesiology*, *40*, 536–540.

McGrady, E. M., MacDonald, A. G. (1988). Effect of preoperative administration of water on gastric volume and pH. *British Journal of Anaesthesia*, *60*, 803–805.

Mendelson, C. L. (1946). The aspiration of stomach contents into the lungs during obstetric anesthesia. *American Journal of Obstetrics and Gynecology*, *52*, 191–205.

Merkel, G., Eger, E. I. (1963). A comparative study of halothane and halopropane anesthesia, including method for determining equipotency. *Anesthesiology*, *24*, 346–350.

Miller, M., Wishart, N. Y., Nimmo, W. (1983). Gastric contents at induction of anesthesia: is a 4-hour fast necessary? *British Journal of Anaesthesia*, *55*, 1185–1188.

Miller, R. D., Way, W. L. (1977). Inhibition of succinylcholine-induced increased intragastric pressure by nondepolarizing muscle relaxants and lidocaine. *Anesthesiology*, *34*, 185–188.

Miller, R. D., Way, W. L., Hickey, R. L. (1968). Inhibition of succinylcholine-induced increased intraocular pressure by nondepolarizing muscle relaxants. *Anesthesiology*, *29*, 123–126.

Mohler, H., Okada, T. (1977). Benzodiazepine receptor: demonstration of the central nervous system. *Science*, *198*, 849–851.

Mohler, H., Richards, J. G. (1988). The benzodiazepine receptor: a pharmacological control element of brain function. *European Journal of Anaesthesiology*, *2*, 15–24.

Moldenhauer, C. C., et al. (1985). Nalbuphine antagonism of ventilatory depression following high-dose fentanyl anesthesia. *Anesthesiology*, *62*, 637–640.

Mora, C. T., Torgman, M., White, P. F. (1989). Effects of diazepam and flumazenil on sedation and hypoxic ventilating response. *Anesthesia & Analgesia*, *68*, 473–478.

Morgan, M. (1984). Control of intragastric pH and volume. *British Journal of Anaesthesia*, *56*, 47–57.

Muzi, M., et al. (1992). Venodilation contributes to propofol-mediated hypotension in humans. *Anesthesia & Analgesia*, *74*, 877–883.

Nussmeier, N. A., Arlund, C., Slogoff, S. (1986). Neuropsychiatric complications after cardiopulmonary bypass: cerebral protection by a barbiturate. *Anaesthesiology*, *64*, 165–170.

Olsson, G. I., Hallen, B., Hambraeus, J. K. (1986). Aspiration during anesthesia: a computer-aided study of 185,358 anesthestics. *Acta Anaesthesiologica Scandinavica*, *30*, 84–92.

Ong, B. Y., Palahniuk, R. J., Cumming, M. (1978). Gastric volume and pH in outpatients. *Canadian Anesthetists Society Journal*, *25*, 36–39.

Owen, H., Spence, A. A. (1984). Etomidate. *British Journal of Anaesthesia*, *56*, 555–557.

Prys-Roberts, C. (1987). Anaesthesia: a practical or impossible construct. *British Journal of Anaesthesia*, *59*, 1341–1346.

Reeves, J. G., et al (1985). Midazolam pharmacology and uses. *Anesthesiology*, *63*, 310–324.

Reich, D. L., Silvay, G. (1989). Ketamine: an update on the first twenty-five years of clinical experience. *Canadian Journal of Anaesthesia*, *36*, 186–187.

Roberts, R. B., Shirley, M. A. (1974). Reducing the risk of acid aspiration during cesarean section. *Anesthesia & Analgesia*, *53*, 859–868.

Saidman, L. J., Eger, E. I. (1964). Effect of nitrous oxide and of narcotic premedication on the alveolar concentration of halothane required for anesthesia. *Anesthesiology*, *25*, 302–304.

Salmenpera, M., Korttila, K., Kilma, T. (1980). Reduction of the risk of acid pulmonary aspiration in anesthetized patients after cimetidine premedication. *Acta Anaesthesiologica Scandinavica*, *24*, 25–30.

Savarese, J. J., et al. (1988). The clinical neuromuscular pharmacology of mivacurium chloride: a short-acting nondepolarizing ester neuromuscular blocking drug. *Anesthesiology*, *32*, 161–164.

Savarese, J. J., Ali, H. H., Antonio, R. P. (1977). The clinical pharmacology of metocurine: dimethyl tubocurarine revisited. *Anesthesiology*, *47*, 277–284.

Scott, D. B., et al. (1972). Factors affecting plasma levels of lignocaine and prilocaine. *British Journal of Anaesthesia*, *44*, 1040–1049.

Sebel, P. S., Lowdon, J. D. (1989). Propofol: a new intravenous anesthetic. *Anesthesiology*, *71*, 260–277.

Shevde, K., Trivedi, N. (1991). Effects of clear liquids on gastric volume and pH in healthy volunteers. *Anesthesia & Analgesia*, *72*, 528–531.

Smith, T. C., Wollman, H. (1985). History and principles of anesthesiology. In: Goodman, A. G., Gillman, L. S., eds. *The Pharmacological Basis of Therapeutics*. 7th ed. New York: Macmillan Publishing Co. (pp. 260–262).

Spivey, W. H. (1992). Flumazenil and seizures: analysis of 43 cases. *Clinical Therapeutics*, *14*, 292–305.

Sutton, T. S., et al. (1991). Fluoride metabolites after prolonged exposure of volunteers and patients to desflurane. *Anesthesia & Analgesia*, *73*, 180–185.

Takeshita, H., Okuda, Y., Sari, A. (1972). The effects of ketamine on cerebral circulation and metabolism in man. *Anesthesiology*, *36*, 69–75.

Teabeaut, J. R. (1952). Aspiration of gastric contents: an experimental study. *American Journal of Pathology*, *28*, 51–62.

Vaughan, R. W., Bauer, S., Wise, L. (1975). Volume and pH of gastric juice in obese patients. *Anesthesiology*, *43*, 686–689.

Vaught, J. L., Rothman, B. B., Westfall, T. C. (1982). Mu and delta receptors: Their role in analgesia and in the differential effects of opioid peptides on analgesia. *Life Science*, *30*, 1443–1455.

Wagner, R. L., et al. (1984). Inhibition of adrenal steroidogenesis by the anesthetic etomidate. *New England Journal of Medicine*, *310*, 1415–1421.

Wangler, M. A., Kilpatrick, D. S. (1985). Aminophylline is an antagonist of lorazepam. *Anesthesia & Analgesia, 64,* 834–836.

Weber, L., Hirschman, C. A. (1979). Cimetidine for prophylaxis of aspiration pneumonitis: comparison of intramuscular or oral dosage schedules. *Anesthesia & Analgesia, 58,* 426–427.

Weir, P. M., et al. (1993). Propofol infusion and the incidence of emesis in pediatric outpatient strabismus surgery. *Anesthesia & Analgesia, 76,* 760–764.

White, P. F., et al. (1989). Benzodiazepine antagonism does not provoke a stress response. *Anesthesiology, 70,* 636–639.

White, P. F., et al. (1982). Ketamine: its pharmacology and therapeutic uses. *Anesthesiology, 56,* 119–136.

Whitman, J. G. (1990). Resedation. *Acta Anesthesiologica Scandinavica, 92,* 70–74.

Practice Scenario 1
Anesthesia and Perioperative Nursing

by Martha March, RN, BSN

Susan Sink is admitted to the ambulatory surgical center for arthroscopy of the left knee. The patient is 5 feet 6 inches tall, weighs 130 pounds, and has had no previous hospitalizations or surgical procedures. She is single and lives with a roommate. The patient has no allergies and takes no prescription drugs. The patient has taken aspirin 4 times a day for 4 months, as prescribed by her physician. There is no family history of chronic or debilitating diseases. The patient has requested to be fully alert during the procedure. She has stated that she does not want spinal anesthesia. The surgeon has agreed to do the procedure with a knee block, which he will perform. The nurse will be responsible for monitoring the patient during the procedure and for administering intravenous sedation.

PERIOPERATIVE INTERPRETATION

Based upon what you have just learned in this chapter, as an experienced perioperative nurse, you would consider the following in the care of this patient.

1. Assessment
   - Based on your knowledge of this procedure and the surgeon's technique, a supine position with both knees flexed will be used. The right knee poses a problem for proper alignment. Special attention should be given to the nonoperative knee.
   - Since the patient prefers to be awake, extra comfort measures should be considered, including maintaining a quiet environment and preserving the patient's privacy.
   - Knowing that local anesthetics and sedatives will be used during the procedure, the nurse should be aware of the expected reactions, maximum doses, adverse reactions, and any special nursing considerations with their use.
   - The use of aspirin for an extended period could interfere with the normal blood coagulation.
   - Since the circulating nurse will be responsible

for monitoring the patient during the procedure, additional help will be needed during the procedure to allow the nurse to stay with the patient.

NURSING DIAGNOSES

High risk for anxiety related to awareness of surroundings during local anesthesia

High risk for hemorrhage related to prolonged use of aspirin

High risk for injury related to positioning and manipulation during surgery

2. Planning
   - Procure padding and positioning aids before the patient enters the operating room to allow the nurse to remain with the patient during induction and positioning.
   - Check with the surgeon regarding the desired local anesthetics and the intravenous sedative that will be used. Review the dosage and side effects before administration.
   - Review the preoperative laboratory results, including clotting time. Report to the surgeon any abnormal results and the prolonged use of aspirin.
   - Plan measures to reduce traffic through the room during the procedure and inform the scrub person that the patient will be awake during the procedure. Introduce the patient to the members of the surgical team when the patient enters the room.
   - Inform the charge nurse of the need for additional personnel, preferably a second registered nurse, to participate in circulating nurse responsibilities so the assigned nurse can stay with the patient and monitor vital signs.

3. Implementation
   - Position the patient on the operating room bed before the knee block is administered to allow the patient to verbalize any areas of discomfort.
   - Check the peripheral pulses in the lower ex-

tremities before positioning the patient and again after positioning to insure adequate perfusion of distal tissues.

- Start the patient's intravenous line, with the fluids ordered by the surgeon, using aseptic technique and personal protective equipment, such as goggles.
- Assess the patient's vital signs and oxygen saturation level before the administration of the local anesthetics and sedatives to establish a base line. During the procedure, monitor the vital signs and oxygen saturation level at least every 15 minutes. Report to the surgeon any abnormal readings or adverse patient reactions during the procedure.
- Provide oxygen therapy as ordered by the surgeon or as the patient's condition requires.
- Monitor traffic in and through the operating room to preserve the patient's privacy and afford a quiet environment for the patient during the procedure.
- Document on the intraoperative record the patient's vital signs and oxygen saturation level; the type, dose, and amount of local anesthetics and sedatives administered; and the observed patient outcomes.

4. Evaluation
- Observe for signs and symptoms of anesthesia-induced central nervous system (CNS) toxicity: tinnitus, lightheadedness, confusion, circumoral numbness, convulsions, unconsciousness, generalized CNS depression, and respiratory arrest.
- Assess the patient for any bruises or reddened areas due to the surgical position.
- Assess the peripheral pulses of the lower extremities at the conclusion of the surgery to compare with the preoperative base line.
- Communicate to the postoperative nurse the surgical procedure, the local anesthetics and sedatives used, and the patient's current vital signs and oxygen saturation level.

Practice Scenario 2
Anesthesia and Perioperative Nursing

by Willa Abbott, RN, BSN

John Deck, age 32, is admitted to the operating room for a lumbar laminectomy. He currently has a definite weakness in the left leg and has started to walk with a slight limp. The patient is 6 feet 6 inches tall and weighs 230 pounds. The patient has had no previous hospitalizations and no previous surgical procedures. Mr. Deck is married and lives with his wife and two children who are 3 and 6 years old. The patient has no allergies and takes no prescription drugs. The patient takes Advil 2 to 3 times a day for pain. The patient recalls that a younger brother's tonsillectomy was canceled and rescheduled for a later day. He does not recall the reason, but thought that it was because of a "high fever."

PERIOPERATIVE INTERPRETATION

Based on what you have just learned in this chapter, as an experienced perioperative nurse, you would consider the following in the care of this patient.

1. Assessment
   - Based on your knowledge of this procedure and the surgeon's technique, a prone position will be used.
   - The patient's height poses a potential problem for proper body alignment. Special attention should be given to the potential for the patient's feet to dangle off the operating room bed resulting in further injury to the feet.
   - Using your knowledge of the anatomic structures, the respiratory system has the potential for airway problems owing to the prone position.
   - Based on the memory of the patient regarding his brother's surgery being cancelled for a "high fever," explore the possibility of malignant hyperthermia in this patient. This surgery cannot be delayed for the proper muscle biopsy owing to the possible nerve damage from the herniated disc and definite weakness in the left leg.

NURSING DIAGNOSES

Decreased respiratory excursion related to the surgical position

High risk for injury related to surgical position and patient's body size

High risk for malignant hyperthermia related to possible family history

2. Planning
   - Evaluate the patient's memory regarding the events of his brother's surgery for family history of malignant hyperthermia. Review the protocol for malignant hyperthermia.
   - Discuss with the surgeon and anesthesiologist the possibility of malignant hyperthermia. Anesthetic agents other than those that trigger the syndrome should be used.
   - Procure the necessary supplies to treat malignant hyperthermia should it develop (at least 36 vials of dantrolene, ice, temperature monitoring and cooling devices) and refrigerate at least 3,000 ml of desired intravenous solution. Alert the charge nurse that additional personnel may be needed in the event malignant hyperthermia occurs.
   - Procure all the needed positioning aids including head support, two armboards, chest rolls, pillows, footboard, and blankets.
   - Arrange for additional assistance to turn the patient from the stretcher to the operating room bed after induction of anesthesia.

3. Implementation
   - Since the patient will be anesthetized on the stretcher, be sure that the stretcher is locked. Stand next to the patient during induction to assist the anesthesiologist and comfort the patient.
   - Use at least 4 people to log-roll the patient from the stretcher to the OR bed.
   - Have the positioning aids readily available when

the patient is placed on the OR bed to facilitate the positioning process.

- Coordinate with the anesthesiologist the temperature monitoring devices used and insert and secure the probes.
- Assess the patient's peripheral pulses before and after positioning to insure distal tissue perfusion.
- Keep stretcher immediately available during the surgical procedure to facilitate returning the patient to the supine position for extubation or in case of cardiac arrest or development of malignant hyperthermia.
- Monitor the patient's body temperature continually in conjunction with the end tidal CO_2 level.
- Document on the intraoperative record the position and aids used, temperature monitoring interventions, other nursing interventions, and patient outcomes.

4. Evaluation:
- Assess the patient's skin integrity for bruises and reddened areas caused by the surgical position.
- Assess the patient's peripheral pulses after returning the patient to the supine position to compare them with the preoperative base line.
- Convey to the post-anesthesia care unit nurse the intraoperative nursing interventions and outcomes and the possibility for malignant hyperthermia.
- Transport the malignant hyperthermia treatment supplies to the PACU in the event the patient develops the syndrome in the postoperative period.
- If an episode of malignant hyperthermia occurs, make sure that it is reported to the North American Malignant Hyperthermia Registry.

Chapter Eight

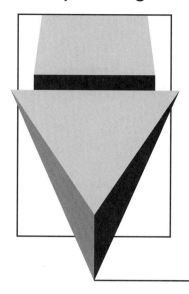

Surgical Patient Intraoperative Positioning

Mae Taylor Moss, RN, MSN, MS • Sheila A. O'Connor, RN, MS, CNS, CNOR

Prerequisite Knowledge   The learner should review human anatomy and physiology and proper body mechanics prior to reading this chapter. Chapter content is correlated with several AORN recommended practices. These recommended practices may be considered a prerequisite to beginning the chapter or a refresher upon completion of this chapter.

Recommended Practices for Documentation of Perioperative Nursing Care

Recommended Practices for Positioning the Surgical Patient

Chapter Outline

Learning Objectives

1. State the major considerations required in the practice of safe body mechanics.

2. State the preliminary considerations in positioning the surgical patient.

3. Describe the general impact of surgical positioning on the musculoskeletal, neurosensory, circulatory, respiratory, and integumentary systems.

4. Discuss the perioperative nurse's responsibilities in positioning the surgical patient.

5. List the major components in the evaluation of positioning techniques.

6. Discuss the physiologic impact of surgical positioning on the geriatric, obese, and malnourished patient.

Surgical positioning is defined as "moving and securing human anatomy into place, allowing the best exposure of the surgical site, and the least compromise in both physiological functions and mechanical stresses, in joints and other body parts" (Gruendemann, 1987).

The Association of Operating Room Nurses' *Standards and Recommended Practices for Perioperative Nursing* (AORN, 1994) provides guidelines specific to the perioperative nurse and the management of the patient undergoing surgical intervention. These guidelines recognize a variety of practice settings in which surgery may be performed and emphasize the collaboration of nursing, anesthesia, and surgery personnel to facilitate a positive outcome and the return of the client to a life-style consistent with his or her preoperative health status. The AORN's *Recommended Practices for Positioning the Surgical Patient* (AORN, 1994) recognizes the importance of the nursing process in patient positioning. These recommended practices provide guidelines for perioperative assessment, planning, implementation, and evaluation of surgical positioning. In addition, they espouse the development of clinically based agency policies and procedures that establish authority, responsibility, and accountability for the process of positioning.

Terminology

The perioperative nurse must have an understanding of the terms used to describe the different anatomic planes. This facilitates successful communication with the surgeon and the anesthesia staff while, at the same time, enhancing the perioperative nurse's ability to carry out successful positioning efforts and to achieve positive patient outcomes. The following terms are frequently employed when discussing the relationship of a positioning device to the limbs or surface area of the body.

Anterior: Situated in front of or in the forward part of, affecting the forward part of an organ, toward the head end of the body; in official anatomic nomenclature, used in reference to the ventral or belly surface of the body

Posterior: Situated in the back part of, or affecting the back part of an organ; in official anatomic nomenclature, used in reference to the back or dorsal surface of the body

Medial: Pertaining to the middle; closer to the medial plane or the midline of a body or structure (Fig. 8–1)

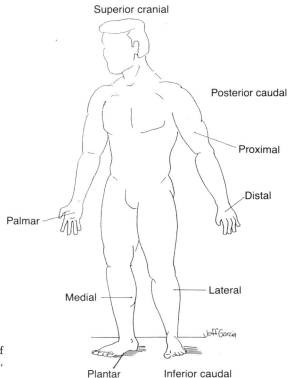

FIGURE 8–1. Anterior View (Courtesy of Jeff Garcia, Houston, Texas, and AORN, Denver, Colorado)

Lateral: Denoting a position farther from the medial plane or midline of the body or of a structure (see Fig. 8–1)

Proximal: Nearest; closer to any point of reference; opposed to distal (see Fig. 8–1)

Distal: Remote; farther from any point of reference; opposed to proximal (see Fig. 8–1)

Range of motion: The amount of joint mobility accomplished by a patient without pain. Since full range of motion is the greatest amount of motion possible in a joint, normal range of motion is accomplished within the limits of full range of motion. In an effort to prevent injury during positioning, the perioperative nurse should have a knowledge of the terminology that defines the body's range of motion.

Abduction: The withdrawal of a part from the axis of the body; the act of turning outward (Fig. 8–2)

Adduction: The act of drawing toward a center or toward a medial line (see Fig. 8–2)

Circumduction: The active or passive circulatory movement of limb (Fig. 8–3)

Dorsiflexion: Backward flexion or bending, as of the hand or foot (Fig. 8–4)

Plantarflexion: Pertaining to bending the sole of the foot downward (see Fig. 8–4)

Flexion: The act of bending or condition of being bent (Fig. 8–5)

Extension: The movement by which the two ends of any part are pulled asunder; a movement that brings the members of a limb into or toward a straight condition (see Fig. 8–5)

Hyperextension: Extreme or excessive extension of a limb or part (Fig. 8–6)

External rotation: The process of turning a joint outward (Fig. 8–7)

Internal rotation: The process of turning a joint inward (see Fig. 8–7)

Inversion: A turning inward, inside out, upside down, or other reversal of the normal relation of a part (Fig. 8–8)

Eversion: A turning outward or inside out (see Fig. 8–8)

Pronation: The act of assuming the prone position, or the state of being prone; applied to the hand, the act of turning the palm backward (posteriorly) or downward, performed by medial rotation of the forearm; applied to the foot,

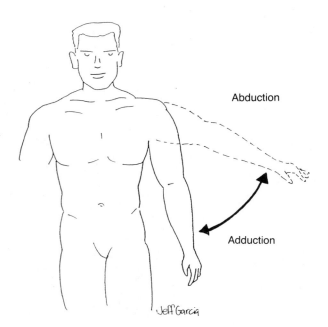

Abduction

Adduction

FIGURE 8–2. Abduction/Adduction (Courtesy of Jeff Garcia, Houston, Texas, and AORN, Denver, Colorado)

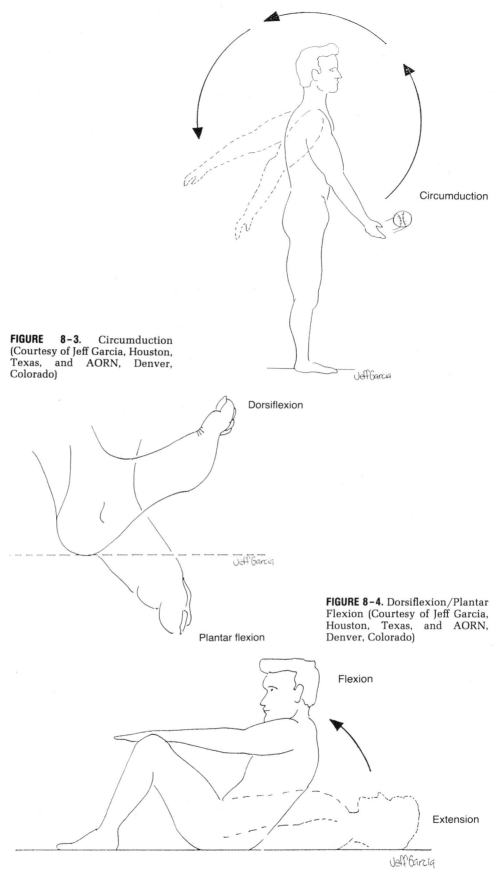

FIGURE 8–3. Circumduction (Courtesy of Jeff Garcia, Houston, Texas, and AORN, Denver, Colorado)

Dorsiflexion

FIGURE 8–4. Dorsiflexion/Plantar Flexion (Courtesy of Jeff Garcia, Houston, Texas, and AORN, Denver, Colorado)

Plantar flexion

Flexion

Extension

FIGURE 8–5. Flexion/Extension (Courtesy of Jeff Garcia, Houston, Texas, and AORN, Denver, Colorado)

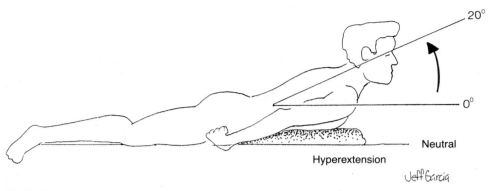

FIGURE 8–6. Hyperextension (Courtesy of Jeff Garcia, Houston, Texas, and AORN, Denver, Colorado)

a combination of eversion and abduction movements taking place in the tarsal and metatarsal joints and resulting in lowering of the medial margin of the foot, hence of the longitudinal arch (Fig. 8–9)

Supination: The act of assuming the supine position, or the state of being supine; applied to the hand, the act of turning the palm forward (anteriorly) or upward, performed by lateral rotation of the forearm; applied to the foot, it generally implies movement resulting in raising of the medial margin of the foot, hence of the longitudinal arch (see Fig. 8–9)

Rotation: The process of turning on an axis; movement of a body about its axis (Fig. 8–10)

General Considerations

BODY MECHANICS

The strain of the lumbar muscle group has been identified as the most common injury in occupational settings. Injury to this area impacts the person's ability to bend forward, backward, and sideways. There is also a decrease in the ability to rotate the lower back and hips from left to right and right to left. In order

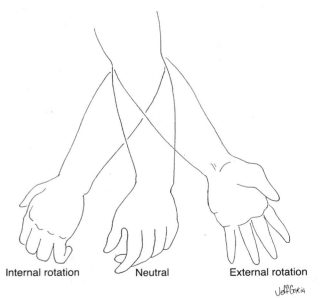

Internal rotation   Neutral   External rotation

FIGURE 8–7. Internal/External Rotation (Courtesy of Jeff Garcia, Houston, Texas, and AORN, Denver, Colorado)

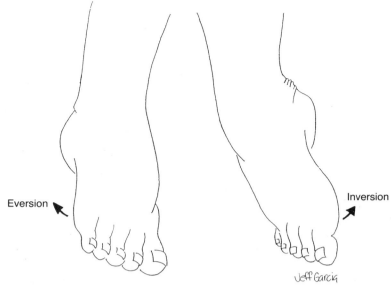

FIGURE 8-8. Eversion/Inversion (Courtesy of Jeff Garcia, Houston, Texas, and AORN, Denver, Colorado)

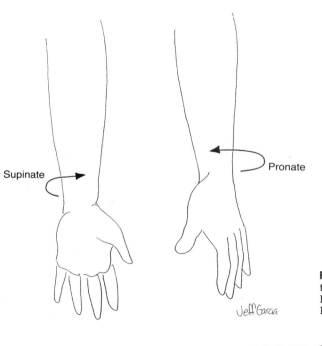

FIGURE 8-9. Supination/Pronation (Courtesy of Jeff Garcia, Houston, Texas, and AORN, Denver, Colorado)

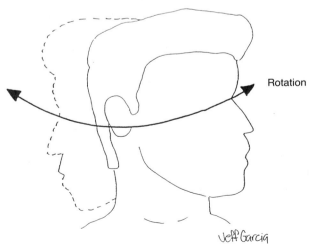

FIGURE 8-10. Rotation (Courtesy of Jeff Garcia, Houston, Texas, and AORN, Denver, Colorado)

to address proper body mechanics, it is necessary to view body mechanics from the prospective of the nursing process. This includes assessing the object to be moved and planning the transfer of the object; the actual implementation of lifting the object; and, finally, the evaluation of the correct use of body mechanics.

Assessment

Assessment in relation to body mechanics must consider the nature of the object to be lifted. The patient who is unable to assist during the transfer and/or process of surgical positioning requires at least four persons to assist, regardless of the patient's height or weight. The patient should be as close to the lifter's center of gravity as possible when being transferred from stretcher to OR bed. The center of gravity is defined as the point at which its mass is centered (Fuerst, 1974). The lifter's body should be positioned in such a way as to require the use of multiple muscle groups. The maximum weight that can be safely lifted is 35% more than a lifter's body weight. In planning transfer techniques and surgical positioning for patients, the perioperative nurse should develop goals directed at promoting correct patient body alignment during the lifting process and reducing the risk to the musculoskeletal system of both patient and lifter. Providing an obstacle-free pathway for lifting and transferring the patient involves the removal of excess linen and clutter. Whenever appropriate, explanations to the patient about the ensuing process not only enhance understanding but also increase cooperation.

When ready to transfer the patient, the perioperative nurse and the support staff should stand as close to the patient as possible. Maintenance of appropriate alignment of head and neck with the vertebrae is essential prior to the actual process of lifting the patient. In so doing, the risk of injury to the lifter's lumbar vertebrae and muscle group is diminished. During lifting, providing a base of support and lowering the center of gravity to the patient also facilitate better body balance, reducing the risk of falling and enabling muscle groups to work together. Evaluation is based upon the avoidance of strain on the musculoskeletal system. This is accomplished through assessment of the effectiveness of correct lifting techniques, and the subsequent feedback that safe lifting techniques were employed.

Safety of both patient and nurse is the primary consideration in transfer from stretcher to OR bed. Self-injury is prevented when the perioperative nurse employs proper body mechanics and maintains erect posture. The perioperative nurse, through initial assessment of the surgical patient, should note any motor deficits that the patient may have, the patient's ability to assist in transfer, and the patient's height and weight.

As with body mechanics, transfer techniques require the perioperative nurse to conceptualize the nursing process in order to be successful. Assessment must address the following criteria:

- Physiologic capacity to transfer—This consists of an assessment of muscle strength, joint mobility and contracture formation, paralysis or paresis, bone continuity, and upper arm strength of the surgical patient.
- The presence of weakness, dizziness, or postural hypertension
- The surgical patient's sensory status
- The patient's level of comfort
- The patient's cognitive status—It is most important that not only the perioperative nurse, but also the surgical patient, recognizes physical deficits and limitations to movement that can impact transfer from the stretcher to the OR bed. The patient's ability to appropriately respond and to follow verbal instructions is essential.

Planning

Based upon the perioperative nurse's assessment of the patient's status, the process of planning the transfer of the patient from the stretcher to the OR bed commences. The appropriate number of staff needed to assist with the transfer is planned for in this phase. Additionally, based upon the patient's cognitive status, the transfer procedure is explained and assistance from the surgical patient is sought. Planning promotes the safe transfer of the patient; facilitates proper techniques to avoid injury to the nurse and client; and promotes cooperation from the patient, thus reducing his or her anxiety level.

Implementation

Based upon the assessment and planning components of the nursing process, implementation of the transfer process from stretcher to OR bed is facilitated. For a safe transfer, both OR bed and stretcher must be locked. If the patient is able to assist in the process, there must be personnel standing on the opposite side of the OR bed as the patient is moving. There should also be staff standing next to the stretcher to render assistance, if needed, to the patient during the transfer.

Evaluation

To evaluate the success of the transfer process, the perioperative nurse must evaluate the patient for the following once the transfer is complete:

- Maintenance of correct body alignment on the OR bed and the presence of any pressure points on the skin
- Tolerance of the transfer activity
- Behavioral response to the transfer

The ability of the patient to participate in the transfer is influenced by the patient's level of mobility, ability to follow directions, and psychosocial factors. Positive patient outcomes are measured in terms of verbalization of comfort, absence of pressure points and peripheral nerve damage, and preservation of musculoskeletal functions.

PRELIMINARY POSITIONING CONSIDERATIONS

The perioperative nurse plays a vital role in safe positioning. Positioning of the patient is dependent upon the surgical procedures and how much exposure is required at the operative field. Positioning is also dependent upon the surgeon's preference, the patient's condition, and the surgeon's idiosyncrasies. Although most of this information is available on preference cards, the operating room nurse should, in all cases, collaborate with the surgeon and the anesthesiologist.

As stated previously, the patient's body must remain in physiologic alignment throughout the process of transfer and surgical positioning. In terms of surgical positioning, the needs of the anesthesiologist are driven by the maintenance of the patient's airway. Positioning should not commence without the approval and/or consent of the anesthesiologist or the nurse anesthetist, since any sudden movement may displace the airway. During any episode of positioning, the anesthesiologist and/or nurse anesthetist must be given time to recheck the endotracheal tube for placement. Additionally, the integrity of all lines must be noted. No abrupt position changes should be made to ensure hemodynamic stability of the patient. Since muscle relaxants are frequently given, care should be taken so as not to hyperextend any muscle group. In certain cases, it may be feasible to position the patient prior to the administration of anesthesia. This helps the circulating nurse in determining patient comfort and is often used for the lithotomy position, although in most cases, the patient is sedated following transfer to the OR bed. Throughout the positioning process, attention must be given to the maintenance of patient privacy. Consideration of the patient's needs from the patient's perspective helps insure the achievement of desired outcomes.

Positioning aids and equipment must be organized and conveniently located to ensure a smooth and safe process. This requires the circulating nurse to check the positioning equipment for function, safety, and cleanliness prior to use. All pieces of equipment should be organized so that they are readily available. The perioperative nurse must be mindful of conditions such as arthritis deformans, which can restrict patient movement, or cardiac pathology, which may inhibit a patient's ability to breathe while lying flat. Care should also be given to patients with hip prostheses. Severe flexion and adduction must be avoided in favor of slow, smooth movements. A thorough assessment of patient comfort prior to induction, with special attention given to those areas most prone to injury, greatly contributes to the prevention of peripheral neuropathy and/or pressure necrosis.

Adequate numbers of personnel during positioning must be planned for to prevent injury to the patient. The importance of the collaborative effort of surgeon and anesthesiologist in assessing the patient preoperatively cannot be over-emphasized. This does much to facilitate a safe and an uneventful surgical experience. However, the operating room nurse must also perform an assessment to determine the presence of implanted surgical devices, disease processes, or other considerations that may impact upon the ability to position the patient for surgery. Other factors that should be included in the assessment are the size of the patient; the site of the operation; and the patient's age, height, and weight. The art of patient transfer is an important nursing skill that requires knowledge of good body mechanics and good posture, awareness of the safety of the client as well as the staff, and organizational skills.

FREQUENTLY USED POSITIONING DEVICES

The numbers and shapes of positioning devices can sometimes be overwhelming to the novice perioperative nurse. For that reason, a compendium of some of the more frequently used equipment, indications, and contraindications for use is presented in Table 8-1.

PHYSIOLOGIC IMPACT OF POSITIONING

Musculoskeletal Considerations

Throughout the process of positioning, the musculoskeletal system of the patient is subjected to an exaggerated range of motion. Normally, pain and pressure receptors guard against the unnatural stretching and twisting of ligaments, tendons, and muscles. Opposing muscle groups also function in this capacity. With the use of anesthesia and muscle relaxants, pain and pressure receptors are depressed, resulting in the loss of tone and leading to exaggerated muscle relaxation. Bony prominences located in the head, thorax, upper extremities, and lower extremities are susceptible to excessive rubbing and pressure as a result of surgical positioning. Preventive measures that should be implemented by the perioperative nurse include pillow placement under the lower back and knees to enhance lumbar concavity, placement of foam under the heels, and silicone gel pads and/or foam under the head. The gel or foam pad at the head allows the strap muscles to relax and prevents cervical strain. Any possibility of rubbing or prolonged pressure should be guarded against. Patient contact with any metal device should also be avoided.

Neurosensory Considerations

The administration of anesthetic agents results in nervous system depression. The amount of neurosensory depression is dependent upon the type of anesthesia (i.e., regional, general, or nerve block). The perioperative nurse must be cognizant of the impact that prolonged pressure and stretching may have on peripheral nerves. As a patient advocate, the nurse must be aware that when nervous system depression takes place the body's compensatory actions are no longer possible. Failure to reverse pressure to peripheral nerves may result in anything from minor sensory motor loss to permanent paralysis. Frequent injuries to the peripheral nerves occur at the divisions of the brachial plexus, ulnar, radial, peritoneal, sciatic, and facial nerves. If the patient is improperly positioned, these nerves may be compromised. What is equally tragic is the compromise of peripheral nerves caused by members of the surgical team leaning on the patient during the operative procedure — or leaning against the armboard, causing the patient's arm to be hyperabducted.

Preventive initiatives include the adequate support of extremities during positioning and the padding of extremities once final positioning has been achieved. All equipment coming in contact with the extremities must also be padded. The forearm should never be allowed to hang over the side of the operative bed, since this may result in the compression of the radial nerve against the humerus. Positions, such as the modified Fowler's, which cause most of the patient's weight to be placed on the dorsum of the body, require extra padding on the buttocks and the small of the back. Prolonged pressure on the dorsum potentiates sciatic nerve damage. In positions in which a kidney rest is not utilized, it is important that the mattresses of the OR bed are positioned in such a way that the patient does not lie in a depression.

Circulatory Considerations

The circulatory system is the system most dramatically affected by positioning. Adequate circulation is necessary to maintain blood pressure, to facilitate venous return, to prevent thrombus formation, and to prevent circulatory disturbances. Compensatory mechanisms for maintaining blood pressure are obtunded with both general and regional anesthesia. Since muscle relaxants are administered during general anesthesia, venous return is diminished owing to the presence of decreased muscle tone. As a result of dilated vascular beds, venous pooling of dependent areas results in decreased cardiac output, circulatory volume, and systemic perfusion. This effect causes the blood pressure to drop. Negative pressure that aids in venous circulation is also diminished with reduced respiratory effort, particularly in ventilator-assisted respiration. As a result, all movement associated with surgical positioning must be slow and gentle. This practice can decrease the likelihood of significant physiologic disturbances. A general rule is to always ask the attending anesthesiologist and/or anesthetist before initiating patient positioning.

Abdominal pressure can restrict venous return to the vena cava, resulting in decreased blood pressure and cardiac output. Obliteration of the vena cava may also result from tension applied to the midsection of the abdomen when in the lateral or kidney position or from the use of deep retractors. Pressure on the vena cava results in hypotension, with venous pooling in the extremities further complicating this situation. Patient repositioning may be required to improve venous flow to the heart. Pressure on the vena cava, as well as on the femoral veins, may also reduce venous return and may occur when the patient is in the prone position. Deep and superficial veins of the lower extremities, such as the saphenous vein, are susceptible to compromise during anesthesia. Since anesthesia relaxes the muscular lining of vessels, resulting in venous pooling, even the most com-

Text continued on page 268

TABLE 8–1. **FREQUENTLY USED POSITIONING DEVICES**

DEVICE	INDICATIONS	PRECAUTIONS
Allen stirrups (Figure A)	May be used for all procedures where the lithotomy position is required; adjustable to any position; locking control prevents patient injury	May result in nerve pressure due to excessive abduction and hyperextension; may cause pressure areas
Axillary roll (Figure B)	Indicated for use in the lateral position; helps to prevent pressure on the axillary peripheral nerves	Potential for slippage once the patient is positioned
Candy cane stirrups (Figure C)	For use when increased exposure to the perineal and/or rectal areas is required	May result in nerve pressure due to uncontrolled abduction and hyperextension; may result in pressure points or thermal injury from the leg resting against the metal portion of the stirrup; not versatile.
Elevated armboard (Figures D and E)	Used in the lateral position for procedures such as thoracotomy and total hip replacement; eliminates ulnar nerve pressure; balances arm in an anatomically correct position	Potential for arm slippage; must avoid contact with any exposed metal from the device; can produce pressure areas.
Foam pads (Figure F)	Used to pad and protect bony prominences and peripheral nerves	Should be discarded after use; potential for pooling of solutions when used in proximity to the surgical site.

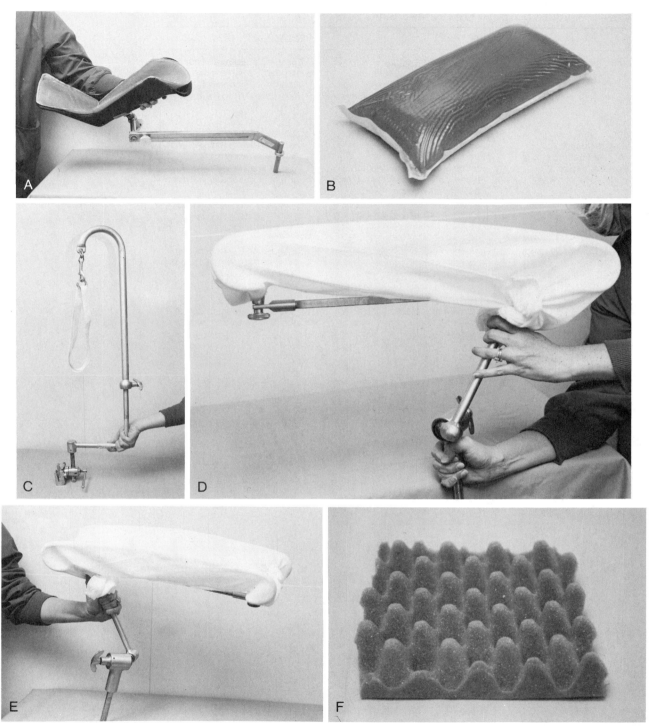

Table continued on following page

TABLE 8-1. **FREQUENTLY USED POSITIONING DEVICES** *Continued*

DEVICE	INDICATIONS	PRECAUTIONS
Footboard (Figure G)	Prevents patient slippage when in the supine and reverse Trendelenburg positions; also indicated for use with patients over 6 feet tall to add length to the OR bed	Footboard must be adequately padded; must take care to appropriately position footboard in relationship to the patient's height
Gel pads: Table pad (Figure H) Donut head pad (Figure I) Chest rolls (Figure J)	Used to prevent decubitus ulcers by evenly distributing perpendicular pressure, reducing tangential pressure (shear forces), and dissipating heat; supports any weight; transfers even, exact temperature when using a heating blanket; won't absorb odors or body fluids	Must not come directly in contact with the skin in patients with already compromised skin integrity, as these pads have the potential to adhere
Kidney rest (part of OR bed) (Figure K)	Used for better exposure and access in kidney procedures	Must position the patient's flank over the kidney rest for optimal utilization; must ensure that kidney rest does not impinge on ribs or iliac crest
Knee stirrups (Figure L)	For use in procedures requiring low lithotomy position, such as cystoscopy	May result in pressure on the popliteal fossa; not versatile

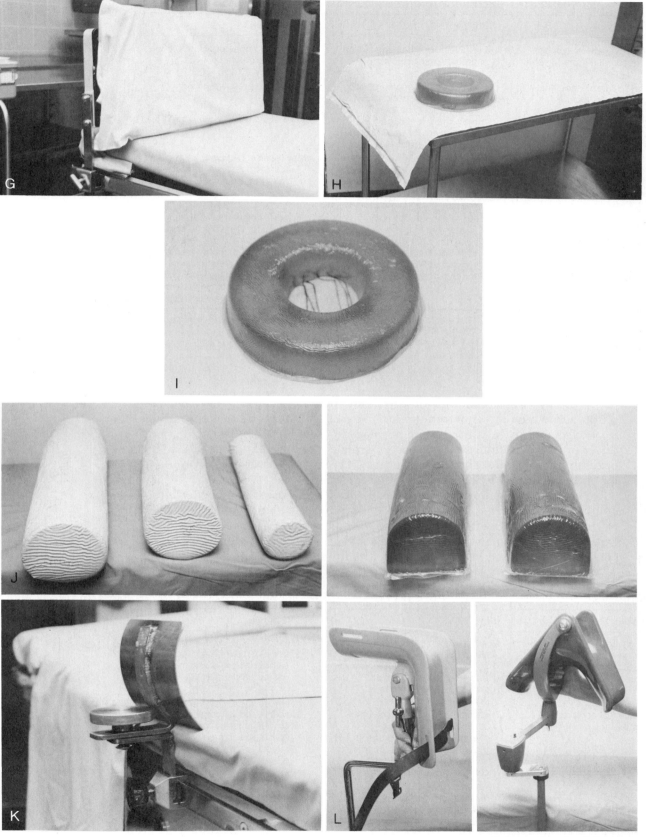

Table continued on following page

TABLE 8–1. **FREQUENTLY USED POSITIONING DEVICES** *Continued*

DEVICE	INDICATIONS	PRECAUTIONS
Mayfield general purpose headrest (Figure M, *left*)	For use in supine or semisitting procedures, including craniotomy	May exert undue pressure on head and unprotected ears
Mayfield horseshoe headrest (Figure M, *middle*)	Permits various angled positions of the head or neck; allows both vertical and lateral movement for proper positioning; for use in supine and prone positions	May cause pressure points
Mayfield modified skull clamp (Figure M, *right*)	For rigid skeletal fixation for the supine, prone, lateral, or sitting positions; rotates 360 degrees for flexibility in positioning of the pins around critical areas	May result in bleeding at the pin sites; increased potential for neck hyperextension
Olympic Vac-Pac (suction beanbag) (Figure N)	Used to support the body or extremities in the desired position; most frequently used in the lateral position; can be molded to the body's contour for enhanced exposure	Pressure points and/or shearing may occur if a wrinkled sheet is placed between the patient and Vac-Pac; skin irritation may be caused if the patient's skin is wet when placed in Vac-Pac; must ensure the patient is not resting on the inflation valve of Vac-Pac

Photographs courtesy of Gus Salinas, St. Luke's Episcopal Hospital, Houston, Texas. Olympic Vac-Pac courtesy of Ohio Medical Instrument Company, Cincinnati, Ohio.

mon surgical position can contribute to venous pooling because of the dependent position in which lower extremities are frequently placed. Venous thrombosis may be caused by pressure from a misplaced pillow or safety belt, which produces pressure on the popliteal space. Assessment of peripheral pulses should occur prior to and after placement of limbs in the surgical position. See Table 8–2 for equipment used to insure adequate circulation.

The external iliac artery is responsible for the perfusion of blood to the abdominal wall, external genitalia, and lower limbs. In the lithotomy position, pressure is exerted by the thighs on the abdomen, compressing this vessel and causing blood to pool in the trunk of the body. In order to allow the body to compensate for increased venous return in the lithotomy position, legs should be

TABLE 8–2. **EQUIPMENT TO INSURE ADEQUATE CIRCULATION**

DEVICE	INDICATIONS	PRECAUTIONS
4", 6" Ace wraps Anti-embolism (TED) stockings	May be used in patients with a history of phlebitis, superficial veins, and varicosities; indicated for use in lengthy surgical procedures where venous pooling may occur	Must be applied in a wrinkle-free fashion; must be applied to the same level bilaterally; must ensure proper fit
Sequential compression stockings	Particularly useful in the reverse Trendelenburg position; alternating pressure prevents thrombus formation secondary to venous pooling; provides consistent pressure	Nipples used for connecting the stockings to the machine can cause pressure points, if not adequately padded; must use proper stocking size
Pillows	Used to provide support and to maintain physiologic alignment; also used for padding and body stabilization	Can predispose patients to thrombus formation; when used to elevate the lower legs, as in the prone position, footdrop and undue pressure to the toes should be assessed

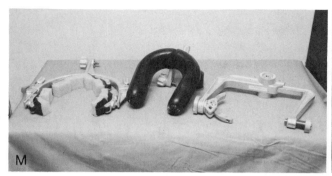 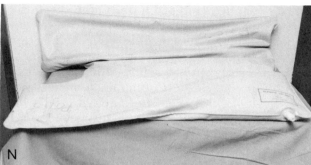

raised slowly and simultaneously. When removing the legs from the lithotomy position, the legs should be moved simultaneously. This allows the body to compensate for shifting blood volume, since 500 to 600 milliliters of venous blood can potentially drain into the legs, resulting in hypotension.

The subclavian and axillary arteries may also become occluded when the arm is hyperabducted to an angle greater than 90 degrees. This hyperabduction may cause injury to the arteries (Kneedler, 1989). Circulation in the radial or brachial pulses should be checked periodically by the perioperative nurse when armboards are in place. Compromised patients, such as obese and cardiac patients, are more prone to the effects that positioning has on the circulatory system. Any patient in poor cardiac status will be a greater anesthetic risk in most positions. Patients 100 pounds or more overweight demonstrate variations in circulatory function.

The inferior vena cava can be occluded secondarily to surgical positioning, leading to decreased venous return. Consequently blood pools in the lower extremities. Through hyperextension and/or twisting of a limb, vessels may be occluded through compression of the bony structures. Preventive measures include the snug application of restraining devices and safety straps. Tight restraining devices restrict blood flow. Additional padding over bony prominences and axillary rolls further prevent circulatory compromise. Support devices, such as pillows, may be necessary to prevent pressure from being exerted on the inferior vena cava.

Respiratory Considerations

Patient positioning during surgical procedures tends to compromise lung compliance owing to the force exerted on the diaphragm. This force shortens the lung along its long axis and results in decreased lung capacity. The chief consideration of positioning with regard to the respiratory system should be to provide proper shoulder alignment and unrestricted chest wall expansion in order to enhance vital lung capacity. The body weight of an anesthetized patient can compress the diameter of the chest, further reducing lung capacity (Smith, 1978). Hypotension due to positioning reduces available blood for oxygenation. Chronic respiratory diseases also complicate respiration and oxygenation.

The vital capacity of the lungs decreases in the supine position. Although inspiratory chest excursions are not significantly compromised, pressure from the abdominal viscera tends to hinder diaphragmatic excursions. The prone position is most likely to compromise normal respiratory movement, as normal diaphragmatic movement is restricted by a compressed abdominal wall. As a result, tidal volume is limited and increased airway pressure is required to ventilate. Improper prone positioning results in hypoventilation because abdominal wall movement is restricted. As the lungs inflate, the entire back rises. This causes a continuous movement at the operative site. In the lateral position, gas exchange ratios in the lungs are affected. Gravitational force causes the lower lung to receive more blood from the right side of the heart. However, the mediastinal compression and the weight of visceral contents on the diaphragm result in less residual air. Restriction of the lower chest wall in the lateral position also causes pooling of secretions in the lower lung.

Integumentary Considerations

Ischemic tissue necrosis develops over bony prominences unless sufficient padding is applied over those areas that are particularly susceptible, such as the heels, elbows, and sacrum. Constant mechanical pressure from skin or linen folds also results in reduced tissue perfusion. The pulling of linen from under the patient during positioning may lead to injury such as tissue shearing. Dependent areas with scar tissue should be considered as potential problem areas because of their decreased tissue perfusion. In surgical procedures lasting more than 3 hours, repositioning patients as frequently as the procedure dictates is indicated. However, this is not a substitute for the adequate padding of bony prominences and positioning devices prior to prepping and draping the patient.

THE PERIOPERATIVE NURSE'S ROLE

Preoperative Planning and Assessment

Through the operating room nurse's initial patient assessment, plans for intraoperative positioning have already begun. Patient demographics must be considered. Age is a key factor that is often the chief indicator of skin turgor and condition. Age also plays a role in the predetermination of positioning dilemmas, since the care of these patients may be complicated by arthritis, peripheral vascular disease, previous surgeries (which may have included a total joint replacement), and decreased sensorium. In all cases, skin status must be inspected for preexisting conditions, such as reddened areas and decubiti. Existing medical conditions must also be noted.

In patients with diabetes and peripheral vascular disease, circulation is already compromised; therefore, special attention must be given to the patient's extremities to prevent further compromise through the exertion of undue pressure. Previous surgical procedures, such as skin grafts and amputation, make intraoperative positioning problematic. Patients who have undergone amputation have increased restriction of movement depending upon the site of the amputation. Above-the-knee amputation can make placing the patient in the lithotomy position extremely difficult and visualization of the operative site limited.

Burn patients who have undergone multiple skin graftings are extremely challenging for the perioperative nurse. Adhesions from the burns cause restriction of movement, and areas that have received skin grafts have limited vascularity.

Body build has a profound effect upon positioning. Obese patients are not only susceptible to respiratory complications but are also prone to vascular compromise from the folding of skin during positioning. In these cases, the perioperative nurse must not only be the advocate for the patient but also for the staff by ensuring that appropriate numbers of personnel are available for positioning. Malnourished patients can also be difficult as bony prominences tend to be closer to the surface, creating an increased incidence of pressure areas. This may also hold true for the debilitated patient, who may already be compromised as a result of an extended institutional stay.

An integral part of the preoperative phase has to do with planning for sufficient numbers of personnel. With the exception of the dorsal recumbent positioning, most positioning configurations require three or more support staff persons. The perioperative nurse's role as an advocate does not begin and end with patient care. The nurse must also be acutely aware of, and be an advocate for, the welfare and safety requirements of peers and subordinates. Failure to make this provision not only results in potential patient injury but also in potential injury to valuable staff members. Consequently, perioperative outcomes cannot be measured only by the success of the surgical procedure and the benefit to the patient, but also by the thoughtful assessment and planning of personnel support aimed at providing a positive positioning outcome.

Positioning devices commonly used include pillows, headrests, silicone gel pads, eggcrate mattresses, armboards, safety straps, shoulder braces, footboards, stirrups and their modifications, axillary rolls, chest rolls, and donut headpads. These devices must be applied appropriately, and their use should be carefully monitored by the perioperative nurse (see Table 8–1).

Assessment of patient needs must also include a knowledge and an understanding of the surgical procedure. The operative schedule must be checked for any special requests the surgeon may have, as well as for the location of the operative site. The consent, as part of the patient interview process, must also be checked for accuracy of operative site and location. During the preoperative interview, the perioperative nurse can determine discrepancies in the consent by assessment of the patient's knowledge of the procedure to be performed.

Collaboration with physicians is also key to successful positioning. Many times the surgeon can provide the perioperative nurse with much insight into positioning needs and can be of great help during the actual process.

The Nursing Diagnosis and Its Implications

The nursing diagnosis for surgical positioning is the high risk for injury related to sustained pressure to certain areas during surgery (Meeker, 1991). This is consistent with AORN's *Patient Outcome Standards for Perioperative Nursing*, which states that the goal of the perioperative nurse is a patient who is free from injury related to positioning; extraneous objects; or chemical, physical, and electrical hazards. The plan of care for the surgical patient should begin with the patient assessment. Prior to the patient's entry into the operating room, all positioning devices must be gathered. They must be checked for cleanliness and safety and should be located to ensure quick access. Although the nursing diagnosis is patient-specific, the operating room nurse must also be acutely aware of the potential for staff injuries related to poor body mechanics and to inappropriate numbers of assistants being available during the positioning.

Individual patient problems must be considered when developing the surgical plan of care specific to positioning. Patients with spinal cord trauma, quadriplegia, and hemiplegia require special consideration. In these cases, there is a dramatic loss in the neuromuscular sensorium that interferes with the patient's ability to compensate. Mobility in the geriatric patient can be problematic in positioning, particularly when there have been previous total joint procedures or when there has been a history of arthritis. The uncomplicated pediatric patient has special requirements that must be considered during surgical intervention. Airway integrity is of special note. Infants 4 weeks old and younger are nose breathers; therefore, any nasal obstruction can result in respiratory distress. Since airway cartilage is soft, hyperextension of the neck may also result in airway obstruction. The tongue can easily block the airway of a child, since the tongue in children is larger than in adults. The cricoid cartilage in children is soft; therefore, uncuffed endotracheal tubes are inserted. In these cases, the perioperative nurse must be constantly aware of the possible dislodging of the tube due to excessive movement. In addition, infants and children are prone to significant loss of body temperature with exposed skin surface. Care must be taken during positioning to preserve the child's core temperature.

The Preoperative Interview

Communication is extremely important when preparing a patient for surgery. The perioperative nurse should answer any questions and explain the sequence of events the patient is about to undergo. This communication is especially important once the patient is brought into the operating room where the surgical procedure will be performed. Apprehension can be reduced by explaining to the patient what is about to happen before it happens. In this way, the perioperative nurse can solicit the most assistance from the patient. It is optimal to attempt to position the patient while he/she is awake. In so doing, the patient is able to indicate to the perioperative nurse any ideas of pressure, any stretching or overextension of limbs, and any generalized discomfort. If this technique is employed, the perioperative nurse must plan a detailed explanation of how the patient can help and what is about to transpire during this process. With the assessment of pre-existing skin conditions, the perioperative nurse can minimize potential pressure points and anticipate areas susceptible to venous pooling. The potential for decreased vascular perfusion is enhanced in patients with peripheral vascular disease, cardiac pathology, and multiple skin grafts.

In all cases, evaluation should begin at the time of patient assessment. This allows the perioperative nurse to predict potential outcomes related to surgical positioning. Documentation on the perioperative nursing record should illustrate all of the components of a thorough assessment and planning strategy. Again, pre-existing conditions rendering the body's compensatory mechanism at risk must be documented on the perioperative assessment, and the perioperative nursing care plan should reflect an anticipated outcome. The surgical position, as well as any position aids, must also be thoroughly documented.

INDICATIONS FOR CONSIDERATION IN SURGICAL POSITIONING

Surgical positioning can be best facilitated through the nursing process: assessment, planning, implementation, and evaluation. Each of the components, as they relate to surgical positioning, is discussed under each respective heading. Since evaluation of surgical positioning examines consistent outcomes pertinent to all styles of surgical positioning, evaluation is discussed in general terms at the end of this section.

SUPINE

Definition

The supine (dorsal recumbent) position is the most natural and common position of the body (Fig. 8–11). Anesthesia is initiated in this position, with modification

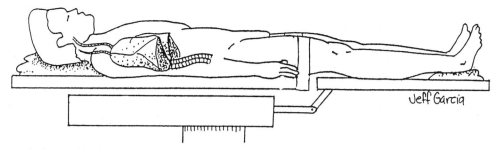

FIGURE 8–11. Supine Position (Courtesy of Jeff Garcia, Houston, Texas, and AORN, Denver, Colorado)

usually taking place after the patient has been intubated and stabilized. Surgical procedures requiring the patient to be placed in the supine position include laparoscopy, cholecystectomy, colon resection, hernia repair, breast biopsy, and modified radical mastectomy; head and neck surgeries requiring the supine position include thyroidectomy, parotidectomy, and radical neck dissection.

Equipment

- Pillow or headrest
- Padding
    Gel pads
    Eggcrate mattresses
    Donut rolls
- Armboards
- Safety belt
- Footboard

Assessment

Care should be taken to avoid compromise of the axillary neurovascular bundle in the dorsal recumbent position. Bony prominences that need special attention include the occiput, elbows, and heels. Sometimes known as the crucifix position, the dorsal recumbent position, although widely used, is poorly tolerated by the awake immobile patient. The most common nerve injury is to the brachial plexus. Injuries in the supine position are the result of overextending an arm while turning the head and neck in the direction opposite to the arm. Extending and suspending the arm straight from the wrist also adds pressure to the brachial plexus (Kneedler, 1989). Sensory loss in the arm and shoulder girdle are the result of injury to the brachial plexus. Radial and brachial pulses should be monitored when the arm is extended for prolonged periods of time.

Planning

The primary concern when placing a patient in the supine position is the protection of bony prominences, peripheral nerves, and blood vessels. A footboard may be indicated to prevent footdrop in the immobilized patient or to add length to the OR bed for the patient who is over 6 feet tall.

Implementation

Ensuring that the OR bed and stretcher are locked, the positioning team will assist the awake patient to the OR bed. If the patient is unconscious or anesthetized, four staff members should be used: one for the legs, one for the head, and one for each side of the patient. The sheet of the stretcher may be utilized as a draw sheet, or the patient may be gently log-rolled to one side and a roller slid underneath the patient and on top of the draw sheet. The patient is then returned to the supine position and rolled over to the OR bed. The patient is then log-rolled to one side on the OR bed, and the roller and/or draw sheet is removed.

In the supine position, the patient is flat with arms secured on armboards with palms down or along the sides of the body. The patient's arms should not at any time contact the metal frame of the OR bed. Electrical burns may occur when cautery is used if any portion of the patient's body is in contact with the metal frame of the OR bed. The palms of the patient's hands should be turned toward the patient. If armboards are in place, the arms should not be abducted beyond the patient's range of motion or 90 degrees. Body alignment is maintained by keeping the legs and hips straight and parallel. They should be on the same horizontal plane as the head and spine. Pillows may be placed under the head to facilitate comfort and respiratory effort. The safety belt should be placed across the thigh approximately 2 inches above the knee, as a safety strap placed directly over or below the knees has little restraining effect on patients waking after anesthesia. There have been incidences in which patients have sustained injuries to themselves owing to incorrectly applied restraints.

Pillows are also placed under the knees to reduce the pressure on the lower back and may also be placed at the curvature of the lumbar spine to promote lumbar concavity. This is especially helpful in older patients. Some operations in the groin and lower extremities require the patient to be frog-legged in the supine position. Positioning remains the same except that the knees are slightly flexed and a pillow is placed beneath each. Since the thighs are externally rotated, special attention should be given to patients with arthritis and joint replacement. With breast, axillary, upper extremity, or hand surgery, the patient is supine with the arm at a right angle to the OR bed. The affected side of the body must be positioned at the edge of the OR bed for easy access. A small pad can be placed under the affected side to facilitate exposure of the operative area.

TRENDELENBURG

Definition

The Trendelenburg position (Fig. 8–12) was first used by Friedreich Trendelenburg in the late 1800s in order to enhance exposure of the urinary bladder, rectum, and vagina by allowing the abdominal contents to gravitate cephalad out of

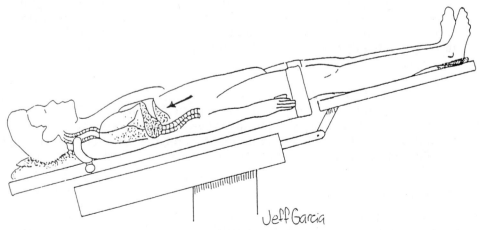

FIGURE 8–12. Trendelenburg Position (Courtesy of Jeff Garcia, Houston, Texas, and AORN, Denver, Colorado)

the pelvis (Barash, 1989). The Trendelenburg position is a variation on the supine position, with the body tilted, with the head down, at an angle of up to 45 degrees.

Equipment

- Padding
    Gel pads
    Eggcrate mattresses
    Donut rolls
- Armboards
- Safety belt
- Padded shoulder braces

Assessment

The perioperative nurse must insure that the brachial neurovascular bundle is not compressed between the clavicle and the first rib in this position (Barash, 1989). Care must be taken during the surgical procedure to insure that pressure is not exerted upon the toes from the Mayo stand. In the Trendelenburg position, respiratory changes are dramatic, and tidal volume is dependent upon the degree of the Trendelenburg position, with vital capacity falling 14.5% below that in the sitting position. This is due to the restrictive effect of the internal organs on ventilation and the subsequent compression of the diaphragm. Although the apex of the lung receives the greatest amount of blood in this position, the alveolar tissue in the base of the lung is the least perfused. Intrathoracic pressure is increased in the Trendelenburg position, causing potential problems in patients with cardiac compensation or in those with increased intracranial and intraocular pressure (Kneedler, 1989).

Planning

The perioperative nurse must be aware that, although this position is a temporary treatment for hypotension, it can result in sustained hypotension as well as increased intrathoracic, intracranial, and intraocular pressure. Optimally, the patient remains in the Trendelenburg position only for a short period of time before being returned to the horizontal position.

Implementation

Transfer of the patient will be the same as that in the supine position. The patient's knees are positioned at the table break of the foot section in the event the legs are lowered. Padded shoulder braces are placed securely against the acromioclavicular joints. In order to maintain the position on the OR bed, the legs may be lowered parallel to the floor to prevent patient slippage toward the head. This also allows more clearance for the Mayo stand above the toes. The patient is returned to the horizontal position prior to transfer to the stretcher.

REVERSE TRENDELENBURG

Definition

Reverse Trendelenburg (Fig. 8–13) displaces the abdominal viscera for upper abdominal surgery and provides the surgeon better visualization of the upper abdomen. In reverse Trendelenburg, the OR bed is positioned to elevate the head higher than the feet. Reverse Trendelenburg is the classic position for surgical procedures in which decreased blood supply to the area of operation is required

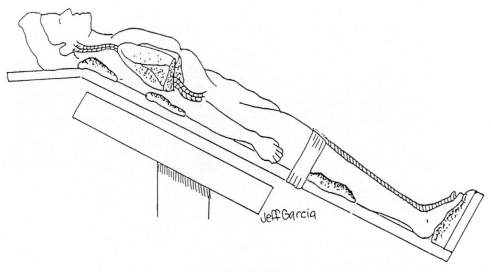

FIGURE 8–13. Reverse Trendelenburg Position (Courtesy of Jeff Garcia, Houston, Texas, and AORN, Denver, Colorado)

but respirations must be facilitated. It can also be used for abdominal cases, such as cholecystectomy and common bile duct exploration, when the abdominal viscera are displaced from the epigastrium, providing better visualization.

Equipment

- Padding
    Gel pads
    Eggcrate mattresses
    Donut rolls
- Armboards
- Safety belt
- Padded footboard

Assessment

Although respirations are less affected in this position, the potential for circulatory compensation is compromised. Reverse Trendelenburg allows for peripheral pooling of as much as several hundred milliliters of blood in the extremities (Kneedler, 1989). Movements out of the reverse Trendelenburg must be done slowly to allow the heart to compensate for changes in the circulating blood volume.

Planning

When planning the reverse Trendelenburg position, the perioperative nurse should be aware that the head of the OR bed will be elevated at an angle of up to 45 degrees. Placing the soles of the patient's feet securely against the padded footboard prevents patient movement on the OR bed.

Implementation

Transfer of the patient will be the same as that in the supine position. As with the supine position, pillows may be placed under the knees and lumbar spine. A padded footboard is essential to prevent the patient from sliding. At the conclusion of the procedure, the patient is returned to the horizontal position prior to transfer to the stretcher.

SITTING POSITION

Definition

The sitting position (Fig. 8–14) is also known as the modified Fowler's position. In the sitting position, the patient is in a semireclining posture on the OR bed. The legs are elevated to the level of the heart with the head flexed ventrally on the neck. This allows for head and neck stabilization during craniotomy and cervical laminectomy.

Equipment

- 2 Stirrup holders
- Foam padding
- Mayfield crossbar adapter
- Mayfield adjustable base unit
- Mayfield skull clamp
- Modified Methodist (Mayfield) headrest
- Pillow
- Footboard

Assessment

The sitting position is the best possible position for respiration since there is no restriction on chest expansion. However, systemic circulation can be greatly compromised. Since most of the body weight rests on ischial tuberosities, the OR bed should be well padded in an effort to avoid pressure areas and sciatic nerve damage, particularly in thin or diabetic individuals. A footboard will support the feet in such a way as to reduce sacral pressure. Since this position results in negative venous pressure in the head and neck, air embolism is of concern. Patient monitoring in this position consists of a central venous line with a Doppler device (Meeker, 1991). The central venous line is used to extract air, which may be carried from the internal or external jugular vein to the heart. The Doppler is employed to provide audible detection of air embolism.

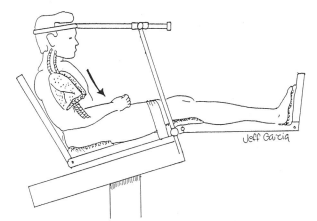

FIGURE 8–14. Sitting Position (Courtesy of Jeff Garcia, Houston, Texas, and AORN, Denver, Colorado)

Planning

Since a patient in the sitting position is prone to air embolism, the perioperative nurse should be prepared to assist anesthesia personnel in the placement of an arterial line or a central venous catheter. Anti-embolism stockings or Ace bandages should be available for application to the patient's legs to facilitate venous return while in the sitting position.

Implementation

Anti-embolism stockings or Ace bandages are applied to the legs. A padded footboard is affixed to the OR bed and positioned snugly against the patient's feet in an effort to prevent footdrop. The safety strap is applied above the knees for safety and to keep the feet in place against the footboard. If the knees are flexed, they are positioned at the lower break of the OR bed. When placing the patient in the sitting position, the perioperative nurse must provide head stabilization until all positioning components are in place. Care must be given at this time to insure that the ears are not impinged by the Mayfield headrest. The nurse maintains the stability of the head until the device is locked into place. Once the head is stabilized in the Mayfield head holder, the head section of the OR bed is removed.

The hands are secured across the patient's legs using a nonabrasive tape. The hands are placed on top of each other and padded with eggcrate mattresses or foam. The padding should extend to the antecubital spaces in an effort to prevent ulnar nerve compression.

LITHOTOMY

Definition

The lithotomy position (Figs. 8–15 to 8–17) originated because Louis XIV of France (the Sun King) had a desire to see his children being born. (Prior to this time, children were born in a birthing chair.) This is the most extreme variation on the dorsal recumbent or supine position. While the patient is supine, the legs are raised and abducted simultaneously, exposing the perineal region. This provides for the surgical approach to the genital and rectal areas. The lithotomy position is utilized in the following surgical procedures: laparoscopy, dilatation and curettage, hysteroscopy, and vaginal hysterectomy. Rectal procedures in which the lithotomy is indicated include hemorrhoidectomy, abdominal perineal resections, and Soave pull-through procedures. Urologic procedures include cystoscopy and urethroscopy.

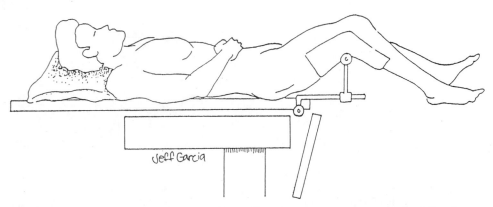

FIGURE 8–15. Lithotomy Position (Courtesy of Jeff Garcia, Houston, Texas, and AORN, Denver, Colorado)

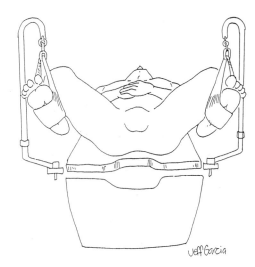

FIGURE 8-16. Lithotomy position using candy cane stirrups (Courtesy of Jeff Garcia, Houston, Texas, and AORN, Denver, Colorado)

Equipment

- Pillow or headrest
- Armboards
- Safety strap
- Stirrups (candy cane, Allen-type, or knee)
- Padding
  Foam
  Gel pads

Assessment

Intra-abdominal pressure against the diaphragm results in decreased respiratory function, leading to a decrease in tidal volume. Gravity plays an important part in circulation of the blood, as the elevated legs cause pooling in the splanchnic region during the surgical procedure. Because of the increased splanchnic volume, blood loss during surgery may not be immediately evident. As the legs are returned to the supine position, there is the potential of 500 milliliters or more of blood diversion occurring, depleting circulating volume and causing blood pressure to fall. Since compensatory mechanisms are depressed by anesthesia, homeostasis may be difficult to achieve. Venous thrombosis results from pressure against the soft tissue of the leg. Lower extremity peripheral pulses should be as-

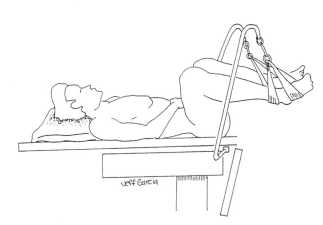

FIGURE 8-17. Lithotomy position using candy cane stirrups (side view) (Courtesy of Jeff Garcia, Houston, Texas, and AORN, Denver, Colorado)

sessed prior to and after positioning to insure circulation. For patients with decreased range of motion in the hip, Allen-type stirrups with knee and foot rests may be required.

Planning

In the lithotomy position, consideration must be given to the predisposition for pressure to be placed on the abdomen, groin, soft tissue structures, peripheral nerves, and lower back. As stated previously, the perioperative nurse should be aware of any decreased range of motion in the patient's hips prior to utilizing this position.

Implementation

To position the patient in lithotomy, both legs are flexed at the knee and hip and are simultaneously elevated by two individuals. Numerous devices, such as candy cane stirrups, Allen-type stirrups, and knee stirrups, are available to achieve the desired position. Devices should be selected based upon the individual patient. Good position is achieved with minimal effort when the perioperative nurse positions the patient's anterior iliac spine on a horizontal plane with the leg holder. The buttocks should be level and at the edge of the break of the OR bed. The height of the stirrups should be compatible with the length of the patient's thigh, and the stirrups must be level with each other. This prevents knee and lumbar pressure. By placing the perineum in line with the longitudinal axis of the bed, patient symmetry in positioning is achieved. The head and neck are supported as previously described. The patient's arms are usually placed on armboards or across the chest. In this case, a folded gown or cover sheet that is tucked beneath the patient may be folded up and over the arms, producing a cradling effect. Folded loosely, the gown or cover sheet is secured with an unsterile towel clip. Care must be taken to insure that the towel clip does not pierce the patient, and the arms must not inhibit chest movement and respiration. In the pediatric patient, the weight of the arms across the chest may create respiratory problems by fatiguing intercostal muscles. If the arms are placed at the patient's side, they are at risk for injury when the foot of the bed is lowered or raised. The patient's feet should be padded prior to securing them in candy cane or Allen-type stirrups in order to prevent pressure on the common peroneal nerve (Fig. 8–18). The lower leg should not come into contact with the leg holders. Obese patients may especially require additional foam or gel padding between the

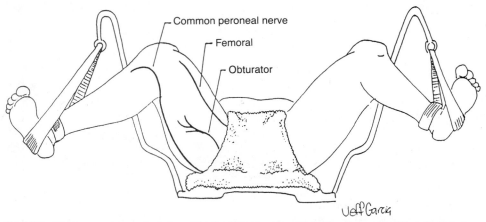

FIGURE 8–18. Nerves commonly injured by the lithotomy position (Courtesy of Jeff Garcia, Houston, Texas, and AORN, Denver, Colorado)

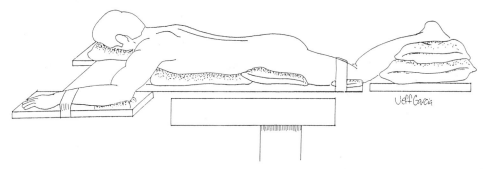

FIGURE 8–19. Prone Position (Courtesy of Jeff Garcia, Houston, Texas, and AORN, Denver, Colorado)

calves and thighs and the metal sections of the stirrups. Since the lithotomy position is an exaggerated one, it is optimal, when appropriate, to have the patient awake while being positioned. This enables the patient to express discomfort or pain, and the perioperative nurse can immediately take appropriate action. Specific care must be taken to preserve the patient's privacy in this position.

When returning the patient to the original supine position, the patient's legs should be lowered slowly and simultaneously by two individuals, with the patient's legs meeting together in the sagittal plane. This allows for minimal torsion stress on the lumbar spine and slows the process of increased vascular volume of the legs to the circulatory system, thereby preventing sudden hypotension.

PRONE POSITION

Definition

When the surgical procedure requires a dorsal approach, the prone position (Fig. 8–19) is indicated. It is most widely chosen for spinal procedures such as laminectomy and spinal fusion. An effective variation on the prone position is to place the patient in a face-down, kneeling position (Fig. 8–20). This position is thought by some to provide the best exposure in laminectomy procedures.

Equipment

- Pillow or headrest
- 2 Armboards (or a laminectomy armboard)
- 2 Chest rolls (or a laminectomy frame)
- Safety strap
- 1 or 2 Pillows
- Padding
    Foam
    Gel pads

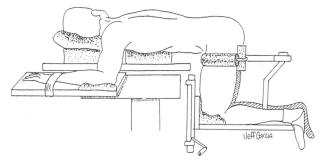

FIGURE 8–20. Prone Position on Andrews Frame (Courtesy of Jeff Garcia, Houston, Texas, and AORN, Denver, Colorado)

Assessment

In the prone position, chest rolls prevent a radical drop in mean arterial pressure. Hypotension is reduced when venous return from the femoral veins and inferior vena cava is uninterrupted. Wrapping the legs in anti-embolism stockings or Ace bandages minimizes venous pooling in distensible vessels and enhances venous return.

In this position, vital capacity can be reduced by 10% and tidal volume by 11%. Restriction of chest movement by the patient's weight is relieved by chest rolls or a laminectomy frame. Respiratory effectiveness facilitates venous flow and enhances blood pressure (Kneedler, 1989). Pressure points are greatest on the chest, knees, ankles, and toes. In this position, additional pressure points can occur at the shoulder and iliac crest.

Planning

Injury to the staff, as well as to the patient, must be avoided. In order to accomplish this, no fewer than four persons are required to transfer the patient from the stretcher to the OR bed. Since the patient is already anesthetized prior to positioning, it is important that proper body mechanics are employed. Proper transfer rests on the transfer of the patient as a unit. The arms and legs must be controlled to prevent problems, such as dislocation of the shoulders and brachial plexus injury. The perioperative nurse must insure that both the OR bed and the stretcher are locked and at approximately the same height to avoid dropping the patient between the stretcher and the OR bed.

Implementation

The patient is anesthetized on the stretcher or bed in the supine position. If the patient is anesthetized in the bed, the perioperative nurse should consider removing the headboard to facilitate intubation. Once the patient is anesthetized and stabilized, the patient's eyes are lubricated and taped. The patient is then positioned prone onto the OR bed. Since maintenance of the airway is a chief consideration, the anesthesiologist directs the turning and the positioning of the patient. The patient should not be moved until the anesthesiologist is ready.

When the patient is prone, the chest and abdomen are stabilized by the laminectomy frame or chest rolls, depending upon the surgeon's preference. If chest rolls are used, they should extend from the shoulders to the iliac crest bilaterally. Breasts and male genitalia should hang free from pressure. Female breasts should be positioned medially to the chest roll to allow for chest expansion and to prevent injury to the soft tissue. The feet should be maintained at a 45-degree angle to the legs and should be supported by pillows in order to prevent pressure on the toes. The head is positioned to the side on a foam or gel-filled pad. Pressure should be avoided to the ears and the eyes. The arms are placed on padded armboards with palms pronated. A safety strap is applied 2 inches above the posterior popliteal space and padded with a blanket.

JACKKNIFE OR KRASKE POSITION

Definition

A variation on the prone position is the jackknife or Kraske position (Fig. 8–21). This position is used to provide access to the sacral, perianal, perineal, and lower alimentary tract. The chief difference between the jackknife and prone positions is the exaggerated flexion of the thighs on the trunk to expose the buttock region.

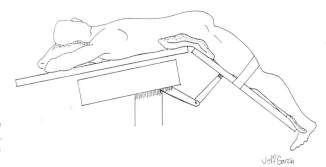

FIGURE 8-21. Jackknife/Kraske Position (Courtesy of Jeff Garcia, Houston, Texas, and AORN, Denver, Colorado)

Equipment

- Pillow or headrest
- 2 Armboards (or a laminectomy armboard)
- 2 Chest rolls (or a laminectomy frame)
- Safety strap
- 1 or 2 Pillows
- Padding
    Foam
    Gel pads
- 3″ Adhesive tape
- Benzoin spray

Assessment

In this position, both respiration and circulation can be jeopardized. As a result of restricted diaphragmatic movement and increased blood volume in the lungs, vital capacity can be reduced by 12.5% (Kneedler, 1989). Cardiac output may be affected as a result of a decrease in stroke volume. Venous pooling in the chest and feet causes a significant drop in the mean arterial pressure. Venous return may also be obstructed by reduced negative intrathoracic pressure. Slow venous return of blood, along with obtunded compensatory mechanisms produced by anesthetics, is the attributed causal factor of decreased mean arterial pressure.

On preoperative assessment, the patient should be assessed for thoracic outlet syndrome and subsequent compression of brachial, iliac, and subclavian vessels near the first rib. This condition requires that the patient's arms be retained by the sides of the trunk. Ventilation can be impaired through the weight of the patient's body, compressing the abdomen and forcing the diaphragm cephalad. Intra-abdominal pressure must exceed or reach venous pressure; otherwise, blood return from the lower extremities and pelvis is obstructed.

Planning

Planning for equipment needs is the same as that for the prone position.

Implementation

The OR bed is flexed at the patient's hips at a 90-degree angle. The patient's hips must be positioned over the central break of the OR bed. Chest rolls may be placed to raise the chest as required. Otherwise, the same positioning considerations are indicated as those in the prone position. In hemorrhoidectomy or pilonidal cystectomy, benzoin is sprayed on the area of the buttocks lateral to the surgical site to enhance the adhesive properties of the tape. Three-inch tape is then applied to the buttocks and secured to the OR bed with gentle traction. This method spreads the buttocks apart, providing exposure to the anal region. The knees must be heavily padded for extremely heavy patients or for those with pathology of the knees. The knee joints are prone to injury in the prone position.

In order to take the patient out of this position, the bed must first be flattened, and the order of steps in moving the patient in the prone position must be reversed. Both the OR bed and stretcher must be in the locked position, with two individuals on the stretcher side ready for the patient to be rolled onto their outstretched arms. The patient is gently lowered and positioned onto the stretcher.

LATERAL POSITION

Definition

Surgical procedures requiring the lateral position (Figs. 8–22 to 8–24) include nephrectomy, thoracotomy, and lobectomy. In the right lateral position the patient is on the right side with the left side up. The left lateral position provides surgical access to the right side.

Equipment

- Pillow or headrest
- Axillary roll
- Armboard
- Elevated armboard (or padded Mayo stand)
- Pillows
- Padding
    Foam
    Gel pads
- Wide adhesive tape
- Padded kidney rest
- Olympic Vac-Pac (suction beanbag)

Assessment

In the process of turning the patient from the supine to the lateral position, injury is possible to the dependent eye or ear. Corneal abrasion can occur if the eyes are not properly lubricated and taped closed. In the lateral position, the weight of the head against an uneven surface may result in contusion of the dependent ear. If the head of the patient is not supported in the lateral position, lateral flexion of the neck may occur. An arthritic cervical spine may be responsible for postopera-

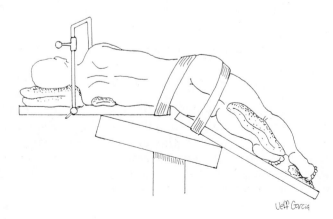

FIGURE 8-22. Lateral Position (Courtesy of Jeff Garcia, Houston, Texas, and AORN, Denver, Colorado)

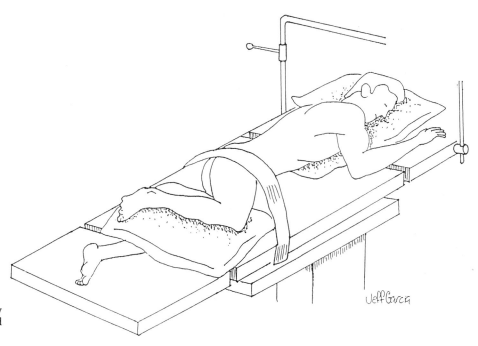

FIGURE 8-23. Lateral Position (Courtesy of Jeff Garcia, Houston, Texas, and AORN, Denver, Colorado)

tive neck pains. A pre-existing cervical disc protrusion may be aggravated unless the head is protected against flexion, extension, or rotation during positioning.

Circumduction of the dependent shoulder can stretch the nerve and result in dull shoulder pain. A supporting pad thick enough to raise the chest off the dependent shoulder should prevent circumduction injury to the suprascapular nerve. Because of restricted expansion of the dependent lung in the lateral position, atelectasis is possible. Flexion of the OR bed on the patient's flank or costal margin can further restrict chest expansion.

Femoral head compression as a result of misplaced restraining tape may result in excessive pressure or aseptic necrosis of the upper hip. Stabilizing tape must be placed across soft tissue on the upper hip in the area between the head of the femur and the crest of the ilium. The common peroneal nerve can be compressed by the weight of the dependent knee against the mattress of the OR bed. Padding the head of the fibula is usually sufficient. If the patient's legs are flexed laterally at the hips and below the level of the patient's head, venous stasis will occur in the lower extremities. Support stockings or Ace bandages can minimize this condition. Lateral flexion of the lower extremities may also obstruct venous return to the inferior vena cava (Barash, 1989).

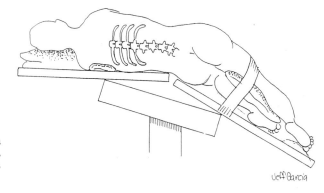

FIGURE 8-24. Lateral Position (Courtesy of Jeff Garcia, Houston, Texas, and AORN, Denver, Colorado)

Gravity tends to shift mediastinal structures in the direction of the dependent chest wall, thus the volume of the dependent lung will be further reduced. Additionally, force from the abdominal contents will be exerted on the dependent diaphragm if the long axis of the trunk is horizontal or the head is lower than the body. The upper chest wall is not as restricted as is the dependent side. There is less vascular congestion because this lung is above the level of the atria. Hyperventilation of the underperfused upper lung and hypoventilation of the congested dependent lung may be the result (Barash, 1989).

Planning

The patient is anesthetized and stabilized on the OR bed. As with the other positions, a four-person team is required. Personnel are positioned at the shoulders, hips, and legs to facilitate positioning. A draw sheet under the patient may also be used by the team.

Implementation

Although the patient may already be on the OR bed when the positioning process begins, in some cases, the transfer of the patient to the OR bed and subsequent positioning may begin following intubation and stabilization of the patient on the stretcher. When ready to position, the assistant at the shoulders and hips brings the patient to the edge of the stretcher. This is accomplished through the utilization of the stretcher sheet as a draw sheet. The assistant located at the shoulder uses his or her arm and hand nearest the patient to cross the chest and grasp the shoulder. The other hand is placed under the near shoulder. The assistant at the hip follows the same technique, crossing the hips and grasping the patient's opposite buttock with the arm and hand nearest the patient, while the other hand is placed under the nearest buttock (Meeker, 1991). The individual handling the legs must stand at the foot of the bed to support and position the legs during transfer. The pillow placed between the legs prevents pressure on the peroneal nerve as well as circulatory complications from excessive pressure from the upper leg. Support must be given to the ankle and foot of the upper leg to prevent footdrop.

The lower arm is positioned with the palm up on a padded armboard, while the upper arm is minimally flexed with the palm down. The lower arm is where the blood pressure cuff should be positioned. Shoulders should be symmetrically aligned, and a small roll or pad should be placed under the dependent axilla to relieve pressure and protect neurovascular structures. It is essential to maintain cervical alignment with the spine. The head should be supported with a pillow between the neck and shoulder to prevent stretching neck muscles, brachial plexus, and to insure maintenance of the patent airway. The elevation of the head is dependent upon the level the lower shoulder keeps with the head of the table. The lower leg is flexed at the hip and knee, keeping the upper leg straight and resting on pillows. Along with other positioning considerations, padding should be placed under both the dependent foot and knee. Positioning of female breasts and male genitalia must be checked after positioning is completed.

Wide adhesive tape may be applied across the hip and secured to the OR bed in an effort to stabilize the patient. The safety strap should be applied 2 inches above the knees and should lie across padded thighs. A padded kidney rest may also be added to stabilize the patient in the lateral position. When transferring he patient to the OR bed, the iliac crest should be positioned near the break of the table to facilitate elevation of the kidney rest. This step will provide increased exposure, as will flexing the OR bed in the middle. Peripheral pulses can be assessed before and after positioning the patient to insure circulation.

SEMISUPINE AND SEMIPRONE POSITION

Definition

The semilateral positions are helpful in reaching anterolateral (semisupine) or posterolateral (semiprone) structures of the trunk (Barash, 1989).

Equipment

- Pillow or headrest
- Axillary roll
- Armboard
- Elevated armboard (or padded Mayo stand)
- Pillows
- Padding
    Foam
    Gel pads
- Wide adhesive tape
- Padded kidney rest
- Sandbag
- Olympic Vac-Pac (suction beanbag)

Assessment

The assessment considerations for these two variations of the lateral position are consistent with the requirements of the traditional lateral position.

Planning

Planning for the semisupine and semiprone positions follows the same considerations as planning for the lateral positions.

Implementation

In the semisupine (Sims) position, support must be provided for the upper arm in order to avoid hyperextension. There should be no traction or compression to the brachial and axillary neurovascular bundles. The dorsal torso and hip should be padded to prevent the patient from slipping back into the supine position. The dependent arm is placed behind the patient in the semisupine position. This is to avoid stress on the shoulder. In order to maintain this position, the dependent lower extremity is straight and the upper leg is flexed at the knee and hip.

A semilateral position, such as the semisupine position described above, can be used for hip surgery by utilizing a sandbag under the affected hip or a suction beanbag under the dependent side to facilitate exposure. Padding of all positioning devices used must be appropriate. Arm positions are dependent upon the degree of lateral position.

Evaluation of Positioning Techniques

Evaluation should begin at the time of the assessment and should focus on desirable patient outcomes. *Standards and Recommended Practices for Perioperative Nursing* (AORN, 1994) should be the guideline to insure optimal patient outcomes. An outcomes management approach is particularly significant during the planning phase of surgical positioning. When the perioperative nurse plans patient care, awareness and knowledge of the patient's expected outcomes are part of the process. Patient outcomes can be a basis for either successful or unsuccessful medical litigation. The doctrine of *res ipse loquitur* provides for the inference of negligence rather than the requirement to submit proof that such negligence occurred. This requires the establishment of three provisions: (1) that the injury would not have occurred in the absence of negligence; (2) that the patient was not responsible for the injury; and (3) that the resultant injury was in the control of the actors. As implied, this doctrine can have a significant impact when addressing medical-legal implications for surgical positioning.

Successful patient outcomes, which are the result of successful surgical intervention, are highly dependent upon adequate exposure through surgical positioning. Patency of the airway, optimal respiratory effort and circulatory status, preservation of nerve integrity, protection of bony prominences from pressure areas, and patient comfort are examples of expected outcomes. Adequate preoperative teaching will in many cases contribute to positive patient outcomes. The perioperative nurse can optimize the likelihood of achieving measurable outcomes by discussing the intended surgical procedure with the patient in a nonthreatening environment conducive to patient and nurse interaction. Detailed and appropriate documentation must begin at assessment and follow through the course of surgical intervention. Further, collaboration between nursing, anesthesia, and surgical staff can help avoid postoperative complications related to positioning.

Consideration of the patient's individual needs also enhances outcome achievement. Special attention should be given to anomalies and physical defects. Modesty must be maintained, regardless of the patient's level of sensorium. Prior to the skin preparation and draping process, the perioperative nurse should observe the patient's final surgical position and determine its adherence to physiologic principles. Documentation must include limitation in range of motion preoperatively, condition of the skin both before and after the surgical procedures, and any special equipment utilized for positioning the patient.

Special Considerations for Surgical Positioning

The perioperative nurse is provided with a number of challenges when interacting with surgical patients. Pre-existing conditions that demand special attention have a direct impact on the perioperative nurse's ability to facilitate smooth, safe, and appropriate surgical positioning. Assessment and planning are critical to the perioperative nurse's ability to adapt positioning to pre-existing disorders. The objective is not to restrict already limited compensatory powers and further impair pathologic physical processes.

THE GERIATRIC PATIENT

The skin of the elderly patient is dry. Peripheral subcutaneous fat has been lost owing to the aging process. Skin integrity may be further compromised owing to the loss of elasticity and turgor. Atherosclerotic changes in the peripheral vascular circulation inhibit the normal process of healing. The elderly patient is predisposed to hematoma and purpura formation, so body parts, particularly limbs, must be handled gently to avoid soft tissue damage.

Poor nutritional status predisposes the skin to even more extensive breakdown. Since bony prominences have less natural padding, the elderly patient is predisposed to increased skin pressure during positioning. Ischemia results from decreased tissue perfusion as a result of peripheral vascular changes. A modified perception of pain and temperature is the result of changes in the central nervous system. As a result, bony prominences require additional padding. The perioperative nurse must thoroughly assess the integumentary system preoperatively, intraoperatively, and postoperatively and document any abnormalities and/or changes.

Osteoporosis, especially in women, leads to musculoskeletal changes in the elderly. Compression fractures of the vertebrae and broken bones are not uncommon. Since curvature of the thoracic spine increases with age, uneven pressure distribution over the thoracic spinous processes in the supine position may occur. The sacral promontory becomes more pronounced, making the sacrum the most common site of decubitus ulcer formation. Generalized loss of muscle bulk, tone, and strength necessitates extra padding. Foam, gel, or sheepskin padding facilitates even pressure distribution.

In the elderly, arthritic and muscular changes limit the range of motion. Peripheral joints, such as the knees and elbows, may require extra support during positioning and lengthy surgical procedures.

The elderly patient who has previously undergone a hip pinning, insertion of a femoral prosthesis, or total hip replacement may be particularly challenging placed in the lithotomy position. Legs should be raised slowly by two people and placed simultaneously into the stirrups. However, in certain cases the patient's range of motion may be so severely limited that surgical personnel may be required to hold the legs rather than placing them in stirrups. When more than the usual amount of abduction is required, one hand can be placed on the lateral hip as the thigh is externally rotated while being flexed. This position will prevent dislocation at the hip and will help alleviate strain on the groin.

Systemic vascular changes are prevalent in elderly patients. Arteriosclerosis increases peripheral vascular resistance. Blood flow to the tissues is diminished. Consequently, oxygen and nutrients supplied to tissues are diminished. Hypotension resulting from certain surgical positions may be problematic, since total blood volume is already lower in the elderly.

The supine, lithotomy, and sitting positions result in venostasis. Warm blankets prevent limbs from becoming cold and help maintain normal body temperature. Generally speaking, since the elderly patient has a decreased choreatic reserve, changes in position should occur slowly to compensate for physiologic response. Decreased subcutaneous tissue may cause peripheral nerves to be very superficial, making them more prone to pressure injury. In all cases, extremities should be handled carefully.

A diabetic elderly patient may have sensory nerve loss due to diabetic neuropathy. The perioperative nurse must make a complete assessment of any sensory or motor deficit. Respiratory problems are common in aged patients. As elasticity of lung tissue decreases, diffusion capacity and compliance in the chest wall are reduced (Agate, 1986). Positions that affect the respiratory system should be carefully evaluated, since vital capacity decreases with age.

THE OBESE PATIENT

Hypertension, diabetes, and cardiovascular disease are health problems to which the obese patient is predisposed, and these conditions impact positioning. A patient whose weight is 20% greater than the norm determined by the established height and weight standards is considered obese. Further, a patient who is 100 pounds over the standard is defined as being morbidly obese (Long, 1985). Although bony prominences do not appear superficial, pressure points in the obese patient must be considered in any surgical position. Since tissue perfusion is necessary to prevent degenerative tissue changes, disease processes commonly found in the obese patent, such as cardiovascular disease and/or diabetes, result in decreased circulation to peripheral areas. This fact, coupled with positioning pressure, can result in decubitus formation. In addition, when prepping the obese patient, care must be taken that the solution does not become trapped in skin folds, possibly causing excoriation.

Because of increased body weight, there is increased strain on joints and ligaments, causing chronic joint and back pain. Even in the supine position, the obese patient is subject to potential problems. Palliative surgical positioning measures may include a lumbar support or a pillow placed behind the thigh superior to the popliteal space. Care must be taken because circulatory impairment can occur when pillows are placed in the popliteal space. When pillows are used for support, they should be arranged so that compression of the popliteal space does not occur.

Positioning changes often result in circulatory volume changes. Venous return to the inferior vena cava is increased in the lithotomy position as a result of raising the legs and placing them in stirrups. Since the obese patient's activity places a greater workload on the heart, the potential danger of circulatory problems in the Trendelenburg position is great because of increased venous return to the heart from the lower extremities, causing the heart to work even harder. In lengthy procedures in which the legs are dependent, Ace bandages or anti-embolism stockings assist in venous return. Lowering the legs results in a 500- to 600-milliliter reduction, owing to the sudden inflow of blood into the extremities. Therefore, extreme changes in positioning must be done slowly to allow for physiologic compensation. When wrapping the legs, care must be taken not to compress the common peroneal nerve. The perioperative nurse must, therefore, assess cardiac function carefully.

Flexion at the groin may cause an obese patient to experience compression of the obturator nerve. Therefore, care should be exercised when placing the obese patient in the lithotomy position. Damage to the obturator nerve may result in weakness or paralysis of the abductors of the thigh. Placing an obese patient's arms at his or her sides on the OR bed is not ideal. This action may result in ulnar or radial nerve damage. Armboards will decrease the likelihood of nerve damage as a result of an arm or elbow protruding off the bed. Placing the arms across the chest also increases the patient's respiratory efforts.

Owing to the increased body weight on the chest and the decreased respiratory capacity, an obese patient may suffer from respiratory problems even when upright. Decreased lung compliance occurs because of excessive fat surrounding the chest. Anesthesia and positioning exacerbate these problems, and ventilatory support is usually required for the obese patient. There is an increased risk of aspiration in any surgical position because of pressure from the abdominal contents against the diaphragm.

THE MALNOURISHED PATIENT

Malnutrition affects the body's ability to deal with emotional and physical stress and wound healing and increases susceptibility to infection. A patient who is in a weakened state is considered to be debilitated. This condition may result from a disease process, an accident, or a self-imposed condition, making the patient prone to infection.

Since these patients may be thin, with poor skin turgor, bony prominences are superficial. There may be existing decubitus ulcers or skin excoriations. Pressure areas must be well padded and the skin gently handled.

The debilitated patient may have contracted joints and/or other limitations to range of motion. Lengthy procedures require footboards, particularly in the hemiplegic or paraplegic, where footdrop is a potential or actual problem. External rotation at the hip may be prevented through the use of a trochanter roll placed from the iliac crest to midthigh on the affected side. The paralyzed patient is particularly vulnerable to dislocation because of loss of muscle tone and mass. Since these patients have a loss of sensation, it is essential that the perioperative nurse make a thorough and complete assessment of the musculoskeletal system, both preoperatively and postoperatively. Dislocations and impairments in skin integrity may not be recognized immediately in the postoperative period.

The debilitated patient is susceptible to venostasis and thrombus formation.

The perioperative nurse must plan for interventions, such as elastic stockings, with those positions that encourage venostasis. Padding the patient's heels gives slight elevation to the calves. Damage to the endothelium of the veins, producing clot formation or loosening existing clots, may result from placing pillows under the calves.

Diminished body fat provides little protection for neural structures. The perioperative nurse must exercise caution when positioning in order to avoid nerve damage. The perioperative assessment should provide information regarding any existing paresthesia. Abnormalities must be documented, and a postoperative evaluation must be performed to assess for any changes.

Atelectasis is a potential in the debilitated patient. There is a decrease in vital capacity along with lung compliance. Positions that increase respiratory effort, such as the prone and Trendelenburg, are not tolerated well. Assessment by the perioperative nurse for cyanosis and respiratory effort and function should be ongoing when caring for the debilitated patient.

Issues for Future Development

With health care reform on the horizon, institutions are being mandated to streamline services and reduce expenses. More and more, surgical procedures are, and will continue to be, moved from a tertiary care setting to a same day surgery or freestanding ambulatory surgery facility. This certainly indicates a limitation in the perioperative nurse's interaction with, and subsequent assessment of, the surgical patient, both preoperatively and postoperatively. Consequently, the nurse's clinical impact must be maximized within a brief period of time. The perioperative nurse's ability to meet this challenge will certainly depend upon his or her positioning expertise. Since postoperative visits, in many cases, will not be feasible, the nurse must have a thorough understanding of the physiologic implications of surgical positioning. This should allow for a proactive patient care approach, which is so necessary in an environment in which the patient is admitted to and discharged from the hospital on the same day.

Gone are the days when health care providers could "make it all better" with a hospital stay. Patient interactions must be decisive and geared toward returning the patient to an optimal level of wellness in the shortest amount of time possible.

REFERENCES

Agate, J. (1986). Common symptoms and complaints. In: Rossman, I. ed. *Clinical Geriatrics.* 3rd ed. Philadelphia: J. B. Lippincott. (pp. 138–149).

Association of Operating Room Nurses. (1994). *Recommended Practices for Positioning the Surgical Patient.* Denver: AORN.

Association of Operating Room Nurses. *Standards and Recommended Practices for Perioperative Nursing.* (1994). Denver: AORN.

Atkinson, L. J. (1992). *Berry and Kohn's Introduction to Operating Room Technique.* 7th ed. New York: McGraw-Hill Book Company.

Barash, P. G., Cullen, B. F., Stoelting, R. K. (1989). *Clinical Anesthesia.* Philadelphia: J. B. Lippincott Company.

Fuerst, E. V., Wolff, L., Weitzel, M H. (1974). *Fundamentals of Nursing.* 5th ed. Philadelphia: J. B. Lippincott Company.

Gruendemann, B. J. (1987). *Positioning Plus.* Chatsworth, California: Devon Industries, Inc.

Kneedler, J. A., Dodge, G. H. (1989). *Perioperative Patient Care.* Boston: Blackwell Scientific Publications, Inc.

Long, B. C., Phipps, W. J. (1985). *Essentials of Medical-Surgical Nursing: A Nursing Process Approach.* St. Louis: C. V. Mosby Company.

Meeker, M. H., Rothrock, J. C. (1991). *Alexander's Care of the Patient in Surgery.* 9th ed. St. Louis: C. V. Mosby Company.

Smith, R. H. (1978). The prone position. In: Martin JT, ed. *Positioning in Anesthesia and Surgery.* Philadelphia: W. B. Saunders Company. (pp. 32–43).

Practice Scenario 1
Surgical Patient Intraoperative Positioning

by Deborah Alpers, RN, MS, CNOR, CNA

SCENARIO

Wayne Henderson is a 36-year-old black male who has been scheduled for a hemorrhoidectomy and rectal fistulectomy on an outpatient basis. He is 5 feet 11 inches tall and weighs 250 pounds. His hemoglobin is low (13 g/dL) owing to rectal bleeding.

Mr. Henderson has a history of asthma, which he developed around the age of 5. He has episodes of difficult breathing approximately six times a year, which are treated with an inhaler at the time of each episode. These episodes are usually initiated during high-stress periods. He does not smoke cigarettes; his alcohol use includes two to four glasses of beer per week. Mr. Henderson's current blood pressure is 138/96, which he controls by taking a daily antihypertension medication.

Mr. Henderson is a high school teacher. He spends most of his day standing and occasionally sitting. His evenings and weekends are spent working on a master's degree in education. He does not participate in a regular exercise program.

PERIOPERATIVE INTERPRETATION

Using what you have just learned in this chapter, as an experienced perioperative nurse you would consider the following in the care of this patient.

1. Assessment
   - Based upon the planned surgical procedure and surgeon preference, the prone position would be used for this patient.
   - The patient's height and weight are factors in safe positioning.
   - The patient's history of asthma, especially during stressful events, may increase the patient's risk for impaired air exchange.
   - The patient's low hemoglobin may also impair respiration and air exchange.
   - The patient's nutritional status and lack of regular exercise program may increase the chance for alteration in tissue perfusion and skin integrity while in the prone position.

   - The patient's hypertension may alter the patient's cardiac output.

NURSING DIAGNOSIS

   - High risk for alteration in tissue perfusion related to prone positioning and body size.
   - High risk for impairment of skin integrity related to prone positioning and imbalanced nutritional status.
   - High risk for impaired gas exchange related to positioning owing to restriction of chest wall expansion, movement of diaphragm, and history of asthma.

2. Planning
   - Schedule adequate personnel for transfer and positioning of patient after anesthesia induction.
   - Secure chest rolls, pillows, and padding to have available in the operating room for patient positioning.
   - Consult with the anesthesiologist on the patient's history in regard to hemoglobin and hematocrit values, history of asthma, and hypertension.

3. Implementation
   - Assess patient's pedal pulses before positioning patient, and after patient is positioned to insure peripheral tissue perfusion.
   - Position patient prone with appropriate number of experienced, knowledgeable personnel to turn patient. Assign specific roles to personnel for turning and positioning. Make sure the patient stretcher or bed is locked before turning the patient.
   - Pad the following areas: head and face, feet, arms (including elbows and wrists), chest, knees, and any other bony prominences. Eyes should be lubricated and taped shut for protection.
   - Chest rolls or pillows are placed under each side of the chest to raise body weight off the chest and facilitate respiration.

- Check genitalia to make sure that they are free of pressure and are hanging free.
- Position the patient's arms at right angles on armboards with palms downward. Care should be taken not to hyperextend the arms or use extreme abduction because this may injure the shoulder girdle and brachial plexus.
- Place the patient's safety strap 2 inches above the knees padded with a blanket.
- Document on the perioperative record the skin condition preoperatively and postoperatively. Also document pre-existing conditions, position and positioning aids used, and patient outcomes.

4. Evaluation
- Assess the patient's skin integrity for color changes, lesions, or breaks in the skin due to prone positioning. Assess for areas of redness on the head, ears, chest, knees, iliac crest, and other areas of the body where pressure points may develop. Check the temperature of the feet and the color of the toes.
- Assess the patient's peripheral pulses to insure continued tissue perfusion as compared with the patient's baseline.
- Report to PACU nurse regarding skin integrity, presence or absence of pedal pulses, patient's history of asthma, nutritional status, and preoperative hemoglobin and hematocrit levels.

Practice Scenario 2
Surgical Patient Intraoperative Positioning

by Elizabeth M. Edel, RN, MN, CNOR

SCENARIO

Paul Donovan is a 43-year-old male admitted with a diagnosis of persistent low back pain with retained orthopedic hardware. He is scheduled for a repeat decompression laminectomy bilaterally at lumbar 4-5 with Luque plates and screws. He has had a previous failed posterior fusion that resulted in continued pain and left leg weakness. The patient is 5 feet 8 inches tall and weighs 212 pounds. The patient has a history of borderline diabetes. Laboratory values indicate a fasting blood glucose of 133 and a glucose of 139. He smokes one to two packs of cigarettes daily and has a chronic cough. He has a short, thick neck. His current medications include pentazocine (Talwin) 50 mg orally every 4 hours and aspirin 10 grains every 8 hours for the past 6 weeks.

PERIOPERATIVE INTERPRETATION

Using what you have just learned in this chapter, as an experienced perioperative nurse you would consider the following in the care of this patient.

1. Assessment
   - Based on your preoperative assessment and knowledge of the surgical procedure, you know that the prone knee-chest position on the Andrews bed will be used.
   - The patient's short, thick neck is a potential concern for anesthesia intubation.
   - The patient's weight poses a potential problem in placing the patient in the knee-chest position.
   - The chronic back pain and left leg weakness should be considered when placing the patient in the knee-chest position.
   - Prior failed back surgery should also be considered in positioning the patient.
   - The daily use of aspirin could disturb the clotting mechanism and place the patient at risk for excessive bleeding.
   - The patient's smoking history and restriction of the lung expansion on the Andrews bed can potentially compromise the patient's respiratory status.

- The patient's history of borderline diabetes and NPO status may impact his metabolic balance. The morning of surgery preoperative glucose blood level and intravenous fluid therapy should be considered.

NURSING DIAGNOSIS

High risk for injury related to:
- body size
- surgical position
- prior failed back surgery
- decrease in mobility, left leg

Decreased respiratory excursion related to:
- surgical position
- history of smoking
- history of chronic cough

High risk for altered tissue perfusion related to:
- borderline diabetic status

2. Planning
   - Obtain sufficient padding, including chest rolls, knee and skin pads, buttock padding, and extra support for the head, and arms.
   - Consult with the surgeon and anesthesiologist on the daily use of aspirin.
   - Consult with the anesthesiologist on the patient's smoking history, chronic cough, and short, thick neck.
   - Collaborate with the anesthesiologist on planning support for the patient's head in the prone position with repositioning every hour during the surgical procedure.
   - Review the patient's preoperative blood glucose value for abnormal results. Discuss any altered values with the anesthesiologist and obtain supplies for intraoperative glucose monitoring.
   - Plan duties so as to be free to assist the anesthesiologist during the intubation.
   - Coordinate availability of extra personnel to help with positioning the patient in the prone position with a focus on the left leg weakness.

3. Implementation
   - Stay with the patient during the induction and intubation to offer emotional support and assistance considering the patient's short, thick neck.
   - Position the patient insuring that all body parts are padded and provide for maximum respiratory excursion. Insure that the patient's genital area is free and not compromised.
   - Assess the patient's peripheral pulses prior to and after placement in the prone position to ensure adequate circulation to distal tissues.
   - Remind the anesthesiologist to reposition the patient's head every hour.
   - Monitor the patient's blood loss by weighing the surgical sponges and measuring the contents of the suction canisters and recording hourly urine outputs. Report the results to the anesthesiologist and surgeon.
   - Monitor the patient's intraoperative blood glucose level in conjunction with the anesthesiologist.

   - Document on the intraoperative record the nursing interventions used to position the patient, including aids used and measures implemented to insure adequate tissue perfusion during surgery.

4. Evaluation
   - Report to the post-anesthesia care unit nurse the patient's back history, left leg weakness, diabetic status and intraoperative glucose level, smoking history and chronic cough, use of daily aspirin, and status of peripheral pulses.
   - Assess the patient's skin integrity postoperatively for any changes due to the surgical positioning and length of surgery.
   - Assess the patient's peripheral pulses postoperatively and compare to the patient's baseline to insure continued tissue perfusion.

Chapter Nine

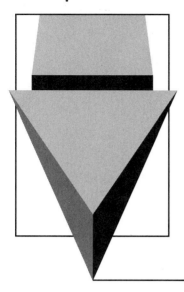

Surgical Wound Management

Donna Wahoff-Stice, RN, MSN, CNOR

Prerequisite Knowledge Prior to beginning this chapter, the learner should review anatomy and physiology, microbiology, and principles of wound healing. Chapter content correlates with several AORN Recommended Practices. These recommended practices may be considered a prerequisite to the chapter or a refresher upon completion of the chapter.

Recommended Practices for Aseptic Technique

Recommended Practices for Documentation of Perioperative Nursing Care

Recommended Practices for Electrosurgery

Recommended Practices for Skin Preparation of Patients

Recommended Practices for Safe Care Through Identification of Potential Hazards in the Surgical Environment

Learning Objectives

1. List the steps in performing a preoperative skin preparation.

2. Describe two techniques for achieving intraoperative hemostasis.

3. Name two absorbable and nonabsorbable sutures with the indications for their use.

4. Differentiate between closed and open wound drainage devices.

5. Assign the appropriate wound classification to uncomplicated surgical cases.

Preoperative Skin Preparation

Intact skin is the body's first line of defense against disease-causing microorganisms. The surgical incision creates a portal of entry for microorganisms. Surgical wound infections are a major source of postoperative morbidity. They account for about a quarter of the total number of nosocomial or hospital-acquired infections (Nichols, 1991). Postoperative wound infection carries consequences for patients and health care facilities. Wound infections can result in increased pain; time lost from work; and increased costs to the patient, facility, and third party payors. The goal of preoperative skin preparation is to reduce the risk of postoperative wound infection.

The human skin cannot be sterilized. However, it can be disinfected using chemical antimicrobial agents. Two types of bacteria, transient and resident microbes, are found on the skin. Transient organisms thrive in the environment created by dirt, sweat, and oil. There is little disagreement within the perioperative nursing community that the concentration of transient organisms on the skin can be effectively reduced by applying an antimicrobial solution (AORN, 1994; Fairchild, 1993; Larson, 1992; Meeker, 1991).

Resident bacteria adhere to epithelial cells. They live and multiply in the skin. Because resident bacteria extend downward between the epithelial cells into hair follicles and glands, they are not easily removed. Resident bacteria continually make their way to the surface of the skin. For this reason it is important that antimicrobial agents applied in the preoperative skin preparation have persistent or residual antimicrobial action.

PREOPERATIVE SKIN ASSESSMENT

Before beginning any surgical prep the perioperative nurse assesses the patient's skin. This assessment guides the nurse in planning nursing interventions. Assessment of the patient's preoperative skin condition sets the base line for postoperative evaluation of the desired outcomes of freedom from infection and injury.

Alterations in nutritional status, such as dehydration, hypovolemia, and extensive time NPO, can affect the texture and tone of the skin. Age and obesity also influence the condition of the skin. The skin of pediatric and geriatric patients is delicate and fragile. The thin delicate skin of infants can be easily injured by the chemicals contained in prep solutions. Similarly, geriatric patients frequently have dry nonresilient skin, which is easily irritated by chemicals and the friction of prepping procedures.

Skin assessment begins with visual inspection, paying careful attention to the surgical incision site. Rashes, bruises, lacerations, burns, or other alterations in the integrity of the skin can influence the choice of prepping agent or the decision to continue with elective surgeries. A skin infection in the area of the planned surgery, for example in the groin of a patient having an elective total hip replacement, could increase the risk of postoperative wound infection. By performing a preoperative skin assessment and consulting with the surgeon regarding abnormal findings, the perioperative nurse reduces the possibility that the patient will be admitted to the operating room and have an anesthetic induced, only to find when the blankets are removed that the patient has a skin infection in the area of the incision, and surgery must be canceled. A cancellation of this nature is detrimental to the patient and results in increased costs for opened unused supplies and wasted operating room time.

Visual inspection of the skin gives the perioperative nurse clues related to underlying physiologic conditions. For example, jaundice can be associated with hepatic disease, and pallor or cyanosis with anemia or inadequate oxygen exchange. These conditions can result in reduced resilience and increased fragility of the skin and increased risk for skin injury and postoperative wound infection.

Visual inspection of the incision site includes the amount of hair present. It has been clearly demonstrated through research that hair removal with a razor causes microabrasions, which are easily colonized by microorganisms, and results in increased rates of postoperative wound infection (Seropian, 1971; Cruse, 1980, Alexander, 1983). Hair is best left at the operative site. Some plastic and craniofacial surgeons, utilizing antimicrobial shampoos before surgery and barrier draping techniques, perform surgery on patients who have a full head of hair.

If the hair is so thick that it interferes with the surgical procedure and the surgeon orders that it be removed, clipping with an electric clipper or using a depilatory cream is preferable to shaving with a razor. Any hair removal must occur in an environment that offers warmth and privacy for the patient, and it must be done by an individual skilled in hair removal. It is undesirable to remove hair in the room where the surgery is to be performed, because dispersal of loose hair carries the potential to contaminate the wound or surgical field.

A patch test to detect sensitivity must be performed before using a depilatory cream. Manufacturers of some depilatory creams may recommend that a patch test be done as much as 24 hours before applying large quantities of the cream, making depilatory use difficult in outpatient surgeries. For hair removal, the depilatory cream is liberally applied to the skin surface, allowed to remain on the skin surface for the time recommended by the manufacturer, and then gently removed. After the hair and depilatory cream are removed, the skin must be thoroughly rinsed to remove any remaining chemicals.

An electric clipper may be the safest and most efficient method of hair removal. Electric clippers are available with both disposable and reusable heads.

PERIOPERATIVE HAIR REMOVAL AND WOUND INFECTION RATE

Seropian and Reynolds (1971) compared two matched groups of patients and showed that the postoperative wound infection rate after use of a depilatory cream was only 0% to 6%, and 5% to 6% in the group having a traditional shave. Cruse and Foord (1980) confirmed the findings of Seropian and Reynolds. They studied 62,939 surgical wounds over a 10-year period. The infection rate in clean wounds when the patient was shaved with a razor was 2.5%. Clean wounds when the hair was clipped with an electric hair clipper rather than shaved with a razor had an infection rate of 1.4%. *The lowest rate of infection, 0.9%, was in patients whose hair was neither clipped nor shaved.*

In spite of these extensive and well-conducted studies, hair is still shaved with a razor for some operating rooms. The overwhelming question is why does this outdated technique continue in perioperative practice? Hallstrom and Beck (1993) reported an evaluation of a planned change in the practice of using a razor for hair removal. At the start of the study, almost all patients in the facility were shaved preoperatively. Analysis of the responses to a pre-intervention questionnaire found that the respondents were well informed about the harmful effects of shaving. However, a pervasive attitude among surgeons was that shaving was good. The researchers shared the results of their study along with information about the harmfulness of shaving to small groups of perioperative staff members. A post-test was administered 16 months later. Attitudes about shaving had shifted from 59.4% thinking shaving was good in the pretest group, versus 30.5% thinking shaving was good in the post-test group. During the term of their study, practices did change. Entire surgical divisions shifted from shaving to clipping. Nursing involvement in the decision to remove hair preoperatively may put a stop to the unsafe practice of perioperative hair removal by shaving.

Disposable heads are intended for single use and are disposed of in a sharps container. Reusable heads must be cleaned after each patient and then sterilized or disinfected before being used again. It is helpful to stretch the skin over the area being clipped to minimize painful pulling of the hair as it is removed. Loose hair must be contained and not permitted to disperse about the patient's bed or the room.

If shaving with a razor is ordered by the surgeon, it must be performed as close to the time of operation as possible. Soaking the hair in soapy water before razor shaving will make the hair softer and easier to remove. Wet hair is also less likely to become dispersed. A clean disposable razor is used. The skin is held taut, and the razor is moved in the direction of the hair growth. Sliding the razor across the skin rather than lifting and setting it down will minimize nicking the skin. Nicks in the skin can increase the risk for wound infection. (Seropian, 1971; Cruse, 1980; Alexander, 1983). The perioperative nurse, as the patient's advocate, can discourage the practice of razor shaving.

Visual inspection of the skin is followed by touching the skin to assess temperature, texture, thickness, turgor, and mobility. By touching the skin, the nurse can determine that, although it appears intact, its fragility increases risk for injury.

The Braden Scale (Braden, 1989) has been designed and tested for use in predicting the risk for development of pressure ulcers (Table 9–1). The scale consists of six subscales: *Sensory perception, Moisture, Activity, Mobility, Nutrition, and Friction and shear.* The time frames in the operating room are not the 24-hour time frames upon which scoring with the Braden Scale is based. Many of the same time factors described in the subscales do exist for surgical patients who are under general or spinal anesthesia for more than 1 or 2 hours, however. When the Braden Scale is applied to the surgical patient under general anesthesia, the scores would be as follows:

		SCORE
Sensory perception	Unconscious	1
Moisture	Occasionally, with prep	3
Activity	Bedfast	1
Mobility	Immobile	1
Nutrition	Variable	1–4
Friction and shear	Potential problem with positioning	2
	Total	9–12

The creators of the Braden Scale consider patients with a score of less than 16 at risk for pressure ulcer development. Perioperative nurses, therefore, must consider the majority of patients in the operating room as being at risk for pressure ulcer development.

Preoperative assessment of the skin is the first step in planning nursing interventions related to both skin preparation and positioning. Preoperative assessment of the skin is essential for comparison with postoperative assessment data and evaluation of the desired outcome of freedom from skin injury.

ANTIMICROBIAL AGENTS FOR PREPPING

The choices of antimicrobial agents and the methods by which agents are applied are highly variable in clinical practice. The agents and methods for preoperative skin preparation are most often chosen by the operating surgeon. Traditionally, the skin has been vigorously scrubbed for 5 to 10 minute with the agent of choice. Surgeons' preferences vary and include wiping with alcohol followed by an antimicrobial scrub; using alcohol to remove the antimicrobial scrub; and using one agent to scrub the skin, followed by an antimicrobial paint, which is then removed with alcohol. Numerous studies have been conducted comparing the effectiveness of

- specific prepping agents
- scrubbing the skin versus painting the agent onto the skin
- plastic incise drapes containing antimicrobials placed over the prepped area
- varying amounts of time spent applying the antimicrobial agents.

In a review of the literature related to the effectiveness of preoperative skin preparations (Jepsen, 1993), it was suggested that conventional preoperative skin preparation techniques may not necessarily be the most effective. Other studies (Alexander, 1985; Rathburn, 1986) have found shorter prepping times, such as 1-minute scrub with 2% iodine in 90% alcohol followed by an application of an antimicrobial adhesive drape, or a 1-minute wipe with isopropyl alcohol followed by the application of an antimicrobial drape to be as effective as 5- to 10-minute scrub preps in reducing microbial counts.

There is no doubt that preoperative skin preparation reduces the potential for postoperative wound infection. Perioperative nurses must consult resource organizations, such as AORN (Association of Operating Room Nurses), APICE (Association for Practitioners in Infection Control and Epidemiology), and CDC (Centers for Disease Control and Prevention), and current research and manufacturers' literature and instructions for assistance in making informed decisions about preoperative skin preparation (Table 9–2).

Considerations in selecting an antimicrobial agent for use in preoperative skin preparation include

- Does this patient have an allergy to a specific antimicrobial? Some patients who are allergic to iodine will also react to povidone-iodine.
- What part of the body is to be prepped?

TABLE 9–1. BRADEN SCALE FOR PREDICTING PRESSURE SORE RISK

Patient's Name _____ Evaluator's Name _____ Date of Assessment

	1	2	3	4	
SENSORY PERCEPTION ability to respond meaningfully to pressure-related discomfort	**1. Completely Limited:** Unresponsive (does not moan, flinch, or grasp) to painful stimuli, due to diminished level of consciousness or sedation. OR limited ability to feel pain over most of body surface.	**2. Very Limited:** Responds only to painful stimuli. Cannot communicate discomfort except by moaning or restlessness. OR has a sensory impairment which limits the ability to feel pain or discomfort over 1/2 of body.	**3. Slightly Limited:** Responds to verbal commands, but cannot always communicate discomfort or need to be turned. OR has some sensory impairment which limits ability to feel pain or discomfort in 1 or 2 extremities.	**4. No Impairment:** Responds to verbal commands. Has no sensory deficit which would limit ability to feel or voice pain or discomfort.	
MOISTURE degree to which skin is exposed to moisture	**1. Constantly Moist:** Skin is kept moist almost constantly by perspiration, urine, etc. Dampness is detected every time patient is moved or turned.	**2. Very Moist:** Skin is often, but not always moist. Linen must be changed at least once a shift.	**3. Occasionally Moist:** Skin is occasionally moist, requiring an extra linen change approximately once a day.	**4. Rarely Moist:** Skin is usually dry, linen only requires changing at routine intervals.	
ACTIVITY degree of physical activity	**1. Bedfast:** Confined to bed.	**2. Chairfast:** Ability to walk severely limited or nonexistent. Cannot bear own weight and/or must be assisted into chair or wheelchair.	**3. Walks Occasionally:** Walks occasionally during day, but for very short distances, with or without assistance. Spends majority of each shift in bed or chair.	**4. Walks Frequently:** Walks outside the room at least twice a day and inside room at least once every 2 hours during waking hours.	

	1	2	3	4
MOBILITY ability to change and control body position	**1. Completely immobile:** Does not make even slight changes in body or extremity position without assistance.	**2. Very Limited:** Makes occasional slight changes in body or extremity position but unable to make frequent or significant changes independently.	**3. Slightly Limited:** Makes frequent though slight changes in body or extremity position independently.	**4. No Limitations:** Makes major and frequent changes in position without assistance.
NUTRITION *usual* food intake pattern	**1. Very Poor:** Never eats a complete meal. Rarely eats more than 1/3 of any food offered. Eats 2 servings or less of protein (meat or dairy products) per day. Takes fluids poorly. Does not take a liquid dietary supplement. OR is NPO and/or maintained on clear liquids or IV's for more than 5 days.	**2. Probably Inadequate:** Rarely eats a complete meal and generally eats only about 1/2 of any food offered. Protein intake includes only 3 servings of meat or dairy products per day. Occasionally will take a dietary supplement. OR receives less than optimum amount of liquid diet or tube feeding.	**3. Adequate:** Eats over half of most meals. Eats a total of 4 servings of protein (meat, dairy products) each day. Occasionally will refuse a meal, but will usually take a supplement if offered. OR is on a tube feeding or TPN regimen which probably meets most of nutritional needs.	**4. Excellent:** Eats most of every meal. Never refuses a meal. Usually eats a total of 4 or more servings of meat and dairy products. Occasionally eats between meals. Does not require supplementation.
FRICTION AND SHEAR	**1. Problem:** Requires moderate to maximum assistance in moving. Complete lifting without sliding against sheets is impossible. Frequently slides down in bed or chair, requiring frequent repositioning with maximum assistance. Spasticity, contractures or agitation leads to almost constant friction.	**2. Potential Problem:** Moves feebly or requires minimum assistance. During a move skin probably slides to some extent against sheets, chair, restraints, or other devices. Maintains relatively good position in chair or bed most of the time but occasionally slides down.	**3. No Apparent Problem:** Moves in bed and in chair independently and has sufficient muscle strength to lift up completely during move. Maintains good position in bed or chair at all times.	

Total Score

© Copyright Barbara Braden and Nancy Bergstrom, 1988
CON–63 (12/88) (Courtesy of Braden and Bergstrom. Reprinted by permission)

TABLE 9-2. **VARIABLES RELATED TO CHOICE OF ANTIMICROBIAL AGENT**

ANTIMICROBIAL AGENT	RAPIDITY OF ACTION	EXCELLENT TO GOOD EFFECTIVENESS	FAIR TO POOR EFFECTIVENESS	RESIDUAL EFFECT	PRECAUTIONS
Alcohol	1 minute	Gram-positive bacteria Gram-negative bacteria Fungi Viruses Mycobacterium tuberculosis		None	Volatile Drying to the skin Use with agents that promote residual antimicrobial activity
Iodine/iodophors	2 minutes	Gram-positive bacteria Gram-negative bacteria Fungi Viruses Mycobacterium tuberculosis		Minimal	Patients allergic to iodine may react to iodophors Can cause skin irritation Rapidly neutralized by organic materials such as blood or sputum Residual effect may be increased when combined with alcohol
Chlorhexidine	Rapid; as little as 15 seconds	Gram-positive bacteria Gram-negative bacteria Viruses	*Mycobacterium tuberculosis* Fungi	6 hours	Ototoxicity
PCMX (chloroxylenol)	Longer than above agents	Gram-positive bacteria	Gram-negative bacteria Fungi Viruses Mycobacterium tuberculosis	Good against gram-positive bacteria	Need further research
Hexachlorophene	Not fast-acting	Gram-positive bacteria	Gram-negative bacteria Fungi Viruses Mycobacterium tuberculosis	Good against gram-positive bacteria	Neurotoxicity Use only on intact skin

Adapted from Larson, 1988; Physician's Desk Reference, 1993; Purdue Frederick, 1989.

Chlorhexidine gluconate (Hibiclens) can result in ototoxicity if instilled into the inner ear. The manufacturer of Betadine, an iodophor, does not recommend using the scrub preparation on mucous membranes, such as the vagina, because it contains detergents. However, Betadine solution can be used in these areas.

- Does the antimicrobial kill gram-positive and gram-negative organisms, spores, viruses, and fungi?
  A broad range of germicidal action is desirable.
- How long does it take for the antimicrobial to work (rapidity of action)?
  Some antimicrobials act in 1 to 2 minutes, others may take 3 to 5 minutes. For how long does the antimicrobial continue to act as a bactericide after it is applied?
  Residual activity is desirable for longer procedures, such as open heart surgery or craniotomy.
- How long does it take to prep with this agent? In the operating room, time is money. If a shorter prep is as effective as a longer more complex prep, using the shorter prep may be cost-effective.

- How much does the prepping agent and associated supplies cost?
An expensive agent or additional supplies needed could negate time saved.

TECHNIQUES FOR SKIN PREPARATION

Skin preparation can begin before the patient is admitted to the health care facility. Depending on the type of surgical procedure to be performed, the surgeon may prescribe antimicrobial showering or shampooing before surgery.

For general anesthesia, the patient is anesthetized and positioned before the prep is started. If the surgery is to be performed using local anesthesia, the patient is positioned before the prep is begun. The circulating nurse verifies with the anesthesiologist that the patient is ready for the final skin prep. The nurse begins by exposing an area wide enough to provide a margin of safety to prevent contamination of the incision site (Fig. 9–1). It is essential that the nurse provide interventions, such as warm blankets, room temperature adjustment, and window shades, to maintain the patient's warmth and privacy. The prepped area must be wide enough to accommodate possible extension of the primary incision, additional secondary incisions, and placement of a wound drain. Drains are placed in a stab wound near the incision, not directly in the surgical incision, as they can be an additional portal of entry for microorganisms. Pulling back draping materials to extend an incision, add an incision site, or place a drain requires that the skin be reprepped and redraped.

An individual surgeon may prefer degreasing of the skin with alcohol or a commercial skin degreaser before the application of other antimicrobial agents. Alcohol rapidly kills most bacteria; however, it has minimal residual antimicrobial action. Degreasing the skin with alcohol improves the adhesion of self-adhering drapes.

Regardless of the choice of agents, the prep is performed in accordance with the principles of aseptic technique (AORN, 1994). An additional principle that applies to skin preparation is *prepping from clean areas to dirty areas*. The site of the surgical incision should be the cleanest area. The prep is, therefore, begun at the incision site. The person performing the prep works outward from the incision site. When the periphery is reached, the sponge is discarded and a new sponge is used (Fig. 9–2). Dripping of solutions from the periphery of the prep area toward the incision may carry microorganisms toward the incision. To prevent this situation, when possible, the incision site is positioned higher than the periphery. For example, if the incision is on the foot, the foot should be held higher than the knee. A second means of reducing occurrences of this form of contamination is to select agents less prone to dripping, such as gels.

An exception to the rule of beginning the prep at the incision site is made if the incision site is considered "dirty." Examples include a stoma, such as a colostomy, the rectum, vagina, or a draining abscess. Starting in an area that con-

PREPPING FOR LAPAROSCOPY

Current literature (Fogg, 1989) suggests that when prepping for laparoscopy, the perineal prep is performed first. The abdomen is prepped second, using a new set. The logic associated with doing the more contaminated perineal area first is that if the abdomen is first, it could become contaminated by aerosolization when the perineal area is scrubbed. This is a question that merits research. If it could be shown that there is minimal difference in microbial counts between the two methods, it would be more cost-effective to prep the cleaner abdomen first and use the same set to continue to prep the perineum.

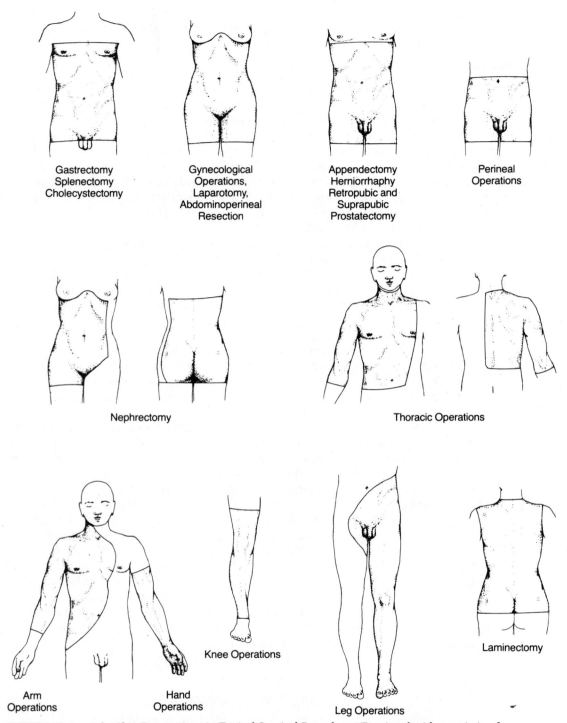

Gastrectomy
Splenectomy
Cholecystectomy

Gynecological
Operations,
Laparotomy,
Abdominoperineal
Resection

Appendectomy
Herniorrhaphy
Retropubic and
Suprapubic
Prostatectomy

Perineal
Operations

Nephrectomy

Thoracic Operations

Arm
Operations

Hand
Operations

Knee Operations

Leg Operations

Laminectomy

FIGURE 9–1. Areas for Skin Preparations in Typical Surgical Procedures (Reprinted with permission from Ethicon, Inc. from *Nursing Care of the Patient in the OR*, Copyright © 1987. Somerville, NJ: Ethicon, Inc.)

tains a large number of microorganisms may introduce bacteria into the surgical wound. In these situations, the cleaner area is done first, and the contaminated or dirty areas are prepped last (Fig. 9–3).

Along with their benefits, antimicrobial prep solutions present a potential hazard to patients. Prepping agents that collect or pool beneath the patient's body or a pneumatic tourniquet cuff can result in injury to the skin, which can result

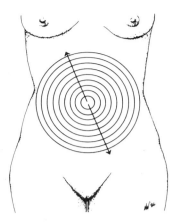

FIGURE 9–2. Prepping motion. Start abdominal prep at the site of incision. Move outward in circular motion. Do not return sponge to center but discard. Repeat the movement from the center outward. (Reprinted with permission from Ethicon, Inc. from *Nursing Care of the Patient in the OR,* Copyright © 1987. Somerville, NJ: Ethicon, Inc.)

in skin loss. In extreme cases of skin injury, debridement and skin grafting may be required. Patients with delicate or frail skin, such as children and the elderly, are especially at risk for injury due to pooled solutions. Towels placed along the boundary of the area to be prepped, around pneumatic tourniquet's cuff, or any location where solutions can pool will absorb the solutions and protect the patient's skin from injury. These towels can be removed at the conclusion of the prep, taking care not to contaminate the area.

Pooled solutions can also interfere with the safe operation of devices, such as the electrosurgical unit and electrocardiograph. The moisture can loosen the electrosurgical dispersive electrode, increasing risk for alternate grounding points. Wet electrocardiograph electrodes can interfere with readable EKG tracings.

Although the perioperative nurse is concerned about maintaining the patient's temperature, overwarming solutions can cause the solutions to become more concentrated, thereby increasing the risk of skin irritation and chemical burns. Solutions can also lose some of their effectiveness when stored at high temperatures (O'Neale, 1990). The issue of a cold solution becomes especially difficult when caring for pediatric and elderly patients, as these patient populations are at increased risk for hypothermia due to decreased subcutaneous fat and increased body surface area (Rothrock, 1990). A potential intervention is to maintain the prep solutions at a temperature that does not exceed 108°F or 42°C. The likelihood that a solution will become concentrated is further decreased if the solution is warmed for as brief a time as possible. However, warming in an autoclave or microwave could result in temperatures above 42°C.

Supplies can be purchased as a disposable kit or prepared and sterilized within the facility. Gauze and foam sponges can be used for applying prep solutions. Counted sponges should never be used for prepping. They can be easily discarded into the trash, resulting in an incorrect sponge count at the conclusion of the surgery.

As previously mentioned, antimicrobial solutions are capable of continued antimicrobial activity after their initial application to the skin. This continued

FIGURE 9–3. Prepping contaminated area. Start vaginal prep at mons pubis. Proceed downward; discard sponge when past anus. Cleanse vagina thoroughly. (Reprinted with permission from Ethicon, Inc. from *Nursing Care of the Patient in the OR,* Copyright © 1987. Somerville, NJ: Ethicon, Inc.)

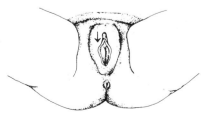

CLEAN VERSUS STERILE PREP KITS

AORN *Standards and Recommended Practices* (1994) state that a sterile prep set be used. In an initial study, Gauthier, O'Fallon, and Coppage (1993) found in 12 healthy volunteers that a clean prep kit was as effective as a sterile prep kit for disinfecting skin with povidone-iodine solutions. The clean prep kit was composed of nonsterile containers, sponges, towels, and exam gloves. Containers were washed in tap water and an enzymatic presoak and cleaner. This is a small study; however, if repeated studies with larger samples produce similar results, a change in practice could result in savings for health care facilities and patients.

ability to kill microbes is called *residual* activity. For greatest residual effect, antimicrobials need to dry on the skin. Removing the antimicrobial solution with saline or alcohol will reduce residual antimicrobial activity.

Many antimicrobial solutions contain alcohol. Alcohol is a flammable liquid and can be ignited by electrosurgical devices and lasers. The use of towels to absorb excess prep solutions and removal of the towels before draping the patient will help prevent skin irritation and remove any excess flammable liquids. Allowing solutions to dry before operating electrosurgical devices and lasers will reduce the risk that solutions containing alcohol will ignite the surgical drapes. Drape materials are fire retardant; however, they will burn.

DOCUMENTATION

Documentation is an essential component of all perioperative nursing care. Complete and accurate charting is the perioperative nurse's best legal defense. Documentation related to the surgical prep occurs in the preoperative, intraoperative, and postoperative phases of the surgical experience. Preoperatively, it is important to document that the perioperative nurse has checked for the presence of allergies, along with specific reactions the patient exhibits to the allergen; and has assessed the skin condition at the site of the proposed surgical incision. If hair removal has occurred, the time, method, and who removed the hair is documented. Intraoperatively, documentation includes the area prepped, the name of the person performing the prep, and all prepping solutions used. Postoperatively, documentation of the skin condition is essential to the evaluation of the expected outcomes for all surgical patients, and for insuring freedom from infection and freedom from injury. The patient's skin must be inspected in the area of the prep and in any areas where prep solutions may possibly have pooled. Associated with this postoperative skin assessment is observation for potential injury associated with surgical positioning.

Surgical Skin Incisions

The purpose of the surgical skin incision is to gain surgical exposure or access to the portion of the body upon which surgery is to be performed. Some factors that influence the surgeon's choice of incision site include ease and speed of reaching the site of surgical intervention and provision for maximum visibility and exposure. Causing as little trauma as possible will minimize postoperative pain and enhance postoperative wound healing.

The size and location of surgical incisions have evolved over time. Advances in endoscopic surgery have replaced large abdominal incisions with a few puncture wounds. These puncture wounds are often located in areas, such as the umbilicus, where they are close to invisible postoperatively. Another incision that serves the purposes of good surgical exposure and cosmetics is a bicoronal or ear-to-ear incision, which can provide access to the entire bony structure of the face while preventing scars on the face.

There are some commonalities to all skin incisions. First, the skin must be incised. Most commonly this is accomplished with the surgical knife, although other methods, such as the electrosurgical device or laser, can be utilized. The second layer encountered is the subcutaneous tissue. The amount of subcutaneous tissue varies with the location of the incision and the patient's size. For example, there is normally more subcutaneous tissue under the skin of the abdomen than in a finger or hand. The third layer encountered is muscle. Muscle is covered by a fibrous layer of fascia. Muscles can be separated by spreading apart and then retracting them. Muscles can also be cut and reapproximated at the time of wound closure. Because muscle is quite vascular, it is preferable to spread muscle rather than cut it if this alternative will provide adequate visibility and access. Cutting muscle also results in more postoperative pain than separating the muscle. Beyond the muscle usually lies the objective of the surgical intervention — the peritoneum containing the major abdominal organs, joint capsules such as the hip or knee, or the pericardium containing the heart. In some parts of the body, access after removing or retracting the muscle layer requires power or other instruments to cut through bone. Examples of these areas are the skull for access to the brain, the ribs for access to the thoracic cavity, and the sternum for access to the heart. Regardless of the surgical site, knowledge of anatomy assists the perioperative nurse in anticipating the wound exposure and closure methods that will be required for a given procedure. Questions the perioperative nurse can ask when planning perioperative nursing care related to wound management include

- On what region of the body will the team be performing surgery — extremity, chest, abdomen?
- Will soft tissue or bone be involved?
- How heavy and tough or delicate will the tissues be?
- How deep will the incision be?

Asking questions such as these will guide the perioperative nurse in planning for positioning and in determining the location of the surgical incision, the area to be prepped, the instruments needed for creating and maintaining the surgical exposure, and the type of suture and wound closure materials required.

INCISION LOCATIONS

Common incision sites of the abdomen are illustrated in Figure 9–4. A good understanding of medical terminology will allow the perioperative nurse to understand the location of most incisions.

GLOSSARY OF INCISIONAL TERMS

Anatomic directions

Superior: Above

Inferior: Below

Distal: Toward the termination or end (e.g., distal femur = above the knee joint)

Proximal: Toward the insertion or beginning (e.g., proximal tibia = below the knee joint)

Median: Middle or midline (usually refers to an abdominal incision; can be classified as upper or lower midline; can refer to above or below the umbilicus.)

FREQUENTLY USED ABDOMINAL INCISIONS

Most abdominal incisions are identified by their location on the surface of the abdomen. A few are referred to by the name of the surgeon who first proclaimed the advantages of each.

BODY LOCATION

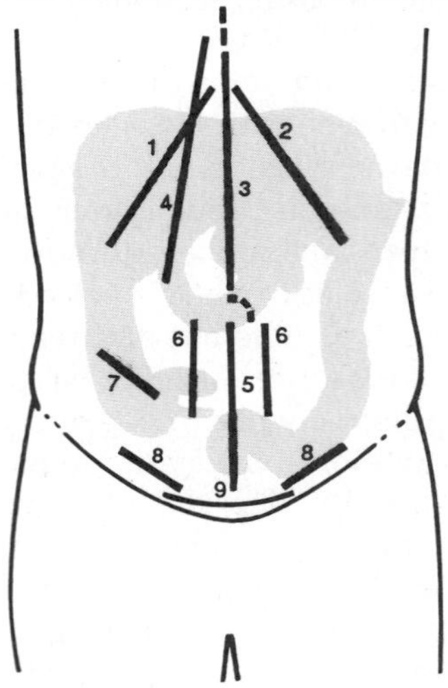

INCISION	USED FOR
1. Right subcostal (Kocher)	Gallbladder and biliary procedures
2. Left subcostal	Splenectomy; high gastric resection
3. Median upper abdominal	Stomach, duodenum, pancreas
4. Right upper paramedian	Stomach, duodenum, pancreas
5. Median lower abdominal	Uterus, adnexa; urinary bladder
6. Right or left lower paramedian	Pelvic structures; colon; abd. exploration
7. McBurney	Appendectomy
8. Left or right oblique inguinal	Hernia repair
9. Transverse suprapubic (Pfannenstiel)	Uterus, tubes, ovaries

FIGURE 9-4. Frequently used abdominal incisions (Copyright © 1978. Davis and Geck. All rights reserved)

Transverse: Across

Lateral: On or toward the side, left or right

Oblique: Slanted or inclined (e.g., inguinal hernia incision and appendectomy. The appendectomy incision is also called McBurney's incision.)

Endoscopic surgery generally requires a minimum of two incisions or puncture wounds (Figs. 9-5 and 9-6). The first puncture wound accommodates the operating scope, which is usually attached to a video camera. The camera allows the surgeon to visualize the surgery on a television monitor rather than through the lens of the laparoscope. Subsequent puncture wounds provide access for instrumentation, such as cutting, suction, grasping, suturing, and stapling devices. As more instrumentation and changes of angle are required for the instrumentation, additional puncture wounds are added.

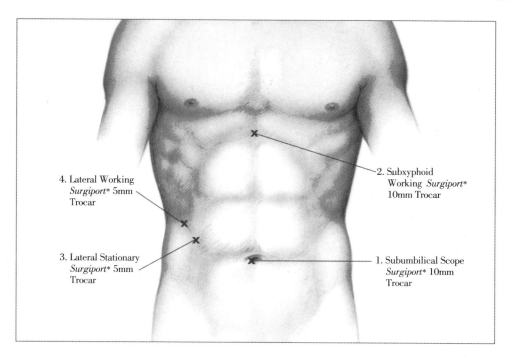

1. The subumbilical scope *Surgiport** 10mm trocar.

2. The subxyphoid working *Surgiport** 10mm trocar.

3. The lateral stationary *Surgiport** 5mm trocar (placed as lateral as possible under direct vision and 1 inch below costal margin).

4. The lateral working *Surgiport** 5mm trocar (placed 1 inch medial to the lateral stationary trocar).

FIGURE 9–5. Trocar Placement for Laparoscopic Cholecystectomy and Operative Cholangiogram (Copyright © 1992, 1994 United States Surgical Corporation. All rights reserved. Reprinted with the permission from United States Surgical Corporation, Norwalk, Connecticut. From Quilici, P. J. 1992. *New Developments in Laparoscopy.* Norwalk, Conn: USSC. p. 20)

Intraoperative Hemostasis, Suture, and Wound Closure

Hemostasis is the arrest and control of bleeding. Historically, the inability to control bleeding was a major obstacle to the evolution of surgical intervention. War injuries and other traumatic wounds, however, required some attempt at hemostasis before a wounded person expired. Archaeologists have found Egyptian mummies dating from 2000 B.C., which bear wounds that have been sewn closed with some type of suture material. However, suture material was not widely used until many centuries later; perhaps because unsterile sutures led to infection. In the early centuries, in addition to manual pressure and tourniquets, more barbaric methods of hemostasis, such as hot irons and hot oil, were employed to cauterize wounds (Fairchild, 1993).

In 1545, a French barber-surgeon, Ambrose Paré, developed a safe method for controlling bleeding, the suture ligature. In this method, a strand of suture is used to tie closed the open end of a severed blood vessel (Fairchild, 1993). This

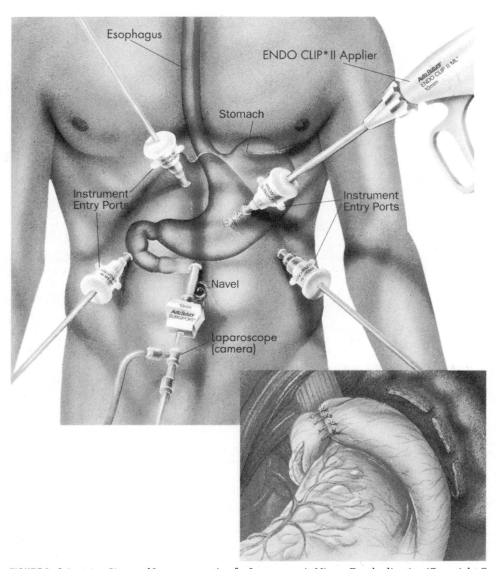

FIGURE 9–6. Incision Sites and Instrumentation for Laparoscopic Nissen Fundoplication (Copyright © 1994 United States Surgical Corporation. All rights reserved. Reprinted with the permission from United States Surgical Corporation, Norwalk, Connecticut. From Quilici, P. J. 1992. *New Developments in Laparoscopy*. Norwalk, Conn: USSC)

technique is still employed today. Additional methods of modern hemostasis include electrosurgery, hemostatic instruments, and chemical agents.

Adequate surgical hemostasis is essential to postoperative wound healing. Masses of clotted blood remaining at the surgical site delay healing and present an ideal medium for the growth of pathogenic microorganisms.

Hemostasis following injury to a blood vessel is a normal physiologic mechanism that consists of a complex sequence of events. First, the vessel constricts with vasospasm. Second, platelets, which normally circulate freely in blood plasma, begin to adhere to the exposed subendothelial layers of the injured vessel wall. Clot formation is the third event in the process of normal hemostasis.

A blood clot consists of a mesh of protein strands. This mesh stabilizes the plug already formed by platelets and continues to collect additional cells. The protein strands of the mesh are made of fibrin. Unlike platelets, which are normally present in plasma, fibrin is not normally present in blood. Fibrin is the result of a coagulation cascade, whereby a series of clotting factors is activated and transformed, resulting in the formation of fibrin (McCance, 1994; Guyton, 1991).

ASSESSMENT

Preoperative assessment is essential to anticipating the potential for bleeding and the methods of hemostasis that are required to control bleeding. Bleeding pathologies can be recognized preoperatively by means of a thorough history and physical examination coupled with laboratory studies. Given sufficient time, normal blood will clot. Excessive bleeding can result from inadequate amounts of any of the many clotting factors involved in the coagulation cascade. Three significant bleeding pathologies are vitamin K deficiency, hemophilia, and thrombocytopenia (platelet deficiency).

Vitamin K is necessary for the formation of four clotting factors involved in the formation of fibrin. Fortunately, vitamin K is continually synthesized in the intestinal tract by bacteria. However, vitamin K deficiency can be anticipated in newborns, because they do not have established intestinal flora. A second cause of vitamin K deficiency is failure of the liver to secrete adequate amounts of bile. Bile is necessary for the absorption of vitamin K, because vitamin K is fat soluble. Vitamin K can be administered by intramuscular injection when vitamin K deficiency is suspected.

The majority of clotting factors are synthesized in the liver. The perioperative nurse, therefore, can anticipate that in pathologies associated with the liver, such as hepatitis, cirrhosis, and carcinoma, the possibility of altered clotting mechanisms exists. Fresh-frozen plasma may be administered before surgery in an effort to correct deficits.

Hemophilia is an inherited bleeding tendency that occurs almost exclusively in males. In 85% of cases, it is caused by a deficiency of factor VIII, which is essential for the formation of fibrin. This bleeding trait can exhibit varying degrees of severity. Assessing for patient and family bleeding tendencies and observing the skin for bruising are methods of preoperative screening. However, most hemophiliacs are identified prior to their need for surgery. Treatment consists of administering the specific factor in which the patient's blood is deficient.

Thrombocytopenia is a condition in which the blood plasma has an inadequate number of platelets. Bleeding does not usually occur until the number of platelets in the blood falls below 50,000 per microliter. Normal levels range from 150,000 to 300,000 platelets per microliter. Preoperative screening for thrombocytopenia includes careful inspection of the skin for small hemorrhagic spots, petechiae, and purpura. Petechiae are small, purplish, hemorrhagic spots on the skin. Purpura are larger and are the result of hemorrhage into the skin. They are initially red, darken to purple, then turn brownish yellow. Laboratory assessment of the platelet count is essential if thrombocytopenia is suspected.

MECHANICAL HEMOSTASIS

The simplest method of applying mechanical hemostasis is to apply pressure on a bleeding site with a gauze sponge. Pneumatic tourniquets are frequently used to obstruct blood flow when surgery is performed on an extremity. The pneumatic tourniquet provides for a bloodless surgical field but does not provide for hemostasis after the tourniquet is released. Vessels must be cauterized and a pressure dressing can be applied to accomplish hemostasis.

The use of bone wax, made of refined beeswax, is another form of mechanical hemostasis. It is particularly effective in controlling bleeding from bone marrow. The bone wax is rolled into small balls and applied to the bleeding marrow with either a finger or the tip of an instrument. Excess bone wax must be removed, because it can interfere with bone healing.

As mentioned earlier, a suture ligature can be utilized to ligate or tie blood vessels. The blood vessel is clamped with surgical instruments, cut, and ligated with suture. Suture ligatures can be applied "free," without a needle, or as a "stick tie," with a needle attached. Larger vessels require a stick tie suture ligature.

The method of hemostasis most frequently chosen to control bleeding in smaller vessels is the electrosurgical unit. It is far less time-consuming to cauterize small vessels with the electrosurgical unit than to clamp, cut, and tie each vessel with a suture ligature.

ELECTROSURGERY

Electrosurgery involves the passing of high energy radio frequency current through the patient's tissue. The tissue is heated and cauterized. The electrosurgical generator is connected to a standard electric outlet and produces high frequency electric energy. This high frequency energy travels through the active electrode to the tissue that the surgeon wishes to cauterize. To perform monopolar electrosurgery safely, it is necessary to have a power generating unit, an active electrode attached to the generator, and a dispersive electrode on the patient and connected to the generator (Fig. 9–7).

Allowing for the high energy radio frequency current to safely pass through the patient's body is a major safety concern. There are three potential sites for patient burns resulting from high energy radio frequency current. The intended site is at the active electrode. One unintended location may be an alternate ground site that forms where the patient is in contact with metal objects, such as electrocardiograph electrodes. Current diversion to a site other than the dispersive electrode can result in patient burns. An isolated electrosurgery generator minimizes current diversion and alternate ground sites.

A second unintended location for high energy radio frequency is under the dispersive electrode, which is intended to return the energy to the generating unit. Current may concentrate owing to poor contact between the patient and

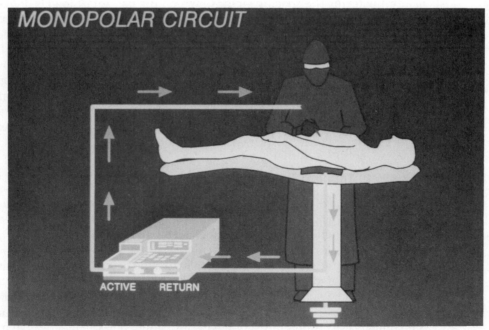

FIGURE 9–7. Monopolar electrosurgical circuit. Electrosurgical energy travels from the electrosurgical generating unit to the active electrode, through the patient's tissue to the dispersive electrode, and returns to the electrosurgical generator. (Courtesy of Valleylab, Inc., Boulder, Colorado)

the dispersive electrode. The dispersive electrode controls where the radio frequency energy exits the patient's body. To reduce the potential for increased temperature and burns at the site where the energy exits the body, the dispersive electrode must provide a large enough surface area for the current to maintain a low density. In order for the dispersive electrode to provide sufficient surface area, its placement must be carefully planned. When placing the dispersive electrode

- Place it as close to the surgical site as possible.
- Place it over a large muscle mass.
- Do not place it over scar tissue.
- Insure that it is in complete contact with the skin. Hair at the dispersive site, moisture from prep solutions, or tension on the cord can reduce dispersive electrode surface area contact.
- Do not include metal implants in the circuit path from active electrode to return electrode. Metal implants can carry a fraction of the electrosurgical energy (Egan, 1994; Pearce, 1986).
- Do not include a pacemaker in the electrical circuit between active and dispersive electrodes.
- Inactivate implantable defibrillators before switching on the electrosurgical unit.

The majority of electrosurgical burns have been caused by a fault condition at the dispersive electrode site, i.e., poor electrical connection between the patient and the dispersive electrode. The causes of poor electrical connection between patient and dispersive electrode are incorrect placement and reduced contact between the dispersive electrode and the patient's skin. Many electrosurgical units have devices that monitor the continuity of the electrical circuit but do not monitor the contact impedance of the dispersive electrode. Valleylab developed the Return Electrode Monitoring Circuit (REM), which measures the dispersive electrode/patient impedance through a current separate from the current being used for electrosurgery. This current travels from the generator, through the cord of the dispersive electrode, to one half of the dispersive electrode, through the patient's tissue, to the other half of the dispersive electrode, and back to the REM monitor in the generator. If the impedance is unacceptable, an inhibit circuit prevents the operation of the electrosurgical generator and causes an alarm to sound (Valleylab, 1986). It is essential that audible alarms *never* be turned off on any electrosurgical unit.

Electrosurgical generators can be utilized with monopolar or bipolar active electrodes. Active electrodes are available in many forms. Most frequently, a monopolar active electrode resembling a pencil is used. Various tips that allow for added length or diameter (needle, ball, loop) are available (Fig. 9–8). Monopolar active electrodes require a dispersive electrode to return the applied electrical energy to the electrosurgical generator (Fig. 9–9).

Bipolar electrosurgery does not require a dispersive electrode to return the electrical energy to the generator. The bipolar active electrode resembles forceps (Fig. 9–10). One tip of the forceps is the active electrode, and the opposing tip functions as the dispersive electrode. Electrical current exits the generator, travels across the bipolar forceps, and returns via the same cord (Fig. 9–11). Because the electrical energy is applied to a small area between the tips of the bipolar forceps, lower wattage is required. Bipolar active electrodes are available in many sizes and types of forceps. Bipolar electrosurgery is frequently used on delicate tissues of the neurologic and cardiovascular systems.

All active electrodes must be protected from inadvertent contact with the patient. An active electrode that is left on the surgical field can be turned on accidentally. If the electrode is accidentally activated while in contact with the patient's skin, the patient can be burned. Any portion of a metal instrument that is

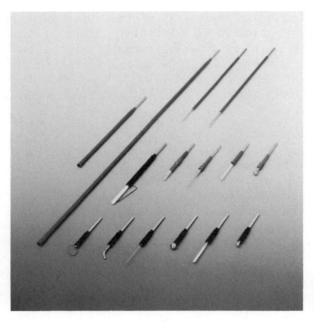

FIGURE 9–8. Active Electrode Tip Examples (Courtesy of Valleylab, Inc., Boulder, Colorado)

not insulated will conduct electrical energy. An active electrode in contact with forceps that are in contact with both the vessel to be cauterized and the patient's skin will burn the patient's skin. An additional hazard is an activated electrode that is in contact with the surgical drapes. The drapes can be ignited. The safest way to handle the active electrode is to keep it clean and dry and sheathed in a nonconductive safety holster in a highly visible area when not in use (AORN, 1994).

TROUBLESHOOTING ALARMS

The first step when an alarm occurs is to check the cords connecting the dispersive and active electrodes to the generator. The second step is to check the dispersive electrode itself. It may have become dislodged if the patient has been repositioned after it was applied. For this reason, it is always advisable to place the dispersive electrode after the patient has been positioned and to check the dis-

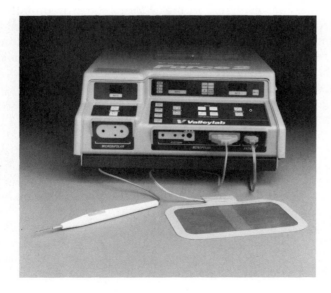

FIGURE 9–9. Electrosurgical Unit with Monopolar Active and Dispersive Electrodes (Courtesy of Valleylab, Inc., Boulder, Colorado)

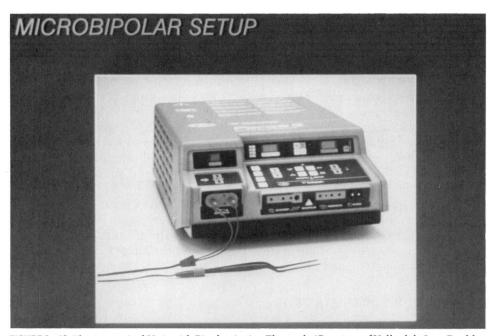

FIGURE 9–10. Electrosurgical Unit with Bipolar Active Electrode (Courtesy of Valleylab, Inc., Boulder, Colorado)

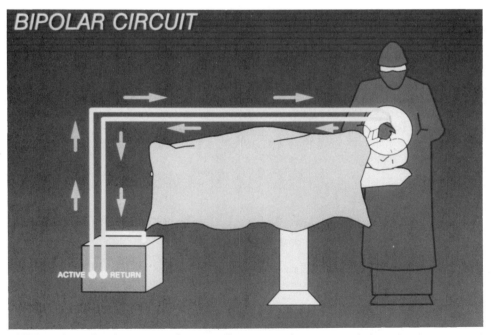

FIGURE 9–11. Bipolar electrosurgical circuit. Electrosurgical energy travels from the electrosurgical generating unit to the active electrode, through the patient's tissue to the opposite side of the forceps which acts as the dispersive electrode, and returns to the electrosurgical generator. (Courtesy of Valleylab, Inc., Boulder, Colorado)

persive electrode if the patient's position has been changed. Prep solutions may have come in contact with the dispersive electrode. The gel on the dispersive electrode may have dried. All of these possibilities are best handled by placing a new dispersive electrode.

If the dispersive electrode does not appear to be causing the alarm, the active electrode can be replaced. Failure to correct the alarm with these measures will require switching to a different electrosurgical generator. The generator that gave the alarm must be sent to the facility's biomedical engineer along with a description of the problem and all active and dispersive electrodes. The contaminated pieces must be contained in plastic and labeled as potentially biohazardous. The biomedical engineer will need all of the involved equipment to determine the cause of the alarm (Table 9–3).

Postoperatively, the dispersive electrode must be removed carefully. By slowly peeling back the pad, irritation to the patient's skin is minimized. It is essential for the perioperative nurse to assess the patient's skin condition at the site of the dispersive electrode at the conclusion of the surgical intervention and to document abnormal findings.

PHARMACOLOGIC HEMOSTASIS

Historically, combinations of crushed roots, bark, leaves, egg yolk, and even dust and cobwebs have been packed into wounds to staunch bleeding. Today, with a better understanding of the mechanisms that cause blood to clot, pharmacologic enhancement of clotting is possible.

Most drugs that promote hemostasis are applied topically (Table 9–4). Fibrin is the basis for the clotting of blood. In the normal clotting cascade, thrombin, in the presence of calcium, acts on fibrinogen, resulting in the conversion of fibrinogen to fibrin. Thrombin can be applied topically to a bleeding area, alone, or absorbed in a second product such as Gelfoam. Products such as Avitine, Instat, and Helistat are composed of collagen, which provides a surface for the aggregation of platelets.

Styptics are chemicals that, when applied topically, assist in achieving hemostasis by causing vasoconstriction. Examples include epinephrine, silver nitrate, and tannic acid. Epinephrine is the most frequently used styptic, and it is

TABLE 9–3. ELECTROSURGICAL SAFETY

Check all cords for fraying or breakage
Check that alarms are activated and functional
Place dispersive electrode as close to surgical site as feasible
Place dispersive electrode over a large muscle mass
Do not place over retained hardware or metal prosthesis
Place dispersive electrode after the patient has been positioned, prior to draping
Remove hair if necessary
Apply to a dry site
Keep the site dry, i.e., prep solutions, irrigation, blood
Check dispersive electrode if patient is repositioned
Keep active electrode from accidental contact with the patient and drapes by utilizing a holder or sheath
Remove the dispersive electrode slowly to minimize skin irritation
Repeated requests from the surgeon for more power may indicate a failure in the safety system
If an alarm occurs
    Check all connections
    Check dispersive electrode and replace if necessary
    Replace active electrode
    Replace electrosurgical generator
    Send generator and all dispersive and active electrodes to biomedical engineer

TABLE 9-4. **HEMOSTATIC AGENTS**

GENERIC/TRADE NAME	ACTION/ABSORPTION	NURSING IMPLICATIONS
Thrombin Thrombostat (Parke-Davis) Thrombogen (Johnson & Johnson)	Catalyzes the conversion of fibrinogen to fibrin Absorbed immediately	Can be dusted on as a powder or reconstituted with saline in dilutions of 100 to 1,000 U.S.P. units per milliliter for soaking other hemostatic agents, or spraying Can be stored in the refrigerator for 3 hours Acts rapidly Washes off easily Does not control arterial bleeding unless combined with other agents Causes intravascular thrombosis if enters the vascular space
Absorbable gelatin sponge Gelfoam, Gelfilm (Upjohn)	Absorbs 45 times its weight in blood for size, and thereby exerts pressure Absorption varies, 1–6 months	Can be cut to desired size Usually soaked in hemostatic agent such as thrombin May cause excessive pressure in confined spaces Accumulation of blood left in place could increase risk of wound infection
Microfibrillar collagen • Avitine (MedChem)	Provides surface for aggregation of platelets Hemostasis occurs in 1–4 minutes Absorbed in approximately 80 days	Very hydrophilic, adheres to any moist surface, i.e., gloves, forceps. Use clean dry forceps, avoid contact with gloves. Moistening with thrombin or saline decreases hemostatic ability. Do not use with autologous blood salvage units. Available as loose powder, compacted sheet, endoscopic applicator
Collagen sponge • Helistat	Platelets aggregate on sheet May be left in situ, absorbs a part of clot	Applied to bleeding site with pressure
Oxidized cellulose Oxycel (Becton & Dickinson) Oxidized regenerated cellulose Surgicel (Johnson & Johnson)	Acts by mechanical mechanism; does not enhance the coagulation cascade to form a gelatinous mass that absorbs 7–8 times its weight in blood May be left in situ, but advisable to remove after clot forms	Available in sheets and pads and can be cut Applied dry May cause excessive pressure in confined spaces Bactericidal against wide range of gram-negative and gram-positive bacteria owing to low pH

Adapted from Johnson & Johnson (1990); Mason (1988); Moak (1991).

contained in many local anesthetics in varying concentrations. Vasoconstriction decreases bleeding as well as the rate at which the local anesthetic is absorbed. Topical epinephrine can be absorbed into gelatin sponges and placed on a bleeding area.

Aminocaproic acid (Amicar) is a systemic agent that acts by inhibiting fibrinolysis. Fibrinolysis, or the dissolution of fibrin by fibrinolysin, can occur when the body is subjected to extreme stress, anoxia, or hypoglycemia. In a fibrinolytic state, the patient's blood is unable to clot. Fibrinolytic bleeding can be a complication of heart surgery or hepatic disease.

SUTURE IN HEMOSTASIS AND WOUND CLOSURE

It is easy for the novice perioperative nurse to become confused by the wide variety of suture available. Gaining a basic understanding of suture entails:

- understanding categories of suture material and their properties
- differentiating the size or gauge of suture
- understanding the types of needles that can be attached to, or used with, a suture.

Manufacturers produce similar products with subtle variations within each category of material. For example, a nonabsorbable monofilament nylon suture is marketed as Ethilon by Ethicon, Dermalon by Davis and Geck, and Monosof by US Surgical Corporation (Table 9–5).

Suture in the surgical environment is employed to ligate blood vessels, create surgical repairs, reapproximate tissues, and close surgical wounds. Characteristics of suture that are desirable include

- minimal tissue reaction and no propensity to encourage wound infection
- high tensile strength (knot-pull strength of the suture)
- ease in handling
- predictable rate of reabsorption.

TABLE 9–5. SUTURE MATERIAL/NAME BY MANUFACTURER

MATERIAL	DAVIS & GECK	ETHICON	U.S. SURGICAL	DEKNATAL
Plain gut Absorbable	Plain	Plain	Plain gut type A	
Chromic gut Absorbable	Chromic	Chromic	Chromic gut type C	
Synthetic Absorbable	Dexon (braided) Maxon (monofilament)	Vicryl (braided) PDS (monofilament)	Polysorb	
Natural Silk Nonabsorbable	Surgical Silk	Surgical Silk (siliconized) Permahand Silk (uncoated)	Sofsilk	
Monofilament Polypropylene Nonabsorbable	Surgilene Novafil	Prolene	Surgipro	Deklene
Nylon Nonabsorbable	Dermalon (monofilament) Surgilon (braided)	Ethilon (monofilament) Nurolon (braided)	Monosof (monofilament) Bralon (braided)	
Polyester Dacron Coated Braided Nonabsorbable	Ticron Polyester (coated) Dacron (uncoated)	Ethibond Extra (coated) Mersilene (uncoated)	Surgidac	Tevdek (high coated) "Silky" Polydek (low coated) "Cottony" Polydek (uncoated)
Polyester Dacron Uncoated Monofilament Nonabsorbable		Mersilene	Surgidac	
316L Stainless Steel Nonabsorbable	Flexon	Ethisteel	Steel	Steel

Reading the outside of the suture package will give the perioperative nurse most of the needed information about the suture inside (Fig. 9–12).

Some key elements are

- name
- type of material
- absorbability
- gauge (diameter or size)
- length
- type & number of needles (if any).

All suture, regardless of the material from which it is made, is available in a range of sizes and tensile strengths. The size of a suture denotes the diameter of the suture material. Imagine a horizontal line with 0 at the center. To the right of the 0, whole numbers 1, 2, 3 and so on denote larger sizes of suture. To the left of the 0, increasing numbers 2-0, 3-0, 4-0 and so on indicate smaller diameters. Hence, the larger the number preceding the 0, the smaller the diameter of the suture. The larger the whole number, the larger the diameter of the suture (Fig. 9–13).

Tensile strength refers to the knot-pull strength of the suture. Knot-pull strength is the amount of resistance a tied knot provides before breaking, not the straight-pull strength of a strand of suture. Minimum knot-pull strengths are specified for each suture size by the United States Pharmacopeia (USP). It is logical that as suture size decreases, so does tensile strength. It follows that a 10-0 suture has less tensile strength than an 8-0 suture, a 0 less than a 1 and so on.

Choice of suture length varies with the application for which the suture is intended. For example, suture for a running or continuous application needs to be longer than suture for interrupted or single stitches. Free ties, precut lengths of suture packaged without a needle, are utilized to ligate blood vessels and to load onto free needles for suturing tissues. Preferences for the length of precut tie will vary with the depth inside the body at which it is being used. For example, a free tie applied deep in the abdomen must be longer than one applied to the hand.

CHARACTERISTICS OF SUTURE MATERIALS

Suture can be classified into two broad categories: absorbable and nonabsorbable. Absorbable suture is capable of being broken down either by the body's enzymes or by hydrolyzation. Nonabsorbable suture remains in the body for as long as 2 years (silk) or indefinitely (steel). Each broad classification of absorbable and nonabsorbable suture includes both natural and synthetic materials. Examples of natural absorbable materials are plain and chromic surgical gut. Silk is a natural nonabsorbable material. Treating absorbable materials can increase their tensile strength and the period of time required for absorption. For example, treating plain surgical gut with chromic salts increases tensile strength retention from 7 to 10 days to 21 to 28 days and absorption time from 70 days to 90 days.

Suture is further characterized as monofilament and multifilament. Monofilament suture is a single strand, which passes easily through tissues and is resistant to fluids soaking into the suture, thereby resisting capillary action. Monofilament sutures tie down easily. These characteristics make monofilament suture well suited for vascular surgery. Monofilament suture can be weakened by crushing or nicking with instruments. This damage may not be visible but can result in the suture's breaking (Ethicon, 1994).

Multifilament suture consists of multiple strands of suture material that are held into a single strand by braiding, twisting, or spinning. Multifilament sutures are more flexible and pliable and have greater tensile strength than monofilament sutures. Because multifilament sutures do absorb body fluids, they are more reactive with body tissues (Ethicon, 1994).

PACKET LABEL INFORMATION

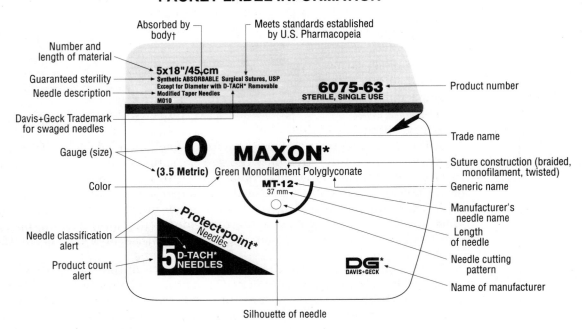

SUTURE BOX LABEL INFORMATION

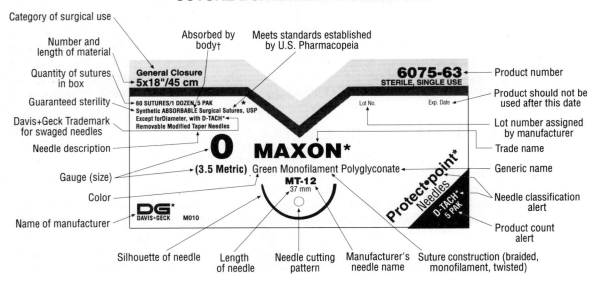

†Suture coating (if any) is designated on this line

FIGURE 9–12. Box Labels for Sutures and Needles (Copyright © 1978. Davis and Geck. All rights reserved.)

SMALLER   **LARGER**

8-0   7-0   6-0   5-0   4-0   3-0   2-0   0   #1   #2   #3

FIGURE 9–13. Suture gauge. To the left of the "0," increasing numbers of "0s" indicate progressively smaller gauge sutures. The larger whole numbers to the right of the "0" indicated larger gauge (diameter) sutures.

Monofilament and multifilament sutures vary in their knot tying characteristics. The coefficient of friction affects the tendency of a knot to loosen after it has been tied; more friction results in a more secure knot. The coefficient of friction of monofilament sutures is relatively low as compared with that of multifilament sutures (Ethicon, 1994). When suture materials such as nylon and polypropylene are tied, it is important that knots are tied flat, that more than one knot is tied, and that the ends are cut longer.

ABSORBABLE SUTURE

Absorbable suture materials are selected for fast-healing tissues, because they have shorter tensile retention and absorption times. *Natural* sources of absorbable suture materials are the submucosa of sheep intestine and the serosa of beef intestine. Plain surgical gut is selected for epidermal suturing where retention of tensile strength for 7 to 10 days is sufficient. Plain surgical gut can be treated with chromium salts to extend the period of tensile strength to 21 to 28 days. Increased tensile strength allows chromic gut to be employed for ligature of large vessels, repair of muscle and fascia, and suturing of mucosal layers, such as in anastomoses in intestinal surgery.

Natural gut suture is contained in a foil package of preserving solution. The suture may be dipped in saline to facilitate handling but should not be left to soak in saline. Excessive handling and rinsing of the suture will decrease its strength. Rinsing is necessary only when surgical gut is being used in the eye. The absorption of natural gut materials is adversely affected by the presence of infection and can lead to wound dehiscence or evisceration. Fever, infection, and protein deficiency may accelerate the absorption of absorbable suture materials (Ethicon, 1994).

Absorbable suture is also manufactured from *synthetic* materials. Synthetic absorbable materials have greater tensile strength and longer absorption periods than treated natural materials. Depending upon the specific synthetic product, 60% to 70% of tensile strength can be maintained for more than 2 weeks. The outside range is 25% tensile strength remaining after 6 weeks for Ethicon's PDS II. This increase in absorption time and tensile strength retention allows for application when infection is present or when increased tensile strength and absorption time are desired (Ethicon, 1994).

NONABSORBABLE SUTURE

Both natural and synthetic materials are employed to manufacture nonabsorbable suture. The most frequent *natural* sources are cotton and silk. Natural long-staple cotton fiber strands are twisted to form smooth multifilament strands of suture. Cotton suture is less frequently used than silk because it is more reactive in tissues. Cotton loses about 50% of its tensile strength in 6 months, but 30% to 40% tensile strength remains after 2 years. Surgical silk is made from threads spun by silkworm larvae. These threads are twisted, braided, or single filament and are available in white, black, or color dyed. Silk ties easily and is generally well tolerated by the body. Silk suture is frequently utilized in gastrointestinal, ophthalmologic, and cardiovascular surgery.

Synthetic nonabsorbable suture materials include nylon, polyester, polypropylene, polyethylene, and surgical steel. Nylon has a very smooth texture and is inert in the body. It is frequently chosen for skin closure and peripheral nerve repair and in plastic surgery and some microvascular surgeries. Polyester suture has a very high tensile strength. It is often coated with Teflon or silicone to ease tying. Polypropylene suture has several advantages. In addition to being nonabsorbable and possessing good tensile strength, polypropylene suture handles like silk, producing minimal tissue trauma as it travels through tissues. This minimal tissue trauma makes polypropylene ideal for applications in vascular surgery. Handling polypropylene suture can be difficult because it has a tendency to kink and return to its packaged shape. The suture must be gently stretched before use. Care must be exercised when stretching suture because overstretching decreases strength and may dislodge swaged needles. Polyethylene suture is soft and pliable. It is utilized in plastic surgery, microsurgery, tendon repair surgery, and cardiovascular surgery.

Surgical steel/wire is inert in the body. It is extremely strong and can be utilized in the presence of infection. Steel is frequently used to wire bone together, such as the sternum following cardiac surgery. Steel can be very difficult to handle and can be a potential hazard to personnel. Some scrub persons double glove when handling steel. Steel kinks easily, and the kinks are difficult to remove, so care must be taken to avoid bending and kinking. Steel placed under tension can exert a sawing action on tissue. Following dehiscence or evisceration, steel can increase the strength of the abdominal closure. Steel can also be employed as a retention suture to reinforce the strength of a wound closure. A heavy needle-holder and wire scissors must be used when working with steel to avoid damage to more delicate instruments.

Increasing numbers of surgical procedures are performed with endoscopic techniques. A range of suture continues to be developed to meet the need for suturing through endoscopic instrumentation. These suture materials have properties similar to traditional sutures.

NEEDLES

Needles provide a mechanism for moving suture through body tissues. Surgical needles are constructed of high quality heat-treated stainless steel to increase their strength and ability to resist breaking. A broken needle left in a wound is a foreign body. Broken needles must be accounted for in their entirety during surgical counts.

A surgical needle consists of three components, the two ends and the shaft between (Fig. 9–14). The leading end or tip can be tapered (noncutting), cutting (cutting edges on both sides, top or bottom), or blunt (does not pierce or cut) (Fig. 9–15). The middle section or shaft determines the shape of the needle. Needles

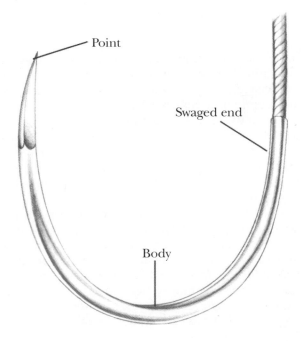

Point

Swaged end

Body

FIGURE 9-14. Needle Components (Reprinted with permission from Ethicon, Inc. from *Wound Closure Manual*, Copyright © 1994)

POINT/BODY SHAPE	APPLICATIONS
Conventional Cutting 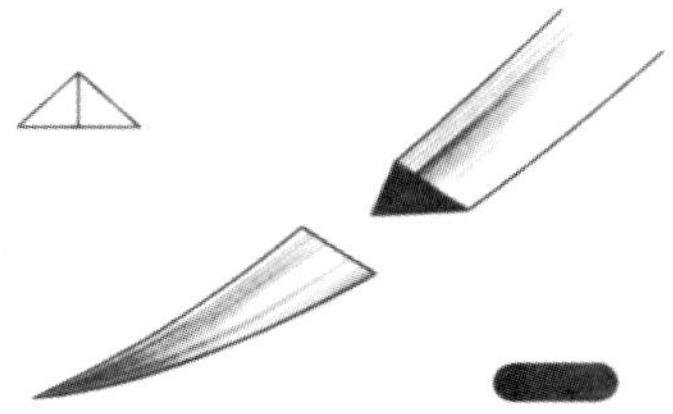	ligament nasal cavity oral cavity pharynx skin tendon
Reverse Cutting 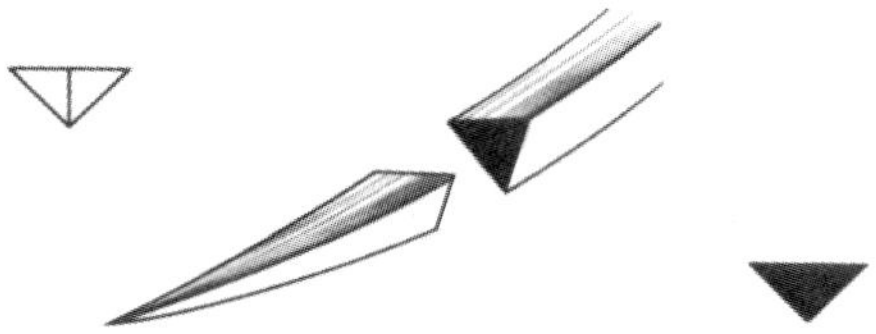	fascia ligament nasal cavity oral mucosa pharynx skin tendon sheath
MICRO-POINT Reverse Cutting Needle 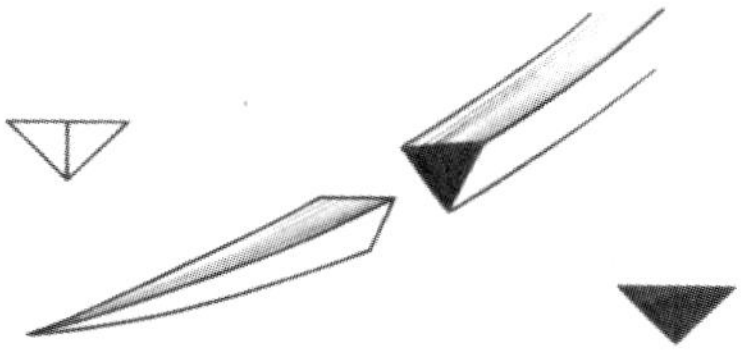	eye
Precision Point Cutting 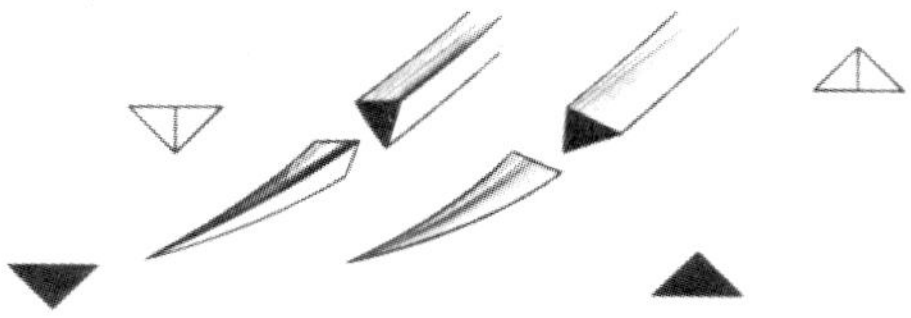	skin (plastic or cosmetic)
Side-cutting Spatula 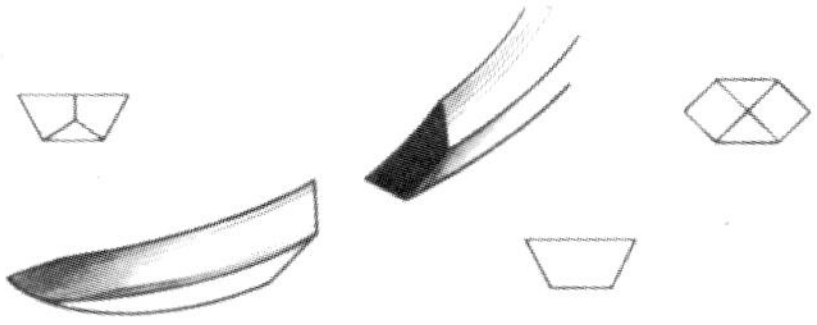	eye (primary application) microsurgery ophthalmic (reconstructive)

FIGURE 9–15. Needle Points and Body Shapes with Typical Applications (Reprinted with permission from Ethicon, Inc. from *Wound Closure Manual*, Copyright © 1994)

Illustration continued on following page

POINT/BODY SHAPE	APPLICATIONS	
TAPERCUT Surgical Needle 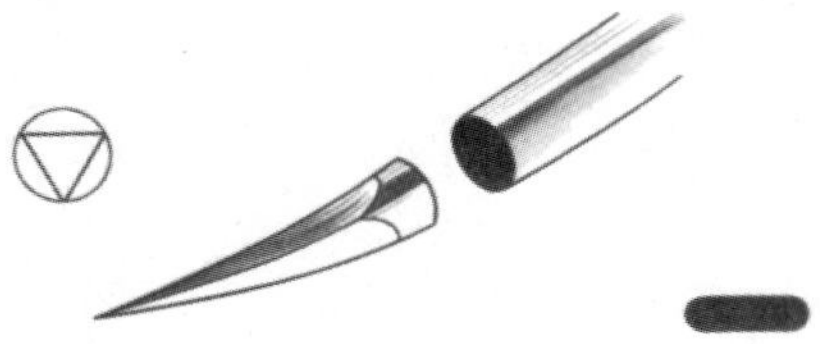	bronchus calcified tissue fascia ligament nasal cavity oral cavity ovary perichondrium periosteum	pharynx tendon trachea uterus vessels (sclerotic)
Taper 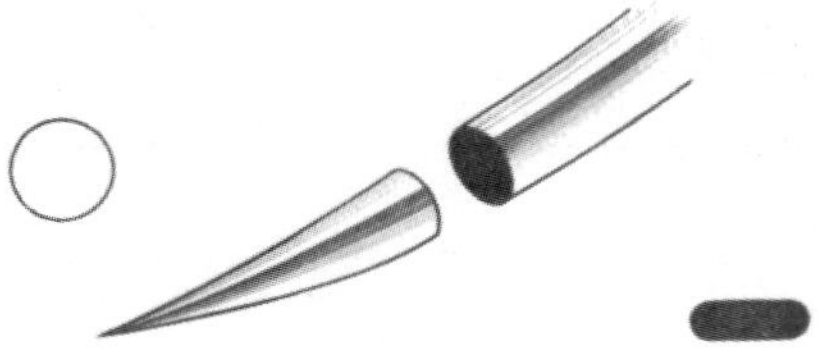	aponeurosis biliary tract dura fascia gastrointestinal tract muscle myocardium nerve peritoneum	pleura subcutaneous fat urogenital tract vessels
Blunt 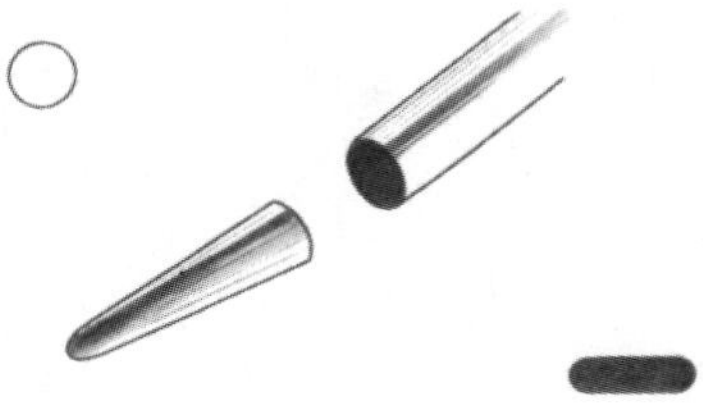	blunt dissection (friable tissue) fascia intestine kidney liver spleen cervix (ligating incompetent cervix)	
CS ULTIMA Ophthalmic Needle 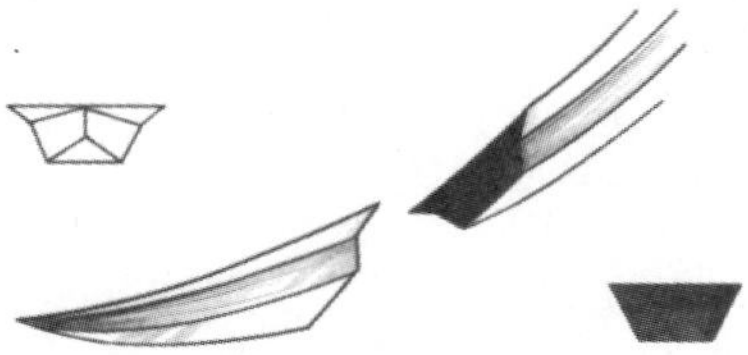	eye (primary application)	
PC PRIME Needle 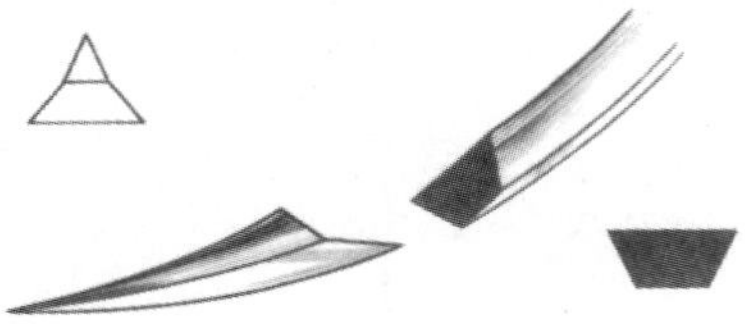	skin (plastic or cosmetic)	

FIGURE 9–15. *Continued*

can be straight like a traditional sewing needle or rounded from a 1/4 to 5/8 circle. The shape of the needle determines its appropriate applications (Fig. 9-16). The body of a needle will usually have a flattened area that allows for secure placement of a needle holder (Fig. 9-17). The end of the needle or eye, where the suture is attached, may not resemble the eye of the traditional needle. The

SHAPE	APPLICATIONS
Straight 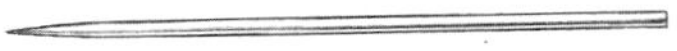	gastrointestinal tract nasal cavity nerve oral cavity pharynx skin tendon vessels
Half-curved 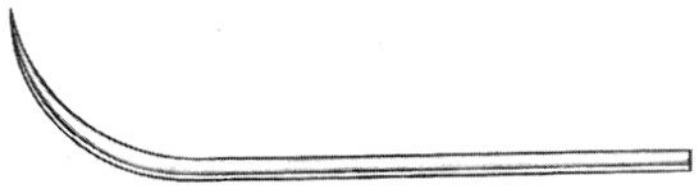	skin (rarely used)
1/4 Circle 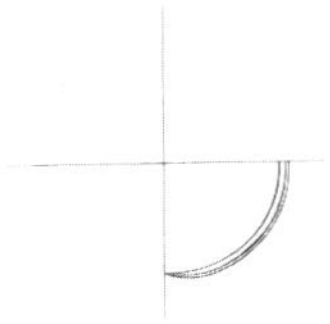	eye (primary application) microsurgery
3/8 Circle 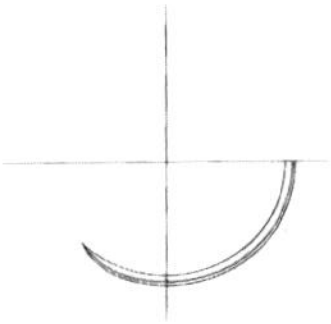	aponeurosis nerve biliary tract perichondrium dura periosteum eye peritoneum fascia pleura gastrointestinal tract tendon muscle urogenital tract myocardium vessels
1/2 Circle 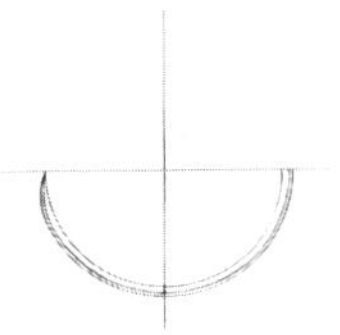	biliary tract pharynx eye pleura gastrointestinal tract respiratory tract muscle skin nasal cavity subcutaneous fat oral cavity urogenital tract pelvis peritoneum
5/8 Circle 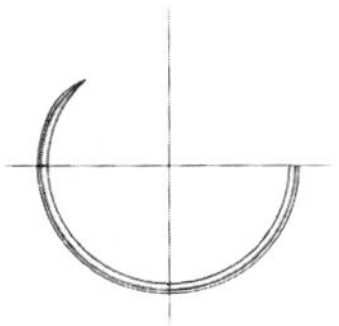	anal (hemorrhoidectomy) cardiovascular system nasal cavity oral cavity pelvis urogenital tract (primary application)
Compound Curved 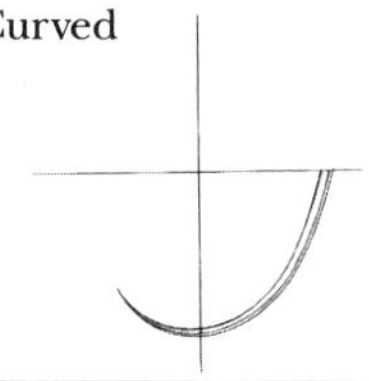	eye (anterior segment)

FIGURE 9-16. Needle Shape and Typical Applications (Reprinted with permission from Ethicon, Inc. from *Wound Closure Manual*, Copyright © 1994)

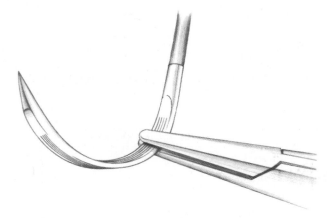

FIGURE 9–17. Arming a Needle Holder Properly (Reprinted with permission from Ethicon, Inc. from *Wound Closure Manual,* Copyright © 1994)

swaged or eyeless needle is the result of joining the suture and needle into a continuous unit (Fig. 9–18).

Various manufacturers have different mechanisms for creating swaged needles, but the result is a continuous unit that minimizes tissue trauma and is simpler to handle. Usually the needle and suture are tightly secured so they do not separate accidentally. In some applications, such as where interrupted stitches are taken, it can be desirable that the needles detach from the sutures with a tug. These needles are called pop-off needles, D-Tach (Davis and Geck), or Controlled Release needles (Ethicon) (Fig. 9–19). This feature can be a great convenience; however, it can also be a great source of irritation if the surgeon is presented with a releasable needle when the suture is intended for reuse or for a running suture line.

Needles fall into two broad categories, tapered and cutting (see Fig. 9–15). Tapered needles have a point on the end of the needle but then are rounded to avoid damage to delicate tissues through which it passes. Common applications for tapered needles are cardiac, vascular, and gastrointestinal surgery. Cutting needles are razor sharp, which permits them to pass through tough fibrous tissues with minimal effort and tissue trauma. There are several types of cutting needles. The conventional cutting needle has three cutting edges, two opposing cutting edges at the sides, and a third facing up on the inside of the needle curve. The reverse cutting needle differs from the conventional cutting needle in that the third cutting edge is on the outer curve of the needle. This design has the advantage of placing the direction of the cut away from the edge of the wound. As the suture is tied, pressure is exerted on the tissue edge closest to the wound. Cutting this edge can lead to suture tearing into the wound.

Specialized needles have been designed for microsurgical procedures. These needles are very finely honed for extreme sharpness and precision. These needles are frequently selected for ophthalmic and plastic surgeries and in microsurgery. Spatula or side-cutting needles have been specifically designed for ophthalmic applications. These needles are flat on the bottom and cut only on the sides. This allows the needle to pierce the tough scleral or corneal tissue and glide between the thin layers.

Needles vary in size according to the application. Careful thought about the type and location of tissues to be sutured, reference to resources such as preference lists, and consultation with surgical team members will guide the perioperative nurse in appropriate suture and needle selection.

HANDLING OF SUTURE AND NEEDLES

Suture must be prepared in advance to assure a smooth surgical course. However, to control costs, only suture that is certain to be used or is essential to have

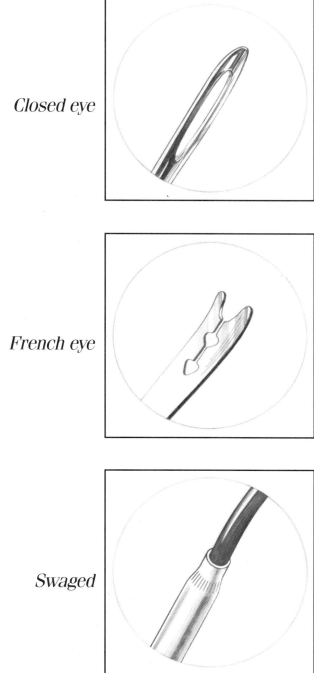

Closed eye

French eye

Swaged

FIGURE 9-18. Needle Eyes (Reprinted with permission from Ethicon, Inc. from *Wound Closure Manual*, Copyright © 1994)

immediately available for large bleeding vessels should be opened. Anticipation, careful utilization of physician's preference sheets, and consultation with other members of the surgical team will facilitate preparedness and minimize waste.

The scrubbed person must develop a system for indexing and storing suture on the back table. Some preferences are to stack the suture by size and type of suture material or in the order of anticipated need. Needles must be counted before making the skin incision, and an accurate count must be maintained throughout the surgical procedure. Maintaining this tally is the responsibility of

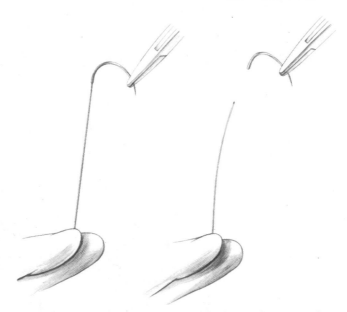

CONTROL RELEASE *Needle Suture*

Holding the needle securely in the needle-holder, the suture should be grasped securely and pulled straight and taut. The needle will be released with a straight tug of the needleholder.

FIGURE 9–19. Control Release Needle Suture (Reprinted with permission from Ethicon, Inc. from *Wound Closure Manual*, Copyright © 1994)

both the circulating nurse and the scrub person. Saving opened suture packets in a sterile trash container on the back table can facilitate the determination of which size needle is missing in the event of an incorrect needle count.

Needles must always be handled carefully to avoid puncturing surgical gloves. Manufacturers are working to develop a blunt tip needle, which will present less potential for injury to the surgical team. An example is the Ethiguard needle manufactured by Ethicon. Most sutures that are used with a needle come with the needle attached. Many sutures can be loaded or armed in the package in which they are supplied (Fig. 9–20). The scrub person who opens the suture package must verify that the number of needles previously counted are indeed contained within the package. The needle holder is attached nearest the eye, about one third of the total length of the needle shaft away from the eye end (see Figs. 9–17 and 9–20). The suture is gently pulled from the package, avoiding undue tension on the connection between needle and suture.

Suture that must be threaded is passed through the closed eye of a needle. If a suture loses its needle part way through a running suture line, a French eye needle can be reattached to the suture. A French eye needle is open at the top unlike the closed loop of a standard needle (Fig. 9–21).

A needle holder is passed with the handle first. The needle faces the surgeon's opposite thumb or chin. Only an unused needle should be passed hand to hand. However, the clean needle can still contaminate the surgeon or nurse by puncturing a contaminated glove. It is preferable that all sharps be passed with a no-touch technique. The needle holder can be placed in position for use in a basin or on a magnetic instrument mat to be picked up by the surgeon. The needle is then returned to the scrub person in a similar manner.

Passing sutures to the surgeon on an exchange basis whenever possible will facilitate needle counting. Mounting two sutures and interchanging them will facilitate the flow of the surgical procedure. At times it is necessary for a needle and suture to remain in tissue to be tied later. These sutures are tagged with a mosquito clamp. If the suture is delicate, it may be desirable to have a clamp with rubber protectors on the tips to protect the suture from damage. To facilitate an accurate needle count, returned needles are immediately placed into a container

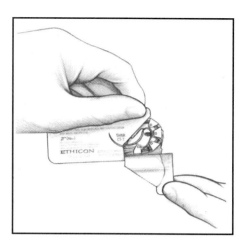

1. Grasp the package with thumb and forefinger and tear down and to the left.

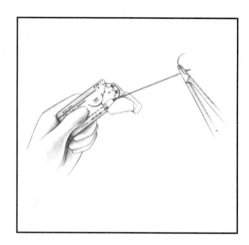

2. Clamp the needleholder approximately three-fourths of the distance from the needle point. *Do not clamp the swaged area.* Gently pull the suture to the right in a straight line.

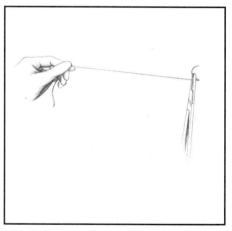

3. Additional suture straightening should be minimal. If the strand must be straightened, hold the armed needleholder and gently pull the strand making certain not to disarm the needle from the suture.

FIGURE 9-20. Opening Suture Package and Arming the Needle (Reprinted with permission from Ethicon, Inc. from *Wound Closure Manual*, Copyright © 1994)

that allows for easy visual inspection during the closing counts and prevents accidental movement and loss.

Needles, like all sharps, are a potential source of inoculation of the health care worker with contaminated body fluids. All members of the surgical team must give careful thought and attention to the handling of needles for their own protection and the protection of all the members of the surgical team.

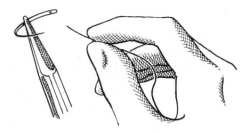

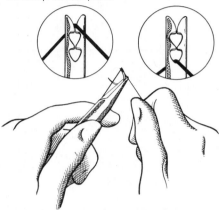

If eyed needle is threaded from inside curvature, take care to avoid pricking glove on sharp needle point.

Holding suture strand taut with left hand, bring strand down over top and spring into eye. Pull through about 3".

FIGURE 9-21. Threading a French Eye Needle (Copyright © 1978. Davis and Geck. All rights reserved)

STAPLING DEVICES

Staples present a quick and efficient alternative to sutures and ligatures. Single stainless steel and titanium clips, applied in pairs, can replace suture ligatures when dissecting blood vessels. Titanium must be used when MRI will be used for future diagnosis. MRI utilizes powerful magnets, which can cause movement in metals, such as stainless steel, which are capable of creating their own magnetic fields. An example of an adverse consequence of this movement during MRI is the torque on a cerebral aneurysm clip causing a tear to the artery to which it has been applied.

When applying standard ligating clips, two clips are placed on a vessel, and the vessel is divided between the ligating clips. Absorbable clip materials are also available. Ligating clips are available in sizes ranging from 2.6 mm open and 3.4 mm closed to 6.2 mm open and 12.5 mm closed. These clips are mounted by the scrubbed person on a reusable applier of the appropriate size. United States Surgical Corporation manufactures a device, the LDS, with which two staples ligate the vessel, and simultaneously, a knife in the LDS divides the vessel between the staples (Fig. 9-22).

Staples can also replace a sutured intestinal anastomosis (Figs. 9-23, 9-24, and 9-25). They can be utilized when performing a pneumonectomy or lobectomy. The advantages of staples are that they produce airtight and leakproof anastomoses and are timesaving devices. However, they are expensive, and the operator must be familiar with their use and operation. Completely disposable stapling devices are more expensive than reusable devices, but potential problems with disassembly, cleaning, and reassembly of complex nondisposable instruments are avoided. An incorrectly assembled stapler can misfire, and incorrectly placed staples are difficult to remove.

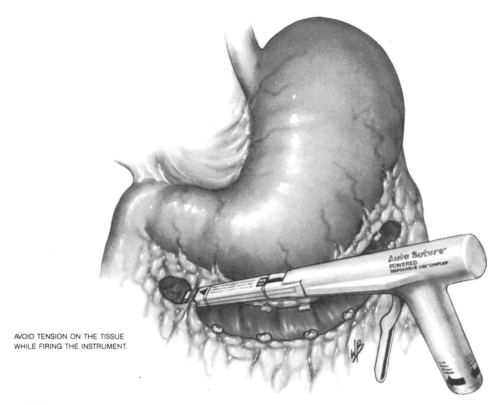

AVOID TENSION ON THE TISSUE
WHILE FIRING THE INSTRUMENT.

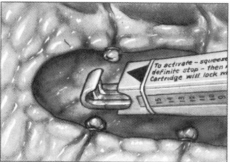

ASSURE THAT THE TISSUE AND STAPLES
ARE FREE OF THE CARTRIDGE PRIOR
TO REMOVING THE INSTRUMENT.

FIGURE 9–22. Disposable vessel ligation device. Disposable stapling device is used to mobilize the stomach by ligating and dividing the omental vessels. The tissue to be ligated is slipped into the jaw of the LDS instrument. Two staples ligate the vessel and a knife blade divides the vessel between the staples. (Copyright © 1988, 1994 United States Surgical Corporation. All rights reserved. Reprinted with the permission from United States Surgical Corporation from Stapling Techniques: General Surgery with Auto Suture Instruments. 3rd ed. Norwalk, Conn: USSC. 1988)

Staples can also be utilized to close the skin (Fig. 9–26). Skin staples are fast and, when applied correctly, leave a good cosmetic result. The application of skin staples requires that both cuticular and subcuticular layer be everted. The assistant, utilizing two sets of forceps or Allis clamps, holds the skin edges slightly raised, and the stapler is applied over the midline of the incision. Skin staples are supplied preloaded in regular and wide widths. It is important to consider the length of the skin incision and select an appropriate number of staples. Dressing a wound closed with staples requires a smooth textured dressing, such as Telfa, as staples will snag in gauze sponges. About 5 to 7 days postsurgery, staples are removed with a staple removal instrument.

If a running suture is selected for subcuticular skin closure as in some plastic and pediatric surgeries, the skin edges are approximated with surgical adhesive

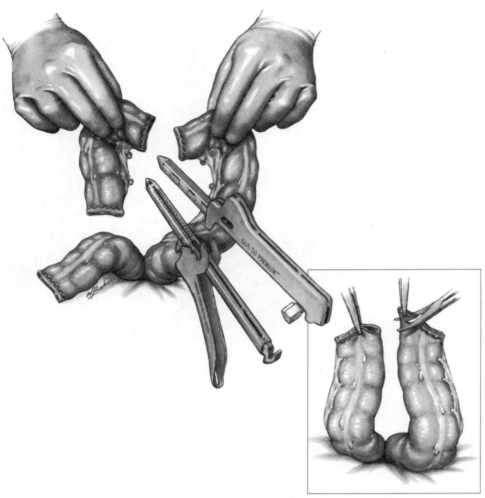

FIGURE 9-23. Creating a functional end-to-end anastomosis using stapling devices. A bowel resection is first performed using two applications of the GIA instrument. The instrument is placed around the bowel at the point of transection in a scissor-like fashion. The GIA is closed and the staples are fired. A double staggered staple line is placed on the patient side and a second double staggered staple line is placed on the specimen side; simultaneously, a knife blade in the GIA transects the bowel between the two double staple lines. The GIA is applied twice, proximal and distal to the portion of bowel to be resected. To use the GIA to perform the anastomosis (inset photograph), the antimesenteric corner of the staple line is excised from the proximal and distal bowel. (Copyright © 1988, 1994 United States Surgical Corporation. All rights reserved. Reprinted with the permission from United States Surgical Corporation from Stapling Techniques: General Surgery with Auto Suture® Instruments. 3rd ed. Norwalk, Conn: USSC. 1988)

strips (Fig. 9-27). These strips are supplied in widths from 1/8th inch to 2 inches. Cutting these strips allows length and width to be customized to the incision. This method of skin closure is preferred in pediatric surgery because there are no skin sutures or staples to be removed postoperatively.

Postoperative Wound Drainage and Dressings

DRAINS

The purpose of draining a surgical wound postoperatively is to evacuate body fluids or air, which, if allowed to accumulate, could be harmful to the patient. Examples include chest tubes to evacuate air from the thoracic cavity and per-

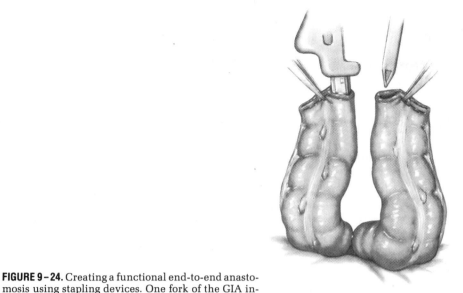

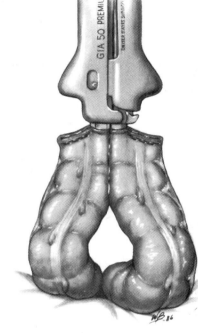

INSERT THE FORKS FULLY TO
ENSURE MAXIMUM STOMAL SIZE.

FIGURE 9–24. Creating a functional end-to-end anastomosis using stapling devices. One fork of the GIA instrument is inserted into each of the antimesenteric borders of the proximal and distal bowel lumens. The instrument is closed and the staples are fired. Two double staggered staple lines join the bowel; simultaneously, the knife blade divides between the two double staple lines creating a stoma. (Copyright © 1988, 1994 United States Surgical Corporation. All rights reserved. Reprinted with the permission of United States Surgical Corporation from Stapling Techniques: General Surgery with Auto Suture® Instruments. 3rd ed. Norwalk, Conn: USSC. 1988)

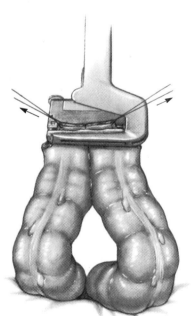

CARE MUST BE TAKEN TO OVERLAP THE
ENDS OF THE PREVIOUS STAPLE LINES.

AVOID DIRECT APPOSITION OF THE
ANASTOMOTIC STAPLE LINES.

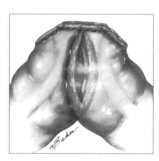

AN ANCHOR SUTURE MAY BE PLACED
AT THE BASE OF THE ANASTOMOSIS
FOR ADDITIONAL SECURITY.

FIGURE 9–25. Creating a functional end-to-end anastomosis using stapling devices. The TA 55 instrument is used to close the now common opening. A traction suture is used at each end of the bowel. The jaws of the instrument are placed over the area to be stapled, taking care to incorporate all previous suture lines and layers of the bowel. The staples are fired and prior to removing the instrument the surgeon excises redundant tissue. The inset photograph demonstrates the completed anastomosis. (Copyright © 1988, 1994 United States Surgical Corporation. All rights reserved. Reprinted with the permission of United States Surgical Corporation from Stapling Techniques: General Surgery with Auto Suture® Instruments. 3rd ed. Norwalk, Conn: USSC. 1988)

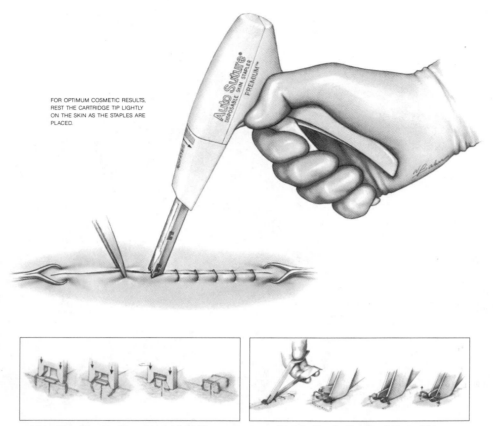

FOR OPTIMUM COSMETIC RESULTS,
REST THE CARTRIDGE TIP LIGHTLY
ON THE SKIN AS THE STAPLES ARE
PLACED.

How Skin Staples Form and Hold Tissue   Simple Staple Removal From Skin

FIGURE 9–26. Skin Stapling Device. (Copyright © 1988, 1994 United States Surgical Corporation. All rights reserved. Reprinted with the permission of United States Surgical Corporation from Stapling Techniques: General Surgery with Auto Suture® Instruments. 3rd ed. Norwalk, Conn: USSC. 1988)

forated drains to remove blood and fluids from the abdomen, hip, and other cavities. Accumulated body fluids are an ideal culture medium for microorganisms.

A wide range of devices is available for draining surgical wounds. They function by gravity or mechanical means, such as suction. The most simple of drains is the Penrose drain. This drain is a soft flat tube of latex. Owing to its flexibilty, it can be easily placed in the abdomen. When placing a Penrose drain, a stab wound is made adjacent to the incision with the surgical knife. With a clamp, the drain is then passed from inside the body cavity to the outside. The purpose of not pulling the drain from outside to inside is to reduce the number of microorganisms that would be introduced from the skin. A suture or sterile safety pin may be placed on the drain to keep it from slipping into the wound. A Penrose drain is not a closed drainage system and is a potential pathway by which microorganisms can enter the surgical wound. Strict aseptic technique must be practiced when changing a dressing containing any type of drain.

A second type of open drain is the T tube. This T-shaped round rubber tube can be placed in the common bile duct after cholecystectomy or common bile duct exploration. Bile and any remaining stone fragments can exit the body through this tube. Attaching a drainage bag to the T tube creates a closed system.

Closed drainage systems employ a catheter or tube that is placed inside the body cavity. These catheters come in a variety of shapes and sizes. They can be round or flat, open at only the end, or perforated along a portion of the length. Externally the catheter or tube is sutured in place and connected to a device that, when compressed (air removed) and attached to the catheter, will exert gentle

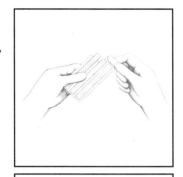

1. Using sterile technique, remove card from sleeve and tear off tab.

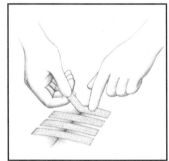

2. Peel off tapes as needed in a diagonal direction.

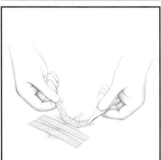

3. Apply tapes at 1/8 inch intervals as needed to complete wound apposition. *Make sure the skin surface is dry before applying each tape.*

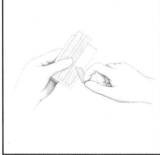

4. When healing is judged to be adequate, remove each tape by peeling off each half from the outside toward the wound margin. Then, gently lift the tape away from the wound surface.

FIGURE 9–27. Skin Closure Tapes (Reprinted with permission from Ethicon, Inc. from *Wound Closure Manual*, Copyright © 1994)

suction on the drainage catheter. Catheters collect wound drainage, allow for accurate tally of the amount of drainage, and decrease bacterial contamination. Trade names for some of these drains include J-Vac, Hemovac, and Jackson-Pratt.

Salem sump catheters are utilized when a large volume of drainage is expected. This catheter is a double lumen device. The outer lumen is perforated and prevents adjacent structures, such as bowel wall, from being sucked into and occluding the principal lumen. Catheters such as this are connected to continuous or intermittent external suction.

A large variety of catheters and tubes are available for urinary drainage. Foley catheters are available in a wide range of diameters and balloon sizes.

Three-way Foley catheters allow for both drainage and irrigation following transurethral resection of the prostate (TURP).

Following thoracic surgery, a chest tube is placed to assist in reinflation of the lung and drainage of fluid. Chest tubes must be connected to suction as soon as the chest is closed. Several manufacturers produce closed drainage devices that allow for underwater seal, drainage collection, and control of centimeters of suction.

Drainage devices that are designed to both collect blood and allow for reinfusion of the collected blood are available. Strict aseptic technique is essential when handling these devices. Reinfusion drainage systems can only be employed on clean surgical wounds, such as in some cardiac and orthopedic surgeries; they are never employed on surgery involving the gastrointestinal tract. The period of time between beginning the collection of blood and reinfusion is stated by the manufacturer.

The perioperative nurse can anticipate the need for postoperative wound drainage based upon the location of the surgery, the amount of drainage expected, and the amount of oozing and bleeding during the surgery. Ideally the drain is available for placement prior to wound closure. The drain should be selected and opened before the first closing sponge count.

It is imperative that the type, size, and location of any drains and the amount of drainage be documented by the perioperative nurse. This information will assist the post-anesthesia care nurse in assessing and planning for immediate postoperative care.

DRESSINGS

Applying dressings is the final step in the surgical procedure. A protective dressing assists in preventing postoperative wound contamination. The type and composition of the dressing is influenced by factors such as

- presence of a wound drain.
- anticipated amount of drainage.
- need for continued hemostasis, edema reduction, i.e., pressure dressing.
- need for additional support, splinting, or immobilization.
- need for protection from contamination and trauma.
- patient's need for physical, aesthetic, and psychologic comfort.
- type of skin closure.
- need for frequent postoperative dressing changes.
- need for direct visual inspection of the suture line.
- physician preference.
- availability and cost of dressing materials.

Starting at the incision site, the choice of the first dressing layer is influenced by the type of skin closure. If staples have been used on the skin, a nonadherent dressing such as Telfa is essential. A nonadherent dressing is an ideal first layer over most surgical incisions because it will not stick to the wound during postoperative dressing changes. The second and third layers depend on the amount of drainage anticipated from the wound. A standard abdominal wound is covered by 4 × 4 gauze sponges and thick absorbent pad.

Dressings must be sterile to protect from bacterial contamination. The perioperative nurse must anticipate the specific type of dressing material that will be needed so that it will be immediately available for application when the skin is closed. A good time for the circulating nurse to begin assembling dressings is immediately after the first closing sponge count.

Counted or x-ray detectable sponges must never be utilized in the postoperative wound dressing. This practice reduces the risk for incorrect counts and misinterpretation of postoperative x-ray studies. Because dressings consist of nonradiopaque sponges, they should not be placed upon the sterile field until the final closing count is completed. This practice will reduce the risk of a nonradiopaque sponge being left in the surgical wound.

The sterile dressing is prepared by the scrubbed person. The area surrounding the wound is first cleaned by the scrubbed person with sterile water and unused sponges. The area is thoroughly dried, and the dressing is then applied by the scrubbed person before removing the surgical drapes. The circulating nurse or team member wearing noncontaminated gloves applies tape to secure and seal the dressing. If large amounts of drainage and frequent dressing changes are anticipated, Montgomery straps can be applied instead of tape. Montgomery straps are adhesive at one end (applied at wound edges) and tie over the dressing to hold it in place. An analogy is tying a shoelace over the tongue of the shoe.

Pressure dressings provide for continued hemostasis and reduction of postoperative edema. They are frequently employed in orthopedic surgery. When a pneumatic tourniquet has been utilized, some surgeons apply a pressure dressing before releasing the tourniquet. A variety of dressing materials similar to an elastic bandage with an adhesive side are available for creating a pressure dressing.

Immobilization of the surgical site can be accomplished in several ways. A splint can be fashioned from plaster or fiberglass, or the entire extremity can be casted. Joints such as the knee can be immobilized in splints that can be adjusted for the desired degree of flexion and extension. The key for the perioperative nurse is to anticipate the need for these specialized materials and to see that they are available in the appropriate sizes and numbers at the appropriate time.

Some dressings will need to provide an added measure of protection for the surgical wound. A prime example of this type of dressing is a hand dressing. It is sometimes necessary that the hand be maintained in a physiologic, relaxed, supported position. After covering the surgical wound with a nonadhesive dressing, fluffed materials, such as gauze or cotton, are placed between each finger, and the palm is filled with similar material. The entire hand is then wrapped in a rolled gauze or elastic bandage. A splint of plaster or fiberglass can also be applied for support.

In some situations, it is desirable that the wound be frequently observed but the dressing not necessarily changed. In these situations, a transparent, vapor- and oxygen-permeable dressing can be chosen. This type of dressing is frequently chosen for IV sites and central lines. If moderate to large amounts of wound drainage occur, these dressings will not adhere to the skin, and another method of wound dressing is then indicated.

Surgical Wound Classification

A component of continuous quality management in the operating room is tracking the number of postoperative wound infections. The Centers for Disease Control and Prevention (CDC) has developed a four-tiered classification system for surgical wounds (Table 9–6). This classification system reflects the probability of postoperative wound infection based upon characteristics of the wound at the time of operation. The four tiers are clean, clean-contaminated, contaminated, and infected.

Clean Wounds/Class I: Uninfected operative wounds in which no inflammation is encountered and the respiratory, alimentary, genital, and urinary tracts are not entered. These wounds can be drained by a closed drainage system.

Examples: Including, but not limited to, elective surgeries such as hernia repair,

TABLE 9-6. **CDC WOUND CLASSIFICATIONS**

CLASSIFICATION	DESCRIPTION
I	Respiratory, alimentary, and genitourinary tracts not entered. No evidence of inflammation. Closed primarily. May use closed drainage system. No breaks in aseptic technique.
II	Surgeries of the respiratory, alimentary, and genitourinary tract. No sign of infection. No breaks in aseptic technique.
III	Open fresh accidental wounds. Major breaks in aseptic technique. Gross spillage from the GI tract.
IV	Old traumatic wounds with devitalized tissue. Existing infection, purulent drainage. Ruptured viscera or appendix.

Adapted from Centers for Disease Control and Prevention.

breast biopsy, total joint replacement, ophthalmic surgery, and open heart surgery

Average risk for infection: 1% to 5% nationally

Clean-contaminated Wounds/Class II: Operative wounds in which the respiratory, alimentary, genital, or urinary tracts are entered under controlled conditions and without unusual conditions or infection present

Examples: Cholecystectomy (no spillage), appendectomy (no inflammation), bronchoscopy, cystoscopy, transurethral resection of prostate (TURP), tonsillectomy, hysterectomy

Average risk for infection: 3% to 11% nationally

Contaminated Wounds/Class III: Surgery involving open, fresh, traumatic wounds or wounds with major breaks in sterile technique or with gross spillage from the GI tract; acute nonpurulent inflammation

Examples: Rectal surgery, traumatic open wounds, spillage of GI contents, inflamed appendix without frank pus

Average risk for infection: 10% to 17% nationally

Infected Wounds/Class IV: Old traumatic wounds with retained devitalized tissue, existing clinical infection, perforated viscera, delayed primary closure. This classification suggests that there was an infectious process present prior to surgery.

Examples: Incision and drainage, perforated viscera, amputations

Average risk for infections: Greater than 27% nationally

The perioperative nurse, in conjunction with the surgeon, is responsible for assigning and documenting the wound classification. The listed definitions are guidelines, and not all surgeries and circumstances are outlined in the examples given. The perioperative nurse must combine knowledge of microbiology and infection control with awareness of the specific surgical procedure to assign an appropriate wound classification. For example, an open fracture that occurred in a horse corral is not specifically listed and carries a very high potential for postoperative infection.

Although the diabetic patient or the patient on steroid therapy presents with an increased risk for postoperative infection, coexisting factors such as these are not included in the assessment of risk for infection in the CDC wound classifications. A major aseptic break during a procedure on a clean wound would require the nurse to reclassify the wound as clean-contaminated (class II). Only wound-related factors are included.

Wound Healing

The skin forms a protective barrier against invading microorganisms. A wound is any disruption in the skin. Surgical intervention, whether through a small puncture wound or a large abdominal incision, represents a breach in the protective barrier of the skin. Normal wound healing follows a predictable sequence.

PHASES OF WOUND HEALING

Wound healing begins immediately when a tissue is injured. The processes of coagulation described earlier in this chapter are a first step in wound healing as platelets reach the site of injury. Three phases of wound healing can be identified: inflammation, proliferation, and maturation. Although there is some overlap in these phases, it is important to understand the cascade or sequence of these events.

INFLAMMATION PHASE

The inflammation phase begins with the injury and lasts approximately 5 days. Inflammation is characterized by an initial vascular component, which involves vasoconstriction and release of chemical mediators. The chemicals of inflammation, prostaglandins, histamine, and kinins, stimulate the migration of polymorphonuclear leukocytes and macrophages to the damaged tissues. These leukocytes naturally debride the damaged tissues. During this phase, the wound is dependent on suture closure materials for strength (Ethicon, 1994; Rote, 1994).

PROLIFERATION PHASE

The proliferation phase lasts approximately 5 to 14 days. It is characterized by an increase in fibroblasts. As fibroblasts multiply, collagen is deposited in increasing amounts. Collagen is a fibrous insoluble protein found in the skin, bone, ligaments, and cartilage. It is collagen that gives strength to the healing wound.

Concurrent with collagen deposition is the process of angiogenesis or the formation of new blood vessels. Surgical intervention disrupts the blood supply to many structures, and it is essential that there be a blood supply for new and healing tissues.

Granulation tissue is formed by capillaries budding out from existing vessels. New vessels formed through angiogenesis provide nutrients to the regenerating tissues. In a full-thickness surgical wound, granulation tissue fills the wound and provides a surface for epithelialization. Epithelial cells multiply and migrate outward from the wound edges and decrease the size of the wound (Ethicon, 1994; Rote, 1994).

MATURATION PHASE

The maturation phase is the longest phase of wound healing. There is no distinct demarcation between the proliferation and maturation phases. These two phases overlap. The maturation phase can last a year or more. During this phase collagen fibers are remodeled or rearranged. As the collagen cells age, they become less vascular and gain tensile strength. This scar tissue is never as strong as the tissues were before the wound occurred. However, approximately 80% of prewound strength is regained (Ethicon, 1994; Rote, 1994).

How a wound is closed or allowed to close is important to the healing process. There are three types of wound closure/healing: *primary intention*, *secondary intention*, and *delayed primary intention* (tertiary). Most surgical incisions are closed with suture and heal by *primary intention*. For primary intention healing to occur, it is essential that the wound edges be reapproximated.

Secondary intention healing occurs when there is too much tissue loss to allow for reapproximation of the wound edges. This can occur in traumatic wounds with extensive tissue loss. The wound may be left open and allowed to heal from the inner layer to the outward surface. Granulation tissue forms in the wound and closes it by contraction. This is a slow healing process.

Occasionally wounds are not closed immediately after surgery. Closure is delayed to a later time. This is called *delayed primary intention*. The patient may be scheduled for a delayed primary closure or DPC. Often the reason for leaving a wound open is the presence of infection. Leaving the wound open allows for the unobstructed drainage of purulent fluids. When the infection is cleared, the wound edges are reapproximated.

Factors That Influence Wound Healing

Many factors can influence wound healing. Some of these factors can be controlled. Other factors cannot be controlled but can be anticipated.

LOCAL FACTORS

Local factors in wound healing include the presence of debris or necrotic tissue, dead space, hematoma, bacterial contamination, and amount of tissue trauma. Careful surgical technique, preoperative skin preparation, strict aseptic technique, careful handling and retraction of tissues, attention to hemostasis, wound drainage, elimination of dead spaces, and careful reapproximation of tissues with closure can reduce these local factors. Some local factors, such as preoperative infection, cannot be controlled by standard surgical techniques.

SYSTEMIC FACTORS

Underlying physical and metabolic conditions can have a profound effect on healing. In spite of careful attention to the local factors described, systemic factors can and do interfere with wound healing.

Preoperative nutritional status can have a profound effect on wound healing. The regeneration of tissue requires adequate amounts of protein and vitamins, particularly vitamins C, A, B_{10} and B_{12}. Dietary proteins are metabolized to amino acids, which are the building blocks for all protein substances. Therefore adequate dietary protein is essential for normal cell proliferation, fibroplasia, remodeling, and collagen formation. Minerals such as iron, calcium, and zinc are also important for wound healing.

Adequate hydration cannot be overlooked. Water makes up approximately 55% of body weight and is necessary for all physiologic body functions. Healing requires a moist environment.

Adequate oxygenation is also essential to wound healing. Patients with deficient circulation and perfusion will not be able to heal normally. Patients who are in this risk group include diabetics and patients with peripheral vascular disease. Smoking also reduces the availability of oxygen at the tissue level. The exact amount of smoking required to make a difference in wound healing is unknown.

Chronic and debilitating illnesses can influence wound healing. Diabetes was previously mentioned because of its long-term vascular effects. Hyperglycemia leads to a delay in the destruction of microorganisms and increased risk of postoperative wound infection. An inadequate insulin supply will hinder the ability of the body to provide glucose to cells working to repair damaged tissues. Other diseases that can affect wound healing are chronic renal failure, atherosclerosis, chronic obstructive pulmonary disease (COPD), cancer, obesity, and anemia.

The immune status of the patient can have a profound effect on wound healing. The immune response is altered in the very young and elderly. Medications, such as corticosteroids, chemotherapy, and other cancer treatments, can impair the ability of the immune system to respond to injury with infection-fighting white blood cells. Patients immunocompromised by HIV infection are at particular risk for postoperative infection.

It is common practice to give prophylactic antibiotics before surgery. Research has demonstrated that these antibiotics have the greatest effect if given within 2 hours of the skin incision (Classen, 1992). Gram-positive organisms, such as *Staphylococcus aureus*, are the most frequent invaders of surgical wounds. The first generation cephalosporins, such as cephalothin and cefazolin, are highly effective against gram-positive microorganisms. If the surgical site is an extremity, it is essential that the antibiotic be given early enough for the antibiotic to reach adequate tissue levels before the pneumatic tourniquet is inflated.

Stress interferes with the healing process. The exact mechanism is not well understood but is probably related to the release of the stress hormones norepinephrine, epinephrine, and cortisol. Psychologic stress for the surgical patient is not easily reduced; however, conveying caring and concern, explaining the surgical environment and procedures, and assessing for and enhancing existing coping mechanisms can modify some sources of stress for surgical patients.

Issues for Future Development

Perioperative nurses still need to investigate the answers to the questions in the controversy boxes in this chapter. The sacred cow of preoperative hair removal must be further investigated and results must be implemented in daily practice.

The order of steps in the surgical prep is another issue that must be further researched. Should the abdomen or the perineal area be prepped first when a combined skin preparation is necessary? Does aerosolization occur during the skin preparation and contaminate the other area?

During the skin preparation procedure is it necessary to use a sterile prep kit since the antimicrobial solutions are not sterile and the resulting skin area prepped is only surgically clean?

Summary

Surgical wound management is a responsibility of all members of the surgical team. Preoperative assessment of the skin and risk factors for postoperative infection, coupled with careful attention to skin preparation, hemostasis, and wound closure will promote the desired outcomes for all surgical patients — freedom from injury and freedom from infection.

REFERENCES

Alexander, J. W., Aerni, S. Plettner, J. P. (1985). Development of a safe and effective one-minute preoperative skin preparation. *Archives of Surgery, 120*(12), 1357–1361.

Alexander, J. W., Fischer, J. E., Boyahian, M., Palmquist, J., Morris, M. J. (1983). The influence of hairremoval methods on wound infections. *Archives of Surgery, 118*(3), 347–352.

Association of Operating Room Nurses. (1994). *AORN Standards and Recommended Practices for Perioperative Nursing.* Denver: AORN.

Braden, B. J., Bergstrom, N. (1989). Clinical utility of the Braden Scale for predicting pressure sore risk. *Decubitus, 2*(3), 44–46.

Centers for Disease Control. (1988). Guidelines for prevention of surgical wound infections. Atlanta: U.S. Department of Health and Human Services.

Classen, D. C., Burke, J. Pl, et al. (1992). The timing of prophylactic administration of antibiotics and the risk of surgical wound infection. *New England Journal of Medicine, 326*(60), 281–286.

Cruse, P. J., Foord, R. (1980). The epidemiology of wound infection. *Surgical Clinics of North America, 60*(1), 27–40.

Egan, J. (1994). Personal correspondence dated April 29, 1994. Boulder, CO: Valleylab, Inc.

Ethicon, Inc. (1994). *Wound Closure Manual.* Somerville, NJ: Ethicon Inc.

Ethicon (1987). *Nursing Care of the Patient in the OR.* Sommerville, NJ: Ethicon, Inc.

Fairchild, S. S. (1993). *Perioperative Nursing: Principles and Practice.* Boston: Jones and Bartlett.

Fogg, D. M. (1989). *Clinical issues. AORN Journal, 50*(6), 1314–1317.

Gauthier, D. K., O'Fallon, P. T., Coppage, D. (1993). Clean vs sterile surgical skin preparation kits: cost, safety, effectiveness. *AORN Journal, 58*(3), 486–495.

Guyton, A. C. (1991). Blood cells immunity and clotting. In: *Textbook of Medical Physiology.* 8th ed. Philadelphia: W. B. Saunders Co. (pp. 390–399).

Hallstrom R., Beck, S. L. (1993). Implementation of the AORN skin shaving standard: evaluation of a planned change. *AORN Journal, 58*(3), 498–506.

Jepsen, O. B., Bruttomesso, K. A. (1993). The effectiveness of preoperative skin preparations: an integrative review of the literature. *AORN Journal, 58*(3). 477–484.

Johnson & Johnson (1990). *Bleeding in Neurosurgery: Exploring the Challenge of Hemostasis.* Arlington, TX: Johnson & Johnson.

Larson, E. (1992). Skin cleansing. In: Wenzel, R., ed. *Prevention and Control of Nosocomial Infections* Baltimore: Williams & Wilkins. (pp. 250–256).

Larson, E. (1988). Guideline for use of topical antimicrobial agents. *American Journal of Infection Control, 16*(6), 253–266.

Mason (1988). *Hemostatic Mechanisms of Microfibrillar Collagen.* Woburn, MA: MedChem Products, Inc.

McCance, K. L. (1994). Structure and function of the hematologic system. In: McCance, K. L., Huether, S. E., eds. *Pathophysiology: The Biologic Basis for Disease in Adults and Children.* 2nd ed. St. Louis: C. V. Mosby. (pp. 755–783).

Meeker, M. H., Rothrock, J. C. (1991). *Alexander's Care of the Patient in Surgery.* St. Louis: Mosby-Year Book.

Moak, E. (1991). Hemostatic agents: adjuncts to control bleeding. *Today's O.R. Nurse.* November 1991, pp. 6–10.

Nichols, R. N. (1991). Surgical wound infection. *The American Journal of Medicine, 91*(suppl 3B), 545–645.

O'Neale, M. (1990). Clinical issues: warming povidone iodine. *AORN Journal, 52*(5), 1066.

Pearce, J. A. (1986). Burn Hazards. In: Pearce, J. A., *Electrosurgery: Medical Instrumentation and Clinical Engineering.* London: Chapman and Hall Ltd. (pp. 214–218).

Physicians' Desk Reference. (1994). Oradell, NJ: Medical Economics Company Inc.

Purdue, Frederick. (1989). *Betadine: Microbicide.* Norwalk, Conn: Purdue Frederick.

Quilici, P. J. (1992). *New Developments in Laparoscopy.* Norwalk, Conn: United States Surgical Corporation.

Rathburn, A. M., Holland, L. A., Geelhoed, G. W. (1986). Preoperative skin decontamination. *AORN Journal, 449*(1), 62–65.

Rote, N. S. (1994). Inflammation. In: McCance, K. L., Huether, S. E., eds. *Pathophysiology: The Biologic Basis for Disease in Adults and Children.* 2nd ed. St. Louis: C. V. Mosby. (pp. 234–267).

Rothrock, J. C. (1990). *Perioperative Nursing Care Planning.* St. Louis: C. V. Mosby.

Seropian, R., Reynolds, B. M. (1971). Wound infections after preoperative depilatory versus razor preparation. *American Journal of Surgery, 21,* 251–254.

Tollerud, L. (1987). Maintenance of skin integrity. In: Kneedler, J., Dodge, G., eds. *Perioperative Patient Care.* 3rd ed. Boston: Blackwell Scientific Publications. (pp. 201–211).

United States Surgical Corporation. (1992). *USSC Sutures/1992.* Norwalk, Conn: USSC Auto Suture Company.

United States Surgical Corporation. (1988). *Stapling Techniques: General Surgery with Auto Suture Instruments.* Norwalk, Conn: United States Surgical Corporation.

Valleylab (1986). *Engineering Bulletin: The Valleylab Return Electrode Monitoring System.* Boulder, CO: Valleylab, Inc.

Wahoff-Stice, D. M. (1993a). *Preoperative Skin Preparation of Surgical Patients* [videotape]. Danbury Conn: Davis & Geck; Denver: AORN.

Wahoff-Stice, D. M. (1993b). Study Guide for *Preoperative Skin Preparation of Surgical Patients.* Danbury Conn: Davis & Geck; Denver: AORN.

Practice Scenario 1
Surgical Wound Management

by Gayle Drinville-Shank, RN, CNOR

Alex Irvine is a 700-gram, 24-week gestation premature infant with a diagnosis of necrotizing enterocolitis. He is scheduled for a bowel resection and is transported to the operating room in an isolette with overhead warming lights.

PERIOPERATIVE INTERPRETATION

Using what you have just learned in this chapter, as an experienced perioperative nurse, you would consider the following in the care of this patient:

1. Assessment
   - The patient's small size and prematurity place him at risk for
     A. Hypothermia related to
        immature heat-regulating system
        minimal subcutaneous fat
        exposure of abdominal contents during the procedure
        use of cold solutions (prep, sterile irrigating solutions)
     B. Skin injury related to fragile (thin, transparent) skin
     C. Injury related to use of electrocautery due to small body surface area for dispersive pad placement
   - The patient will be placed in a supine position.
   - The patient will be prepped from nipple line to midthigh for a transverse abdominal incision.

NURSING DIAGNOSIS
   - High risk for alteration in body temperature (hypothermia) related to prematurity and environmental exposure
   - High risk for skin injury related to fragile skin and use of electrocautery
   - High risk for infection related to condition diagnosed and surgical intervention

2. Planning
   - Raise the room temperature before the patient enters the operating room.
   - Procure all the supplies necessary to maintain the patient's temperature throughout the surgical procedure, such as a warming blanket, temperature monitoring device, blankets, and stockinette.
   - Procure dispersive pad of appropriate size for the patient's body size.

3. Implementation
   - Increase the temperature in the operating room to 30°C prior to the patient's arrival in the room.
   - Place a warming blanket on the OR bed and set the temperature from 38°C to 40°C.
   - Cover the patient's head and extremities with stockinette to prevent heat loss.
   - Warm all solutions for prepping and irrigation according to the manufacturer's guidelines.
   - Place the temperature monitoring probe on the patient and attach to the monitor.
   - Transfer and position patient using extreme care to not damage the patient's skin.
   - Prior to the skin prep, place washcloths along the patient's body to catch prep solutions, thereby preventing pooling of the solutions under the patient, which might cause skin injury.
   - Prep the patient's skin from nipple to midthigh using aseptic technique, and prepping from clean (incision) to dirty (periphery) areas.
   - Apply and remove all pads and probes with care.
   - Have a warm isolette available at the conclusion of the surgery to place the patient in. Warm blankets instead can be placed over and around the patient during transport.

4. Evaluation
   - Assess and document the patient's temperature at the conclusion of the procedure and compare it with preoperative base line.

- Check the patient's skin for any areas of ecchymosis, abrasions, and allergic reactions, and document the condition of the patient's skin.
- Convey to the post-anesthesia care unit nurse or the newborn ICU nurse information regarding the patient's temperature and heat-conserving measures used intraoperatively, antibiotics given, and the status of the patient's skin. Request that the patient be monitored for signs of postoperative wound infection, such as fever or redness or purulent exudate at the incision site.

Practice Scenario 2
Surgical Wound Management

by Judy Little, RN, BSN, CNOR, CST, CCST

Thirty-four-year-old Ned Dingle is well known to the hospital staff owing to repeat admissions for ulcerative colitis. Recurrent exacerbations of the disease have made necessary one previous surgical procedure. Two years ago, Ned underwent a partial colectomy with colostomy. Ned is 5 feet 10 inches tall and weighs 130 pounds. He has continued to present with problems related to his disease. Manifestations of Cushing's syndrome related to long-term use of steroid therapy are evident. Abdominal pain, chronic diarrhea with severe intermittent bleeding, and malnutrition are the most recent causes for his present admission. Following consultation with Ned and his family, he is scheduled to undergo an ileostomy for control of symptoms.

PERIOPERATIVE INTERPRETATION

Using what you have just learned in this chapter, as an experienced perioperative nurse, you would consider the following in the care of this patient:

1. Assessment
   - Visual evidence of nutritional deprivation is apparent in the gaunt features and multiple bony prominences over the surface of Ned's body.
   - A 16-gauge intravenous catheter has been sutured in place into the left subclavian vein for the administration of hyperalimentation.
   - Ned wears a colostomy bag. The skin around the edge of the bag, although reddened and sloughing, is in a state of healing. The bag contains a small amount of brownish, blood-tinged fluid.
   - The midline incision for this procedure will follow the line of a previous scar from the xiphoid process to pubis. The colostomy stoma will be included in the preparation zone. A hair-removal prep has been requested and povidone-iodine (Betadine) will be the prepping solution of choice.

NURSING DIAGNOSES

High risk for wound infection related to
   diminished nutritional status
   proximity of colostomy stoma to operative site
   immunosuppression related to steroid therapy

High risk for hypothermia related to
   body fat and muscle mass deficits
   degree of body surface exposure planned for this procedure
   environmental requirements in the operating room i.e., room temperature

2. Planning
   - The patient will be placed in a supine position. In order to protect vulnerable areas from pressure injury, the operating bed must be covered with a weight displacement mattress.
   - Blood and body fluid precautions will be observed in the removing and disposing of the colostomy bag prior to the surgical prep.
   - Adhesive remover must be used to remove adhesive residue from the patient's skin around the stoma where the colostomy bag is attached before the prep is begun.
   - Consult with the blood bank regarding blood replacement quantities available for this patient and inform the anesthesiologist of this information. A peripheral infusion site must be accessed in order to facilitate the administration of blood and other drugs and fluids.
   - Discuss perioperative thermoregulatory options with the anesthesiologist. Consider alternatives such as room temperature elevation, warming lights, an external warming device such as insulative blanket, and warmed prepping solutions and irrigants.

3. Implementation
   - Raise the room temperature for the immediate preoperative period.

- Position the patient as planned in supine position. Provide patient with a warm blanket and remain at the bedside until induction and intubation are complete.
- Remove blanket and patient's gown. Check patient's anatomic alignment. Secure the patient on the bed and pad pressure points.
- Don nonsterile gloves and remove the colostomy bag using appropriate precautions. Discard the bag and its contents according to policy. Apply adhesive remover to site around stoma as necessary to remove all residue of adhesive.
- Don sterile gloves and place sterile towels along patient's sides to catch spills and prevent pooling of prepping solution. Begin prep along point of incision, carefully avoiding colostomy stoma. Following the principles of clean to dirty and the procedure outlined in this chapter, continue with prep moving in a circular motion outward toward the periphery. Prep around the stoma until the entire area, nipple to pubis is prepped in this fashion. Beginning at the edge of the mucosa move inward to the orifice of the stoma in the same fashion. When the prep is completed, remove the towels, taking care not to come in contact with the prepped surface of the patient's skin. Be sure no solution has run into the crevices of contact with the dispersive grounding pad or the electrocardiogram electrodes or is pooled beneath the patient.
- Prepping solution is poured into a small basin on the field so that the surgeon may swab the surface of the stoma and isolate it from the incision site with sterile towels.
- Following removal of the bowel, irrigation of the abdominal cavity with warm saline eliminates remaining contaminants. Dirty instruments are discarded and gowns and gloves are changed by the surgical team.
- Using uncontaminated sterile instrumentation, formation of the ileostomy stoma is completed prior to closure of the incision. The cavity is again irrigated with warm saline.
- An ileostomy bag is placed over the new stoma to prevent the now continuous drainage of fecal liquid from coming into contact with the wound site.

4. Evaluation
- The patient's skin is assessed for signs of injury or compromise at pressure points and around the operative and electrosurgical dispersive pad site.
- Assess the patient's body temperature postoperatively and compare with the preoperative base line.
- Verbal report should be given to the post-anesthesia care unit nurse regarding dressing type, drains, and antibiotics given intraoperatively. The perioperative nurse also informs the PACU nurse of the patient's previous steroid therapy, Cushing's syndrome, and the hyperalimentation subclavian line.

Chapter Ten

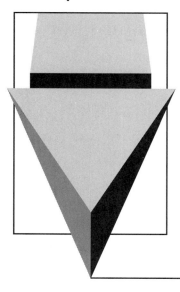

Perioperative Clinical Education

Linda Brazen, RN, MSN, CNOR, C

Prerequisite Knowledge Solid clinical skills and theoretic background knowledge in perioperative nursing are needed.

Chapter Outline

Learning Objectives

1. Define the outcomes of an orientation program.

2. Apply the factors in a learning moment to a teaching/learning milieu for others.

3. Contrast the differences between andragogy and pedagogy.

4. List the steps in designing an educational activity.

Historically, clinical educators were usually senior staff nurses whose sole qualifications were excellent clinical skills. These first educators were neither academically nor experientially prepared to shift from the clinician to educator role and, not surprisingly, often lacked an attitude/aptitude for teaching. Today, education is a service of dynamic organizations as well as one of their mandates, and the challenge for the educator is to meet the ongoing, complex, diverse, and multiple learning needs of the organization's employees. Although a solid clinical background is the background of a service educator, additional knowledge, skills, and expertise in adult education theory and educational design are needed.

Today's educator values the uniqueness of each staff member and works with management to enhance job satisfaction and competency levels and a culture of positive learning in the organization.

Clinical Education

Learning, not patient care, is the direct focus of clinical education; the job of the perioperative service educator, regardless of any formal title or position, is to create the educational experiences that facilitate (1) learning the job's responsibilities, (2) learning about the organization, and (3) learning about one's self in the workplace.

Clinical education as a whole is composed of educational activities commonly known as orientation and in-service programs and may include some continuing education. Each of these activities is its own entity; each has its own outcomes. They are all interrelated in the development of professional practice. In the "big picture" of professional practice, the interrelationship between orientation and other activities is small since the nurse must first become a professional. However, once practice is actualized and operationalized in the work setting, the overlap between in-service training and continuing education is considerable.

The outcome of an *orientation* program is twofold: (1) to identify and clarify role expectations for new staff members in the practice environment, and (2) to socialize new staff members to the norms, practices, attitudes, and values of the practice environment and profession. The outcome of a *preceptorship* program in an orientation program is to facilitate the learning of new staff members within a specific work setting, for example, the operating room or the post-anesthesia care unit. The outcome of an *in-service* activity or program (a series of activities) is to improve the staff's daily working, thinking, and behaving through structured work-related education. The goal of any in-service presentation for professional nurses is improved patient care through better and evolving nursing practice. The outcome of *continuing education* is to enhance the learner's knowledge base and core skills through planned and organized experiences.

Outcome measurement, especially in relation to educational activities, is at an early stage of development today. Outcomes are more than goals; outcomes are results-oriented action-based tools for planning. Goals, on the other hand, are end points of planned activities. The application of outcomes and related measures must be learned and built upon a standards framework. Although there are no standards for clinical education activities, regulatory agencies do suggest minimal guidelines. For example, the Joint Commission on the Accreditation of Healthcare Organizations (JCAHO, 1995) states that

An individual's orientation includes, at least, information about organizational mission, governance, policies, and procedures; department/service policies and procedures, the individual's job description; performance expectation; the organization's plant, technology, and safety management programs, and the individual's safety responsibilities; the organization's infection control program and the individual's role in the prevention of infection; and the organization's quality assessment and improvement activities and the individual's role in these activities.

Accrediting bodies, such as the American Nurses Association (ANA) and the American Nurses Credentialing Center (ANCC), have structure and process standards for nursing staff development and for nursing continuing education. Although the Association of Operating Room Nurses, Inc. (AORN) is neither regulatory nor accrediting, guidelines for orientation are a part of its structure standards. Pursuit of ongoing/life-long learning is part of the AORN's process standards.

The philosophy and the mission of the workplace are the most influential factors in establishing the structure, process, and outcome framework of orientation, in-service training, and continuing education as clinical education activities. Growth and development, for example, is a topic to include in the orientation program for a pediatric care setting; body mechanics is a universal in-service training topic for both support and professional perioperative staff; and, if the workplace services a Hispanic population, Spanish for health care workers is an appropriate continuing education course.

Table 10–1 compares the traditional approach of clinical education with the current approach of clinical service education. Constant health care changes have been a major driving force in catapulting the responsibility for clinical education activities and the role of the service educator to the frontline of practice. In the perioperative setting, the value-based clinical significance (LeFort, 1993) of

TABLE 10–1. **CHARACTERISTICS OF CLINICAL EDUCATION**

TRADITIONAL	CURRENT
Meet continuous basic learning needs (CPR)	Meet intermittent time-sensitive learning needs (tuberculosis update, acquired immunodeficiency syndrome update, personal protective equipment update)
Pre-scheduled times	Just in time, short-term scheduling
Maintain foundational knowledge bases of staff	Facilitate/support the changing organization

potential changes, such as the practice of nurses versus the use of assistive personnel, needs to be validated.

Clinical education, as a whole, is an outcome based activity. The outcomes of the whole as well as the parts (orientation, in-service training, and continuing education) are significant components in quality patient management. Social validation of any nursing practice is based on the following premise that "For change to be clinically significant, it must make an obvious qualitative difference in people's sense of well-being" (LeFort, 1993). The service educator is very significant for future health care scenarios, because of the goals (1) to assess, develop, and maintain competent practitioners and (2) to design outcome based (i.e., learning) clinical education activities.

Clinical Educators

Every educator has a set of basic philosophic beliefs, and these beliefs are carried out in his or her teaching activities. These beliefs have come into the person's life by accident or by intention. They may be self-created, but more often they are created because of life experiences. The intensity of the experience forms the static or dynamic nature of the belief system. The static or dynamic nature of a person's belief system can be summarized by his or her concept of human nature.

- If a person believes that the human race is morally bad, he or she then believes that each learner needs to have their behavior trained.
- If a person believes that the human race is morally good, he or she then believes that each learner needs to have their behavior facilitated.

For any teacher to function effectively, understanding beliefs is not as critical as identifying them. Knowing yourself as a learner is the first step to knowing yourself as a teacher. What the educator identifies as important in a *learning moment* is equally as important to re-create for others. In order to identify a learning moment, ask yourself:

- What was your *most significant* learning experience in the last 6 months?
- When did it occur?
- What was the position or title of those involved?
- What happened during the experience?
- What helped/hindered your learning?
- How did you feel at the conclusion of the experience?

Answers to these questions will help establish the teaching/learning milieu for others.

WHAT IS LEARNING?

Learning, as a concept, can be described in many ways. When learning is used to describe a *product*, the emphasis is on the outcome of the experience, such as the nurse will perform a surgical scrub. When learning is employed to describe a *process*, an attempt is made to account for what happens when a learning experience takes place, such as the nurse will be able to state the steps in a surgical scrub. When learning describes a *function*, the emphasis is on certain important factors that are believed to help produce learning (e.g., change, motivation), such as the nurse will understand the importance of a surgical scrub as part of aseptic practices.

It is suggested that the term *learning* defies precise definition because it is put to multiple uses, with the only common feature of all the definitions being newness. Learning therefore becomes an activity of one who learns. It may be intentional or random; it may involve acquiring information or skills, new attitudes, understandings, or values. It is accompanied by changes in behavior and goes on through life. It seems reasonable to expect that practicing nurses would be able to identify their own learning needs and seek out experiences to meet these needs. Unfortunately, this is not always the case.

The uniqueness of patients lies in the fact that they are human beings. Human beings are complex, dynamic, and individual, and their behaviors are not easily explained, described, or predicted. Nursing practice is also complex and does not lend itself to generalizations. Nurses, therefore, cannot be expected to teach in linear patterns, because their teaching is informed by their practice of nursing. Likewise, nurse learners cannot expect to learn in sequence, as their learning is dependent on their practice. However, the underlying expectation of an educator is for learners to learn, and the underlying expectation of learners is to be taught. Education as an active interchange and exchange of ideas is a concept that needs to be explored.

As children most of us were in a system of formal education. External controls, such as our teachers and/or our age, determined when we were in math class or spelling class, or in third grade or fifth grade. Someone else decided when we would learn to read, what we would read, and when our focus should change from reading to the value of literature. We depended on authorities such as parents and teachers to tell us what was best for us, what we needed, and what we were capable of learning and doing.

- Teacher-centered learning or *pedagogy* is, therefore, what most learners expect of the service educator. For example, a nurse who is new to the operating room practice setting may expect to be taught how to do an inguinal hernia repair, a femoral hernia repair, an umbilical hernia repair, and an incisional hernia repair.
- Content and structure are core values of pedagogy. Teachers and textbooks (content) should tell us, and tell us sequentially [!] (structure), what is right and what is true. What is right and what is true should not deviate from one case or patient to another.
- Motivation to learn is based on a system of reward and punishment. In the perioperative setting, for example, a new learner may expect the entire surgical team to recognize and acknowledge how well he or she did in caring for a patient.

Since the idea of learning is new to most adults, especially those who have been exposed to only traditional educational activities, bridging the gap between their perception of learning and actualizing of learning becomes the first job of the educator. The job of the educator is education through adult teaching and learning principles. Actively engaging learners in the learning process by transforming learning situations in which there is a large amount of information to be learned into formats that incorporate learner participation is the best way to educate adults.

- Learner-centered learning, or andragogy, refers to the art and science of *helping* adults to learn.
- Process is the core value of andragogy as adult learners have a problem to solve or task to accomplish. In order to do so, adults are self-directed to find and participate in educational/improvement experiences.
- Motivation to learn is driven by the internal desire to improve personal ability to function, simplify life, improve relationships, or achieve a goal.

Table 10–2 is a comparison of the pedagogical and the andragogical process concepts of teaching-learning andragogy vs. pedagogy advantages/disadvantages. Lindeman (Davenport, 1985) introduced the idea that adults seem to learn differently than children. Apparently, because he presented this as an idea for educators to consider in practice, he never received the recognition he deserved for identifying the concept.

TABLE 10–2. **BASIC CONCEPTS OF PEDAGOGY AND ANDRAGOGY**

CONCEPT	PEDAGOGY	ANDRAGOGY
Learner	Dependent	Self-directed
Learning experience	A foundation	A resource
Orientation to learn	Subject-centered	Problem-centered
Motivation to learn	Reward/punishment	Incentive/curiosity

. . . in this process, the teacher finds a new function. She/he is no longer the oracle who speaks from the platform of authority, but rather the pointer-out, who also participates in learning in proportion to the vitality and relevancy of his/her facts and experiences.

When Knowles (1973) proposed andragogy as a learner-oriented unifying theory of adult learning, as well as a professional identity for educators and trainers, the concept took on a life of its own. From the 1970s to the present, the controversy, philosophic debate, and critical analysis about the five principles of adult learning that constitute the basis of Knowles' theory have been phenomenal.

Knowles has met the challenges to his ideas with grace and dignity (Table 10–3). Knowles' assumption that the difference between adult and child learners is in the quality and quantity of an adult's experience is the only one that has stood the test of time. An adult's experience is almost always broader than a child's experience. For example, very few 10-year-olds have the experience of being a parent. Children's individual experiences are just as variable. For example, in a group of 10-year-olds, some have traveled the world, while others have not explored beyond their own back yard. The main source of learning is life experience, not teachers.

Knowles also acknowledges that if a person is in an unfamiliar environment, there is a need for structure and content. As the learner accumulates a new foundation of knowledge about the new content area, the learner should take the initiative in learning. The learning experience of the learner is in direct relation to whatever the situation presents. If the learner is challenged, learning will be produced; if the learner is not challenged, he or she will take the initiative to seek out more challenging learning experiences.

Knowles' framework creates a sensitivity to the learner as a person with developmental needs and interests that can be met with educational experiences. Meeting a learner's needs and interests can increase the learner's self-esteem. "Self-esteem is not provable, but it is noticeable" (Bell as cited in Feuer and Geber, 1988).

Self-esteem is a central variable in human behavior. Individuals with positive self-esteem tend to function more effectively in their personal and professional lives. It is very important for service educators to consider a learner's self-esteem because it develops gradually; tends to be fragile in nature; and profoundly affects one's thinking, emotions, values, and goals. Table 10–4 describes self-esteem in terms of learning and teaching concepts.

TABLE 10–3. **ADULT LEARNING: CONTROVERSIAL ISSUES**

Are typical adults truly self-directed or is self-directedness a goal for educators?

Are typical adults ready to learn and oriented to learning because they have a problem to solve or task to accomplish?

Are typical adults motivated to learn because of internal factors such as self-esteem?

Is andragogy more a model of effective instruction than a theory of adult learning?

What is the evidence that proves there are differences between how adults and children learn?

TABLE 10-4. **PROFESSIONAL MATURITY: SELF-ESTEEM AND LEARNING**

DEVELOPMENTAL STAGE	LEARNING	TEACHING METHODS
New nurse learner	Seeks to gain control of the environment by over-learning	Structured and consistent
Nurse learner	Seeks to establish a style based on what works best and is comfortable, or takes risks	Listen, ask questions, discussion
Experienced nurse	Comfortable with current knowledge base; lives according to convictions; potential for learning is high, but is also very influenced by coworkers and colleagues	Explain relationships between old and new concepts/practices; clarify misconceptions; point out similarities and differences in new application of previous learning

The ideal of adult educators is to educate learners who feel successful and enjoy their work in spite of occasional mistakes. To do so, health care service educators, like other adult educators, have a responsibility to reflect on the theoretic frameworks of educational practice. The mutual goal of the teacher and learner in adult education is to create positive and realistic educational encounters that facilitate the adult learner's ability to cope with daily situations.

A learning environment may be highly structured, content-oriented, or flexible; the teaching method may be experiential or didactic. In any case, the adult learner should be informed of the rationale for the learning method. This understanding provides a cognitive map, which will enhance learning ability and influence retention. Adult learners should understand what they are expected to learn in any educational activity, its relevance to their future professional lives, and how the sequence of activities will enable them to learn what it is they need to learn.

Educational activities that include every type of learning experience cannot be planned. It is impossible to account for all student differences. Providing as many learning resources as is feasible, though, increases the likelihood that adult learners will assimilate the required knowledge and skills and creates a more exciting experience.

Adult learners need to be able to adapt their education to a number of real situations. For example, a nurse who has transferred to the operating room from the intensive care unit has the skill to insert Foley catheters. A good rule of thumb for the educator to remember is to respect what a learner already knows but may think is different — because the care activity is occurring in an environment new to that learner.

Most successful adult learners had professional role models who contributed to their image of competence. Education in the clinical setting needs to go beyond an emotional identification with these individuals to actual emulation of their patient care behaviors. Adult learners should be given concrete and systematic opportunities to observe these individuals and study the behaviors that constitute their effectiveness.

Adult learners need practice, supervision, and feedback to determine the adequacy of their performance. They should have opportunities as well to correct deficiencies until the level of mastery specified in the expected outcome is achieved. Supervision and feedback that are evaluative and not judgmental in nature can assist adult learners to become competent practitioners. Adult learners should have adequate opportunities to practice using the knowledge and skills they have learned and should receive feedback on their performance until the expected level of competence is attained.

The motivational desire adult learners bring to the educational activity has much to do with personality and previous learning. Creating an overall positive experience is likely to enhance their level of motivation and their desire to learn.

Adult learners need to have ample opportunity to examine ways of adapting learned knowledge and skills based on the characteristics of a given situation.

The transfer of general nursing and/or didactic learning concepts into actual clinical practice is a definite challenge. Teaching, as well as learning variables is complex and often independent of the educational activity. The two basic approaches to meet the apparently opposing demands of the situation are (1) concept-based learning and (2) behavior-based learning. Table 10–5 compares the concepts involved in these two approaches. A third approach, which has been popular in nursing education since the mid-80s and is still in research in perioperative nursing practice, is that of learning styles/preferences (Goldrick, 1993). The core ideas for each of these approaches are outlined in this section for perioperative educators and perioperative practice learners. Since it is assumed that, as professionals, nurses are involved in formal and informal teaching-learning activities, an awareness of each of these approaches seems germane to day-to-day nursing practice.

TABLE 10–5. DIFFERENCES BETWEEN CONCEPTUAL LEARNING AND BEHAVIORAL LEARNING

CONCEPTUAL	BEHAVIORAL
Concepts are ideas expressed and communicated through words or labels. They are the strands, threads, or underlying themes . . . to shape, organize, and implement a curriculum in some logical focused way . . . . If the meaning of [a concept] is unclear or there are multiple interpretations of them, confusion may result.* **Process concept:** thinking abilities and attitudes or perspectives that are integral to an individual and used to guide his or her actions **Content concept:** relating to knowledge that can be studied, memorized, analyzed, absorbed, and applied	A desired performance is achieved as a result of the learner's participation in an educational activity.
inductive tentative dynamic	deductive firm static
understanding	memorizing
ideas broad deep experiential active questions process strategy	facts narrow surface rote passive answers content tactics
alternatives exploration discovery active	goal prediction dogma reactive
initiative whole brain	directive left brain
life long-term change	job short-term stability
content flexible risk synthesis open imagination	form rigid rules thesis closed common sense

*Valiga, T. M., Bruderle, E. (1994). Concepts included in and critical to nursing curricula: an analysis. *Journal of Nursing Education, 33*(3): 118.

Concept-based learning is an instructional design model that uses the "big picture" approach to transferring knowledge into practice. The term *concept* refers to a set of objects, events, or ideas that are classified and referred to by specific names and/or symbols (Kinnick, 1990). An everyday example of a concept is that common characteristics such as bark, leaves, and branches could be used to define a tree. In perioperative nursing practice, common characteristics such as heat, pressure, and time could be used to define sterilization; common characteristics such as weak fascia, protrusion, and presence of a sac could be used to define hernia.

Each of these concepts has subconcepts that are further defined by additional subconcepts—each more and more discriminating. The core of concept-based learning in perioperative clinical education activities is to (1) name the concept, (2) define the critical characteristics that must be present to identify or classify an example of the concept, and (3) relate the concept to other concepts. In order to *teach* using concept-based learning, the educator provides inductive expository examples, such as cut tissue will bleed; bleeding requires hemostasis; hemostasis can be achieved by (a) clamping, (b) topical agents, (c) electrocoagulation, (d) suturing, or (e) pressure. On the other hand, in concept-based learning, the learner employs inductive statements, such as if it is cut, it will bleed; when it bleeds, the bleeding must be stopped.

The AORN *Preceptor Guide for Perioperative Nursing* (AORN, 1993) and *A Job Analysis* of the National Certification Board: Perioperative Nursing, Inc. (NCB:PNI) are the most common frameworks for concept-based clinical education activities. Each of these documents can reference technical and professional competencies of perioperative nursing. Each has broad, general statements for expectations and describes the behaviors that should be achieved when the concept is grasped. For example, the job analysis item *Patient Protection* is a concept. The publication itemizes both the knowledge and the skill inherent in this concept, such as transferring, positioning, equipment, pharmacology, and emergency support systems. Educators can use the knowledge and skills to create learning experiences; learners can demonstrate behaviors that appropriately show mastery of the concept. Neither the learning experiences nor the actualized behaviors need to be black and white. Therefore, concept-based learning is more nonlinear than the traditional education most of us have experienced.

Behavior-based learning is an educational design approach that utilizes topics and content development to transfer knowledge into practice. Behavior-based learning consists of an activity documentation form developed by the teacher, which is generated by a learning needs assessment, learning objectives, teaching methods/resources, content, and evaluation. Each of these components of behavior-based learning is briefly described in this section. Behavior-based learning is formally structured and planned and is usually didactic in nature. It assumes the learner is dependent on the teacher to identify what is important to learn. The elements of educational design are the tools for logically organizing the teaching experience for an activity, program, or course. Implementing a systematic plan helps to insure that the educational activity will result in the outcome that is desired.

Educational Design

The purpose for designing educational activities is to produce the most effective sequence of instructional techniques and strategies. This planning will help convey the information in a manner that best helps learners accomplish their learning. The emphasis in design should focus on selecting strategies that facilitate learner participation and achievement. The optimal goal is a stimulating and

TABLE 10-6. **TYPES OF NEEDS**

Real need	An objective deficiency of an individual, group, institution, or community in relation to the environment. For example, the ability to maintain a sterile environment is a real need.
Educational need	A need that can be satisfied by a learning experience. It is considered to be a lack, deprivation, or deficiency that tells one what to do in a new situation. For example, an RN who has come from a student experience in an academic setting needs assistance in making the transition from the student to an employee role (orientation).
Real educational need	Refers to specific understanding, skills, and aptitudes that are lacking but are required to obtain a more desirable condition. It can be satisfied by a learning experience. An example is the experienced nurse in the OR who ceases to use principles of asepsis in practice. Upon investigation, the real educational need is not lack of knowledge of asepsis but lack of motivation.
Perceived need	Something regarded as necessary by the person or persons concerned. For example, a nurse asks to observe a procedure rarely performed but which he or she believes will enhance his or her performance.

comfortable learning environment in which everyone involved can benefit from the results of education.

All parts of the design will be intertwined through the process of developing the activity. Once the activity is designed, however, the task is not finished. The design itself will be evaluated by both learners and educators and reshaped for future presentations. The design process must be ongoing.

The initial step in the educational design is an educational process of performance assessment called *learning needs assessment*. Is there a discrepancy between the actual performance and the desired or optimum performance level? If the answer is yes, a learning need may have been identified (Table 10–6). It is easy to fall into the trap of seeing education as the answer to every performance problem. The educator must investigate to determine if a true learning need exists or if the discrepancy is due to some other reason. Even when the discrepancy can be corrected by an educational session, there may be more cost-effective and time-efficient methods.

A learning needs assessment is more than just a "shopping list" of topics that would be good to know, although a shopping list of topics may be what learners generate when asked their interests. A great disservice an educator can do is to ask a presenter to speak about a topic from a list. Instead, the educator must look for trends in the lists, compare the trends with the practice setting, and compare the topics with the desired outcomes of educational activities. If, for example, one of the topics requested is "turnaround time," the educator must ask himself or herself, "Is the nature of this request a time, place, or person request. . . what is our average turnaround time. . . how is it documented. . . is there a policy . . . "

A variety of techniques can be utilized to assess learning needs. Some provide more objective data than others. Not too long ago, in order to assess learning needs at the departmental level, it was not unusual to poll the staff for a list and to rank the topics generated; review patient documentation; or search the literature for upcoming trends, issues, and procedures. However, it has now been suggested (Brown-Stewart, 1993) that learning needs be assessed on the basis of the following:

- Patient populations to be served by the department/unit
- Aspects of care or service to be provided
- Needs of individual staff members
- Information gathered from quality management activities
- Availability of new technologies

- Availability of new or revised care delivery systems
- Findings from staff performance appraisals
- Findings from safety management programs
- Findings from infection control activities
- Findings from peer review activities

In summary, education activities that are not based on the learning needs of the learner are useless. If a policy states that the count section of patient care records is to be signed by both the scrub person and circulator and an audit reveals that this is not being done, it is not likely that the learning need is that people are unaware of the policy. Instead, staff may need a review of time management skills. Alternatively, the system that requires the scrub person to remain gowned and gloved until the patient and the chart leave the room may actually prevent implementation of the policy.

A *learning objective* is the desired outcome or end result of what is to be accomplished when learning has occurred. An objective describes a proposed change in the learner and describes the expected performance. Without clearly defined objectives, the learner has no guide to the expected outcome (behavior). It is also impossible to evaluate the activity, educator, or learner; to make appropriate changes in content; or to choose other learning experiences in order to accomplish the desired results. If objectives are to be useful, they must describe performance in terms of terminal achievements at the end of an activity. Learning objectives are statements of what the learner will be able to accomplish after participating in an educational activity. If a behavior change is accomplished, it can be assumed that the learner has learned.

Objectives are developed from assessed educational learning needs. Directing learning from the educator's perspective of what should be learned does not motivate a learner. Deciding what another person needs to know does not mean that person will be accountable for his or her learning. Adult learners accept responsibility and accountability for learning only if the objective meets a personally identified educational need.

If possible, the objectives should always be written in conjunction with the learners. When learners are able to help develop the objectives, it is more likely that they will be motivated to work toward accomplishment of the objectives, because they reflect their beliefs and expectations. Working with the learner in developing the objective also assures that the objective is individualized.

The first component to consider in developing a learning objective is the *who*, that is, the person who is to perform the change in behavior. When setting an objective, remember to make the objective a statement of learner performance, such as "The learner will be able to . . . ."

The task statement tells what the learner will be able to do once the learning has been completed. The actual task statement behavior must be stated as an action verb that can be clearly and directly measured to determine whether the learner is demonstrating achievement of the objective. For example, the verbs *know*, *understand*, and *believe* cannot accurately refer to mastery, since these behaviors cannot be objectively measured. Verbs such as *define*, *measure*, *draw*, and *list* describe specific actions that the learner will be able to demonstrate. Some behaviors can be measured and others cannot. The following list of verbs indicates some actions that are measurable and some that are not.

Behaviors That Are Not Measurable	Behaviors That Are Measurable
Appreciate	Compare/contrast
Become aware of	Define
Believe	Demonstrate
Communicate	Describe
Enjoy	Design

Table continued on following page

Behaviors That Are Not Measurable	Behaviors That Are Measurable
Increase	Discuss
Implement	Identify
Know	List
Learn	Set up
Motivate	State
Understand	Use

The more accurately the expected *new* performance/behavior is analyzed, the better the different task behaviors can be addressed using appropriate teaching tactics. Keep asking "What is this lesson to accomplish?" or "What is the learner to be able to do?" Common sense helps a person function well in many situations without knowing underlying principles and facts. Conversely, facts can be known, but ignored. For example, a group of nurses can know that patient care planning is a professional responsibility and have the ability to write plans of care, yet not actually write patient plans of care. In this instance, the educational task is to develop positive feelings about patient care planning.

Knowledge and skills checklists assist the educator in assessing the level of knowledge and skills the individual possesses. The educator plans appropriate content based upon the outcome of the assessment.

Content is described as the information (knowledge and/or skills) presented in education activities. The selection of content is an important element in the teaching/learning process. Content reflects the information — the *what* — that a learner needs to know. The content of educational activities includes facts, concepts, principles, and theories that the objectives identify as essential to be included in order to achieve learning. After determining the content that can meet the established learning objectives, it is essential to think about sequence. Sequence is the order in which content is learned. This order cannot be established without taking into consideration that the learners are generally at different experiential levels.

Methodologies/resources enhance or facilitate the learning process. Methods should be chosen that take into consideration the target audience — adult learners; methods should also be adapted to the individual differences of the learners and should take into consideration learning styles. They should stimulate as many of the sensory organs as possible, since retention of learning increases as more senses are stimulated. Given that adults appreciate nonsimulated experiences, educators must strive to facilitate *real patient* practice as much as possible. For example, allowing new learners to perform surgical preps on each other is no different from having student nurses begin their clinical experiences by giving intramuscular injections to each other.

Resources should be selected taking into consideration their availability. For example, are the physical facilities offering the kinds of experiences that are necessary to accomplish the objectives? If the desired resources are not available, the educator has a responsibility to evaluate new techniques, manipulate the facilities, and vary the methods. The creative educator can usually devise unique activities that meet the learners' needs in addition to fulfilling objectives and still obtain the most mileage from physical resources.

Evaluation is one of the most widely discussed topics in educational and health care systems. Evaluating outcomes by measuring whether learners accomplish desired objectives and determining the degree to which the teaching/learning process is successful demonstrate accountability to the process of education. The primary purpose of evaluation is to enhance the learning process not to penalize the learner. Increased attention is being focused on evaluation in relation to the educational activity's return on investment, the application of the skills and knowledge acquired in the activity, and whether the application improves patient care.

Evaluation of educational activities can be formal or informal, ongoing or spontaneous, but it must never be left to chance. The teacher needs to develop and utilize strategies to measure and communicate the learner's competencies. The students need an opportunity to share perceptions and satisfaction with the elements (i.e., educational experiences), since they relate to them from the perspective of the learner. The evaluation provides valuable information that should be collected, compared, and used to design and develop future activities.

- Evaluation is the sum of all the design elements.
- The goal of evaluation is to produce information to use in refinement of the program to assure the desired positive outcomes.

The process of evaluation is not an easy task. When the evaluation is done, it should result in positive actions that will enhance the educational activity. This action may take the form of changing the activity by altering the objectives or the course, identifying changes that are planned, or soliciting input from those expressing interest.

In the 1970s, a new framework for examining the behavior called learning emerged—that of *learning styles*. The assumption underlying the concept of learning styles is that people learn *more* and *better* if taught in the way they *prefer* to learn. Teaching based on learning style, therefore, concentrates on *how* people, as individuals, best process new information in education or training situations. Learning style refers to how people, as individuals, best *process* new information in educational or training situations. An individual's preferences, dispositions, and tendencies can be a cognitive style, which is measured in terms of how many and how well. There are numerous learning style assessment tools available to investigate individual learning styles. All have been used and crossused by researchers to demonstrate the learning style preferences of various groups. Unfortunately, the validity of learning style research has been limited owing to (1) lack of clear and consistent operational definitions, (2) small and homogeneous study samples, and (3) less than rigorous research design. Nonetheless, even with these limitations, there is consensus that educators in all disciplines (1) need an awareness of the concept of learning style, and (2) need to know that learning style can be related to but should not be considered to be a component of educational design.

- Learning style does not reflect degree of intelligence or lack thereof.
- Learning style is not a static prescriptive diagnosis.
- Matching learning style to teaching style to enhance potential has yet to be established.
- The relationship of learning style to cognitive style needs to be investigated.
- The issues involved in cultural diversity have not been related to learning style.
- The influence of the environment on learning seems to be a missing link in the teaching/learning research literature.

PRECEPTORSHIP

Preceptorship has long been accepted as an effective means of orienting new staff to an institution and a new work environment. Clinical preceptors can assist the learner in bridging the gap between theory and practice. Preceptorships offer an individualized approach and, therefore, can be employed with staff of various levels and types of experience, as well as with staff with no previous experience. The *Preceptor Guide for Perioperative Nursing* (AORN, 1993) outlines the following objectives of a preceptor program:

- Efficiently foster the development of an individualized orientation plan based on the needs of the learner. (Rationale: Individualized orientation can eliminate areas already mastered by the preceptee and instead build on the individual's previous experiences and knowledge.)

- Provide a role model for the preceptee. (Rationale: New employees should witness the standard of care that will be required of them. Since one of the qualifications of the preceptor is excellence in nursing practice, the preceptor is in the ideal position to serve as a role model.)
- Assist the preceptee in the socialization process of adjusting to the unit and institution. (Rationale: Belonging or being part of the work group is an important component of job satisfaction and retention.)
- Insure competent nursing care for all patients. (Rationale: Preceptorships provide close working relationships, thus offering the opportunity for the identification of knowledge deficits and corrective action plans.)
- Promote an understanding of how the institutional culture impacts the delivery of patient care. (Rationale: Understanding the institutional culture is part of the process of becoming an effective employee.)

Issues for Development

What motivates learners to learn and what creates excitement about the process of learning continues to be a constant challenge for educators from all disciplines. Instead of a paucity of literature that exists on many similar problems, the concept of learning has been addressed fully in the nursing literature. As a dimension of learning, the concept of learning styles to assess and explain the learning process of both nursing students and practicing nurses has been a popular topic in journals oriented to nursing education, higher education, staff development, continuing education, and even management.

Educators seem to have a strong sense that learners should not be sent out to the world of practice unprepared for the reality of their profession. The problem is that what they need and can use involves a total universe of knowledge. The questions then become what to teach, how much to teach, and in how much time, and how not to let personal preferences or insecurities influence the answers to these questions. Trying to teach everything is not possible and may be self-defeating. As accrediting agencies incorporate their terms of evaluation, outcomes, and objective performances in their standards and criteria, educators must concentrate on differentiating the levels of importance in order to assess competence and productivity.

Education has a tradition that, over time, has become its informal rules as to how teaching is done. However, educators are facing massive changes in the way they perform their jobs. Philosophic and conceptual paradigm shifts are required as knowledge/skill (i.e., competence) rather than instruction is emphasized. The shift from teaching to learning, specifying expected outcomes, identifying learning resources, and stimulating an environment of mutuality (trust/caring/respect), provides a new focus for educators.

Organizational effectiveness, not individual effectiveness, is another new focus since education is part of an organization. Educators must see their mission as not to teach but to link themselves to the organization's productivity and profit. An environment that expects learning, growing, and changing will also facilitate opportunities to do so. The organizations that survive today will be those that are dynamic, not static, systems. Tools and techniques must also be dynamic. The service of education is both a tool and a technique.

RESEARCH IMPLICATIONS FOR CLINICAL EDUCATORS

Once adult education becomes the ultimate focus of the educator, it is best to approach the practice of clinical education as a framework for that learning. What do educators, today and tomorrow, need to study and think about in order to provide the adult learner with the best learning encounters?

Health care educators plan and implement educational encounters to meet a wide range of needs. At one end of the continuum are highly skill-oriented activities such as CPR, fire safety, and equipment operation; at the other end are professional development activities such as decision making, problem solving, and critical thinking. What teaching/learning methods/models work best in a practice environment where the norms are rapid change, ambiguity, uncertainty, and explosive growth of information/technology?

Individual competence is an essential ingredient of an organization's doing the right thing and doing it well. Good results are achieved when competent people work in effective systems. Poor results most often are the product of ineffective systems. The responsibilities of the educator are to contribute to the "big picture" by meeting the learning needs of the staff. The competencies of the educator are as important as the competencies of the adults they teach.

REFERENCES

American Nurses Association. (1992). *Roles and Responsibilities for Nursing Continuing Education and Staff Development Across All Settings.* Kansas City, MO: ANA.

American Nurses Association. (1994). *Standards for Nursing Professional Development: Continuing Education and Staff Development.* ANA: Washington, D.C.

Association of Operating Room Nurses. (1993). *Preceptor Guide for Perioperative Nursing.* Denver: AORN (p 3).

Association of Operating Room Nurses. (1994). Standards and Recommended Practices. Denver: AORN.

Brown-Stewart, P. (1993). Redesigning needs assessment for new JCAHO standards. *Staff Development Insider, 2*(5), 1–3.

Davenport, J., Davenport, J. A. (1985). Knowles or Lindeman: would the real father of American andragogy please stand up? *Lifelong Learning, 9*(4), 4–5, 610.

Davis, A. R. (1988). Developing teaching strategies based on new knowledge. *Journal of Nursing Education, 27*(4), 156–160.

Feuer, D., Geber, B. (1988). Uh-oh . . . Second thoughts about adult learning theory. *Training Magazine, 25*(12), 31–39.

Goldrick, B., Gruendemann, B., Larson, E. (1993). Learning styles and teaching/learning strategy preferences: implications for educating nurses in critical care, the operating room, and infection control. *Heart and Lung, 22*(2), 176–182.

Joint Commission on the Accreditation of Healthcare Organizations. (1995). *Manual for the Accreditation of Health Care Organizations.* Oakbrook, IL: JCAHO.

Joint Commission *Perspectives.* (November/December 1992). Agenda for Change Q & A: The survey process and surveyors. (pp. 13–14).

Joint Commission *Perspectives.* (July/August 1992). Interpretations: Standards for individual competence assessment clarified. (pp. 11–12).

Kinnick, V. (1990). The effect of concept teaching in preparing nursing students for clinical practice. *Journal of Nursing Education, 29*(8), 362–366.

Knowles, M. (1973). *The Adult Learner: A Neglected Species.* Houston: Gulf Publishing Company.

Knowles, M. S. (1980). *The Modern Practice of Adult Education: From Pedagogy to Andragogy.* Chicago: Follett Publishing Company.

Knowles, M. (1984). *Andragogy in Action: Applying Modern Principles of Adult Learning.* San Francisco: Jossey-Bass Publishers.

LeFort, S. M. (1993). The statistical versus clinical significance debate. *Image: Journal of Nursing Scholarship. 25*(1), 57–62.

Leonard, D. J. (1993). Workplace education: adult education in a hospital nursing staff development department. *Journal of Nursing Staff Development, 9*(2), 68–73.

McDaniels, O. B. (1983). Existentialism and pragmatism: the effect of philosophy on methodology of teaching. *Journal of Nursing Education, 22*(2), 62–66.

National Certification Board: Perioperative Nursing, Inc. (1992). *A Job Analysis.* Denver: NCB: PNI.

O'Leary, D. S. (1992). Articles misconstrue Joint Commission's position on quality improvement. Joint Commission *Perspectives, 12*(6), 2.

Thompson, C., Crutchlow, E. (1993). Learning style research: a critical review of the literature and implications for nursing education. *Journal of Professional Nursing, 9*(1), 34–40.

Urden, L D. (1989). Knowledge development in clinical practice. *The Journal of Continuing Education in Nursing, 20*(1), 18–22.

Valiga, T. M., Bruderle, E. (1994). Concepts included in and critical to nursing curricula: an analysis. *Journal of Nursing Education, 33*(3), 118.

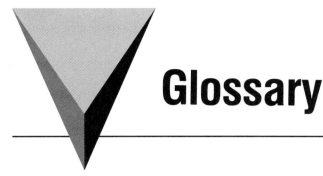

Glossary

Active Electrode Accessory that directs the high energy, radio frequency electrical current flow from an electrosurgery generator to the operative site (*Chapters 5 and 9*)

Allocation Process of distributing resources according to a specified plan (*Chapter 2*)

Andragogy Self-directed learning; i.e., the learner assumes responsibility for the direction and pace of the learning experience; contrast Pedagogy (*Chapter 10*)

Antimicrobial Chemical that acts against microbes to prevent the development of pathogenic activity (*Chapter 9*)

AORN Association of Operating Room Nurses (*Chapter 9*)

APICE Association for Practitioners in Infection Control and Epidemiology (*Chapter 9*)

Approximate To bring the edges of tissues together to promote wound healing after surgery (*Chapter 9*)

Artificial Nails Cosmetic adhesives used to enhance or lengthen natural fingernails (*Chapter 3*)

American Society of Anesthesiologists (ASA) Physical Status Classification of the preoperative status of the surgical patient developed by the ASA and based upon coexisting systemic diseases that could have an impact on the patient's condition while under anesthesia (*Chapter 7*)

Asepsis Absence of microorganisms that cause disease; freedom from infection; exclusion of microorganisms (*Chapter 3*)

Aseptic Technique Method by which the contamination of a sterile field with microorganisms is prevented (*Chapters 3 and 9*)

Assessment Collection and documentation of data about the health status of the patient (*Chapter 6*)

Bacteria Microscopic unicellular organisms that reproduce and are capable of causing disease (*Chapter 9*)

Bactericidal Capable of destroying bacteria (*Chapter 9*)

Behavior-based Learning Educational approach that uses topic and content development to transfer knowledge into practice (*Chapter 10*)

Bioburden Degree of microbial contamination on a device or object prior to sterilization (*Chapter 4*)

Bronchospasm Abnormal narrowing of the bronchi leading to obstruction of the airway due to contractions of the bronchial smooth muscle (*Chapter 7*)

Capacitance Ability of an object to store an electrical charge (*Chapter 7*)

Capnography Continuous monitoring of the percentage of carbon dioxide in exhaled air of mechanically ventilated patients (*Chapter 7*)

Centers for Disease Control and Prevention (CDC) Branch of the Department of Health and Human Services that develops and provides information related to epidemiology and infection control (*Chapter 9*)

Primary chapter references supplied in parentheses. Terms may also appear in other chapters.

Certification   Documented validation of the professional achievement of acknowledged standards of practice and body of knowledge (*Chapter 2*)

Chemical Germicide   Generic term for an agent used to destroy microorganisms; registered with the United States Environmental Protection Agency; this classification includes sporicides, general disinfectants, hospital disinfectants, sanitizers, and other chemicals (*Chapter 3*)

Chemical Indicator   Device to monitor certain parameters of a sterilization process by means of a characteristic color change, including chemically treated paper, pellet sealed in glass tube, and pressure-sensitive tape (*Chapter 3*)

Chronotropic   Influencing the time or rate of an event, such as the heart rate (*Chapter 7*)

Collaboration   Process of working together to achieve defined goals or outcomes (*Chapter 2*)

Collagen   Insoluble fibrous protein in connective tissue, skin, bone, and cartilage; plays an important role in wound healing (*Chapter 9*)

Concept-based Learning   Educational approach that provides the learner with the broad scope and interrelationships of the material to be learned (*Chapter 10*)

Confine and Contain   Principle that recommends that the potential spread of microorganisms be restricted to an area of three feet around the patient to prevent cross-infection of other patients and personnel; microorganisms outside this area should be confined in a leakproof or impervious container or destroyed (*Chapter 3*)

Contamination   Presumed presence of pathogenic microorganisms on or in an object (*Chapter 3*)

Cross Infection   Microorganisms spread from one source to another, e.g., from one person to another (*Chapter 3*)

Current   Rate of flow of electrons through a conductor (*Chapters 5 and 9*)

Data Collection   Gathering of information through interview, physical examination, observation, consultation (with family members or health care professionals), and review of medical records (*Chapter 6*)

Data Organization   Process of grouping collected information in logical patterns or clusters to prevent decision making based upon a single fact (*Chapter 6*)

Decontamination   Process that removes as many microorganisms as possible from an object by physical, mechanical, or chemical means (*Chapter 4*)

Deep Wound Infection   Infection involving the tissues or spaces at or below the fascial layer; generally occurs within 30 days of surgery, but with implants can occur within the year following surgery (*Chapter 9*)

Dehiscence   Splitting open, as in the bursting of a wound (*Chapter 9*)

Disinfection   Process that destroys or inhibits disease-producing microorganisms, excluding spores (*Chapters 3, 4, and 9*)

Dispersive Electrode   Accessory that directs the current flow from the patient back to the electrosurgery generator; also called a "patient plate" (*Chapters 5 and 9*)

Documentation   Recording of the nursing process in the medical record (*Chapter 6*)

Dysphoria   Exaggerated feeling of depression and unrest that is not related to an apparent cause (*Chapter 7*)

Electrosurgery   High radio frequency current used to cut and coagulate tissue (*Chapters 5 and 9*)

Engineering Controls   Physical devices that remove or reduce hazards in the workplace (*Chapter 5*)

Epidemiology   Study of the interrelationships of the host, agent, and environment in disease (*Chapter 9*)

Evaluation   Review of the effectiveness of provided nursing care based upon established goals (*Chapter 6*)

Evisceration   Protrusion of viscera through a cavity wall, often resulting from abdominal wound dehiscence (*Chapter 9*)

Exposure   Measure of the total quantity of radiation reaching a specific point; unit of measure is based upon the amount of ionization produced in air by a specified amount of x-ray or gamma ray energy; radiation exposure may be controlled by shielding, distance, or time (*Chapter 3*)

Fenestration Opening, e.g., the pre-formed opening in a surgical drape (*Chapter 3*)

Fibroblast Cell or corpuscle from which connective tissue develops (*Chapter 9*)

First Intention Healing Close approximation of wound edges to promote healing within hours of surgery (*Chapter 9*)

Fluoroscopy Imaging process in which internal structures are viewed through fluorescence produced on a screen by x-rays transmitted through an object; produces ten times more radiation exposure to humans in one minute than does one x-ray film exposure (*Chapters 3 and 5*)

Generator Machine that produces high energy, radio frequency electrical current (*Chapter 9*)

Germicidal Capable of destroying pathogenic organisms (*Chapter 3*)

Goal Expected outcome of nursing care; what the nurse intends to observe within a defined period of time (*Chapter 6*)

Granulation Fleshy projections formed on the surface of a wound that is not healing by primary intention (*Chapter 9*)

Hands-free Technique Instrument transfer that insures that the scrub person and the surgeon never touch the same sharp instrument at the same time, e.g., instruments can be placed in a neutral zone between the scrub person and the surgeon (*Chapter 3*)

High-level Disinfection Process in which an EPA-registered agent kills vegetative bacteria, tubercle bacilli, some spores, fungi, and lipid and nonlipid viruses through appropriate concentration, submersion, and contact time; manufacturers' recommendations may differ (*Chapter 3*)

Hospital-grade Chemical Germicide Agent that is effective against *Salmonella, Staphylococcus aureus*, and *Pseudomonas aeruginosa* that performs low- or intermediate-level disinfection (*Chapter 3*)

Hypercarbia Increased level of carbon dioxide in the blood (*Chapter 7*)

Implementation One or more nursing activities necessary to accomplish the intended goals of patient care (*Chapter 6*)

Incisional Wound Infection Infection located above the fascial layer in a wound, occurring within 30 days of surgical intervention; also called superficial wound infection (*Chapter 9*)

Infection Invasion of a body or body part by a pathogenic organism; can be local or systemic and often is transmissible (*Chapter 9*)

Infection Control Practices or procedures intended to limit the transmission of microorganisms (*Chapter 9*)

Infectious Waste Debris that is capable of producing a transmissible disease; factors that must be present simultaneously for infection to occur include the presence of a pathogen in sufficient virulence and quantities, portal of entry, and susceptible host (*Chapters 3 and 5*)

Inotropic Influencing the force of an event, e.g., muscle contraction (*Chapter 7*)

In-service Training On-the-job structured educational activities (*Chapter 10*)

Intermediate-level Disinfection Process that inactivates *Mycobacterium tuberculosis*, vegetative bacteria, most viruses, and most fungi but does not necessarily kill bacterial spores (*Chapter 3*)

Intraoperative Phase of the surgical experience that begins when the patient is transferred to the operating room bed and ends when the patient is admitted to the postanesthesia care unit (*Chapters 2 and 6*)

Ionizing Radiation Electromagnetic radiation, such as x-rays, that yields ions as it passes through the body (*Chapter 5*)

Laryngospasm Contraction of the laryngeal muscles (*Chapter 7*)

Laser Acronym for *light amplification by stimulated emission of radiation*; used in surgical procedures (*Chapter 5*)

Laser Plume   Smoke that is generated as tissue is vaporized by a laser (*Chapter 5*)

Learning Objective   Desired outcome or result of an educational experience (*Chapter 10*)

Low-level Disinfection   Process that kills most bacteria, some viruses, and some fungi but that cannot be relied upon to kill resistant microorganisms, such as tubercle bacilli and bacterial spores (*Chapter 3*)

Microabrasion   Minute cuts in the skin that are invisible to the naked eye (*Chapter 9*)

Microbiology   Study of microorganisms, including bacteria, fungi, viruses, and pathogenic protozoa (*Chapter 9*)

Microorganism   Minute (usually microscopic) organism (*Chapter 9*)

Monitored Anesthesia Care (MAC)   Technique in which an anesthesiologist or anesthetist is present to provide adjunct drugs and monitoring for a patient undergoing surgery, usually with local anesthesia (*Chapter 7*)

Myoclonic   Intermittent twitching of the muscles (*Chapter 7*)

Necrosis   Cell death caused by disease or trauma; usually localized (*Chapter 9*)

Non-ionizing Radiation   Type of electromagnetic radiation that does not accumulate in the body; does not require monitoring; and, when properly handled, does not produce any hazard (*Chapter 5*)

Nonwoven   Processed cellulosic and synthetic fibers randomly oriented in a sheet held with binders or a fabric produced by bonding fibers; designed as single-use material (*Chapter 3*)

Nosocomial Infection   Infection originating in a health care facility (*Chapter 9*)

No-touch Technique   Use of an extension instrument, such as a sponge forceps (rather than one's hands), to handle or touch contaminated or sterile objects (*Chapter 3*)

Nursing Diagnosis   Actual or potential health problem that provides a basis for the selection of nursing interventions to achieve desired outcomes for which the nurse is accountable (*Chapter 6*)

Nursing Process   Systematic approach to nursing care that includes assessment, nursing diagnosis, planning, implementation, evaluation, and reassessment (*Chapter 6*)

Occupational Safety and Health Administration (OSHA)   Federal regulatory agency that addresses all aspects of employee safety for most employers (*Chapter 5*)

Opisthotonos   Tetanic spasm in which the head and heels are bent backward, and the body is bowed forward (*Chapter 7*)

Pedagogy   Learning process that is controlled by someone other than the learner; the instructor plans the direction and pace of the learning experience; contrast *Andragogy* (*Chapter 10*)

Perioperative   Activities beginning with the decision for surgical intervention and ending with the postoperative follow-up office evaluation (*Chapter 6*)

Personal Protective Equipment   Specialized equipment or clothing used by individuals to protect themselves from direct exposure to blood or other potentially infectious materials, including gloves, gowns, fluid-resistant aprons, head and foot coverings, face shields or masks, eye protectors, and ventilation devices (mouth pieces, resuscitation bags, and pocket masks) (*Chapters 3 and 5*)

Planning   Mapping out of nursing activities necessary to help the patient achieve specific goals (*Chapter 6*)

Pneumatic Tourniquet   Balloon-like cuff attached to a source of compressed gas or air used to constrict blood vessels to control or prohibit blood flow within the surgical field (*Chapter 9*)

Postoperative   Phase of the surgical experience that begins with admission to the postanesthesia care unit and ends with the resolution of surgical sequelae (*Chapters 2 and 6*)

Potentially Infectious Materials   Any human body fluid to which a health care worker may be exposed in the practice setting, including blood, serum, semen, vaginal secretion, cerebrospinal fluid, synovial fluid, pleural fluid, pericardial fluid, peritoneal fluid, amniotic fluid, saliva, any body fluid visibly contaminated with blood, any unfixed tissue or organ, any HIV cell or tissue culture, and tissue from any animal infected with HIV or HBV (*Chapter 3*)

Preceptor Clinically experienced individual who assists in orienting new employees to a work environment by bridging theory and practice (*Chapter 10*)

Preoperative Phase of the surgical experience that begins when the decision for surgical intervention is made and ends when the patient is transferred to the operating room bed (*Chapters 2 and 6*)

Professional Development Process in which the nurse acquires knowledge, skills, and abilities required to fulfill a defined role in the practice setting (*Chapter 2*)

Pulse Oximetry Continuous noninvasive measurement of the arterial oxygen saturation of the hemoglobin and the heart rate (*Chapter 7*)

Reassessment Review at each stage of the nursing process due to constantly changing patient data (*Chapter 6*)

Recommended Practices Guidelines that represent an optimal level of practice (*Chapter 2*)

Regulated Waste Liquid, semiliquid, or other potentially infectious materials, including contaminated items that, if compressed, would release blood or other infectious materials; items caked with dried blood or other potentially infectious substances; and pathologic and microbiologic debris containing blood and other infectious substances (*Chapter 5*)

Rehydration Process of adding moisture to linen by laundering with water before sterilization (*Chapter 3*)

Resident Microbes Microorganisms that exist in parts of the body, such as epithelial cells of hair follicles and glands, that are not easily removed by scrubbing (*Chapter 9*)

Risk Management Program that seeks to improve the working conditions and the health and safety of patients and employees by enforcing safety procedures, monitoring activities, correcting problems, and documenting incidents for follow-up evaluations (*Chapter 5*)

Safe Medical Devices Act Federal law that mandates the reporting of adverse experiences with medical devices to the United States Food and Drug Administration (*Chapter 5*)

Secondary Intention Healing When wound edges are not reapproximated, the healing occurs from the internal to external surfaces; usually involves granulation (*Chapter 9*)

Shelf Life Length of time a package may be considered sterile (*Chapter 4*)

Sporicide Agent that destroys spores (*Chapter 3*)

Standards Authoritative statements that describe the responsibilities for which nursing practitioners are accountable (*Chapter 2*)

Static Electricity Electrical charge at rest that develops from friction and accumulates on an object (*Chapter 5*)

Sterile Free of microorganisms, including spores (*Chapter 3*)

Sterile Field Area surrounding the incision site that has been prepared for the surgical procedure, including the area over and around the patient, the scrubbed and gowned personnel, and all the furniture covered with sterile drapes (*Chapter 3*)

Sterilization Destruction of all microorganisms on an object (*Chapters 3 and 4*)

Sterilizer Automated processing unit that destroys all microorganisms on a substance by exposure to physical force, such as steam under pressure, and chemical agents, such as ethylene oxide (*Chapter 3*)

Substerile Area Service area between two or more operating rooms, which may be equipped with a flash sterilizer, warming cabinet, supply storage, and small sink (*Chapter 3*)

Sudomotor Stimulating the secretion of sweat (*Chapter 7*)

Surgical Wound Infection Limited to the incision area, although the infection can extend to or originate in deeper structures (*Chapter 9*)

Surgically Clean Sanitized but not sterile; items are rendered surgically clean through the use of chemical, physical, or mechanical processes that reduce the number of microorganisms (*Chapter 3*)

Systemic   Pertaining to the entire body rather than to a single organ or part (*Chapter 9*)

Terminal Cleaning   Performed at the completion of the day's surgical schedule (*Chapter 3*)

Third Intention Healing   When a wound is left open, to be closed at a later time (*Chapter 9*)

Thrombocytopenia   Decrease in the number of blood platelets (less than 150,000 per microliter) (*Chapter 9*)

Transient Microbes   Microorganisms that are loosely attached to the skin and are easily removed by scrubbing (*Chapter 9*)

Universal Precautions   Procedures and practices used to prevent the transfer of microorganisms by controlling the environment, including appropriate handwashing, handling of sharps, trash and linen containment, and wearing of personal protective equipment (*Chapter 3*)

Validate   Process of proving that a concept or practice is well grounded on evidence or principles (*Chapter 2*)

Voltage   Force that moves electrons through material and induces current to flow in one direction (*Chapter 5*)

Washer/Sterilizer   Processing unit that cleans through a spray-force action known as impingement; employs a vigorous agitation bath combined with jet stream air to create underwater turbulence; sterilization cycle follows washing cycle (*Chapter 3*)

Work Practice Controls   Procedures and practices that reduce the likelihood of exposure to hazards by altering the manner in which a task is performed (*Chapter 5*)

Index

Note: Page numbers in *italics* refer to illustrations; page numbers followed by the letter t refer to tables.

DATE DUE

DEMCO 38-297